Textbook of
Applied Sociology
for Nurses

Textbook of Applied Sociology for Nurses

As per the Revised Syllabus

Third Edition

TK Indrani BSc(N)
Ex-Assistant Lecturer
College of Nursing
Sri Ramachandra Medical College and Research Institute
Sri Ramachandra Deemed University
Chennai, Tamil Nadu, India

Alisha Talwar
MSc(N) Medical Surgical (Gastroenterology) Nursing
RN RM BSc(H) Nursing
New Delhi, India

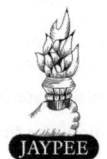

JAYPEE BROTHERS MEDICAL PUBLISHERS
The Health Sciences Publisher
New Delhi | London

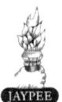 **Jaypee Brothers Medical Publishers (P) Ltd.**

Headquarters
Jaypee Brothers Medical Publishers (P) Ltd
23/23-B, Ansari Road, Daryaganj
New Delhi 110 002, India
Phone: +91-11-23272143, +91-11-23272703
+91-11-23282021, +91-11-23245672
E-mail: jaypee@jaypeebrothers.com

Corporate Office
Jaypee Brothers Medical Publishers (P) Ltd.
4838/24, Ansari Road, Daryaganj
New Delhi 110 002, India
Phone: +91-11-43574357
Fax: +91-11-43574314
E-mail: jaypee@jaypeebrothers.com

Overseas Office
JP Medical Ltd
83 Victoria Street, London
SW1H 0HW (UK)
Phone: +44 20 3170 8910
E-mail: info@jpmedpub.com

EU GPSR Authorised Representative
Logos Europe, 9 rue Nicolas Poussin
17000, La Rochelle, France
Phone: +33 (0) 6 67 93 73 78
E-mail: Contact@logoseurope.eu

Website: www.jaypeebrothers.com
Website: www.jaypeedigital.com

© 2023, Jaypee Brothers Medical Publishers

The views and opinions expressed in this book are solely those of the original contributor(s)/author(s) and do not necessarily represent those of editor(s) and publisher of the book.

All rights reserved. No part of this publication may be reproduced, stored or transmitted in any form or by any means, electronic, mechanical, photocopying, recording or otherwise, without the prior permission in writing of the publishers.

All brand names and product names used in this book are trade names, service marks, trademarks or registered trademarks of their respective owners. The publisher is not associated with any product or vendor mentioned in this book.

Medical knowledge and practice change constantly. This book is designed to provide accurate, authoritative information about the subject matter in question. However, readers are advised to check the most current information available on procedures included and check information from the manufacturer of each product to be administered, to verify the recommended dose, formula, method and duration of administration, adverse effects and contraindications. It is the responsibility of the practitioner to take all appropriate safety precautions. Neither the publisher nor the author(s)/editor(s) assume any liability for any injury and/or damage to persons or property arising from or related to use of material in this book.

This book is sold on the understanding that the publisher is not engaged in providing professional medical services. If such advice or services are required, the services of a competent medical professional should be sought.

Every effort has been made where necessary to contact holders of copyright to obtain permission to reproduce copyright material. If any have been inadvertently overlooked, the publisher will be pleased to make the necessary arrangements at the first opportunity.

Inquiries for bulk sales may be solicited at: jaypee@jaypeebrothers.com

TK Indrani's Textbook of Applied Sociology for Nurses

First Edition   : 1998
Reprints   : 2003, 2005, 2006, 2008
Second Edition   : 2018
Third Edition   : 2023
Reprint   : 2024, **2025**

ISBN: 978-93-5696-109-8

Printed at: Sterling Graphics Pvt. Ltd.

Dedicated to

*M/s Jaypee Brothers Medical Publishers (P) Ltd,
for showing keen interest to publish the book*

PREFACE

With great pleasure and pride, we are presenting the *Textbook of Sociology for Nurses* to our beloved students, which has been drafted as per the revised syllabus. This textbook attempts to meet the educational and professional needs of the students and nurses to strengthen the services to the patients and the society.

The content includes comprehensive coverage of core concepts that will encourage critical thinking and discussion throughout the book. The text is organized using a consistent approach across all the chapters. Each chapter starts with Chapter Outline, Learning Objectives and Key Terms that make the teaching-learning process further easier.

Throughout the book theoretical content have been presented in an integrated approach with an easy and understandable language.

We are sure this textbook would be useful for nursing students and faculty as a ready reference. We wish it would be a great success.

TK Indrani
Alisha Talwar

ACKNOWLEDGMENTS

"Let no man in the world live in delusion, without Guru none can cross over to the other shore"
—**Guru Nanak Dev Ji**—

No one walks alone on the journey of life, just where do you start to thank those that joined you, walked beside you, and helped you along the way continuously urged us to write a book, to put our thoughts down on over the years, those that we have met and worked with have paper, and to share our insights together with the secrets to our continual, positive approach to life and all that life throws at us.

We are greatly and sincerely indebted to Guruji, the Almighty for showering his blessings to complete this book.

We would like to express my gratitude to Shri Jitendar P Vij (Group Chairman), Mr Ankit Vij (Managing Director), Mr MS Mani (Group President), and Dr Madhu Choudhary (Director-Educational Publishing) who are the continual source of inspiration throughout this journey.

We are extremely blessed to have an experienced team comprising of Ms Jitika, Ms Teresa, Ms Dipti, Dr Aditya, and Dr Sakshi who have made the journey of the book effortless by their constant support and encouragement.

We owe our thanks to M/s Jaypee Brothers Medical Publishers (P) Ltd, New Delhi, India especially Ms Pooja Bhandari (Production Head), Ms Sunita Katla (Executive Assistant to Group Chairman and Publishing Manager), Ms Samina Khan (Executive Assistant to Director-Educational Publishing) and Mr Rajesh Sharma (Production Coordinator) for their efforts and support in the completion of this project.

We would also like to sincerely thank Ms Seema Dogra (Cover Visualizer), Mr Kapil Dev Sharma (Typesetter) and Mr Ravi Kumar (Graphic Designer) who added hue and life to the entire book and perfected the script.

CONTENTS

UNIT 1: Introduction to Sociology   1
- Definition of Sociology 2
- Nature of Sociology 3
- Scope of Sociology 6

UNIT 2: Social Structure   15
- Basic Concept of Society, Community, Association, and Institution 16
- Community 26
- Personal Disorganisation 30
- Social Group 32
- According to Cooley's Classification 38
- Other Types of Groups 46
- According to Summer's Classification 48
- According to FH Gidding's Classification 50
- According to Miller's Classification 50
- According to Leopold's Classification 50
- According to Dwight Sanderson's Classification 50
- According to Charles a Ellwood's Classification 51
- According to Tonnie's Classification 51
- According to Park and Burger's Classification 52
- Class (Social Class) 53
- Caste 59
- Socialization 87
- Social Change 93

UNIT 3: Culture   128
- Meaning of Culture 129
- Definition 130
- Nature of Culture 131
- Characteristics of Culture 132
- Elements of Culture 133
- Evolution of Culture 133
- Diversity and Uniformity of Culture 135
- Culture and Socialisation 138
- Transcultural Society 140
- Influence of Culture on Health and Disease 141

UNIT 4: Family and Marriage   148
- Family 149
- Marriage 164
- Legislations on Indian Marriage 173
- Influence of Family and Marriage on Health 178

UNIT 5: Social Stratification   181
- Meaning and Types of Social Stratification 182
- The Indian Caste System: Origin and Features 188
- Social Class System and Status 192
- Status 194
- Social Mobility: Meaning and Types 196
- Race 199
- Racism 204
- Influence of Caste, Class and Race on Health and Health Practices 206

UNIT 6: Social Organization and Disorganization   208
- Social Organization 209
- Voluntary Associations 212
- Social System 215
- Role 217
- Status 219
- Institutions 222

- Social Control 225
- Social Norms 236
- Folkways 238
- Mores 239
- Law 241
- Customs 242
- Fundamental Rights of Individual, Women, and Children 253
- Social Problems 256
- Poverty 257
- Housing 262
- Illiteracy 266
- Prostitution 270
- Food Supplies 276
- Vulnerable Group: Elderly, Handicapped, Social Status of Old People in India 280
- Minority Groups and other Marginalized Groups 289
- Child Abuse 293
- Child Labor 299
- Substance Abuse 302
- Drug Addiction 307
- Alcoholism 310
- Juvenile Deliquency 315
- Crime 321
- HIV/AIDS 325
- Social Welfare Programs in India 329
- Role of Nurse in the Prevention and Eradication of Social Problems 330
- Women Welfare Services in India 331
- Child Welfare Programs in India 333
- Social Welfare Programs for Old People 334

UNIT 7: Clinical Sociology   **338**

- Sociological Strategy for Developing Services for the Abused 343

Index   ***347***

INC SYLLABUS

APPLIED SOCIOLOGY

PLACEMENT: I SEMESTER

THEORY: 3 Credits (60 Hours)

DESCRIPTION: This course is designed to enable the students to develop understanding about basic concepts of sociology and its application in personal and community life, health, illness and nursing.

COMPETENCIES: On completion of the course, the students will be able to:
1. Identify the scope and significance of sociology in nursing.
2. Apply the knowledge of social structure and different culture in a society in identifying social needs of sick clients.
3. Identify the impact of culture on health and illness.
4. Develop understanding about types of family, marriage and its legislation.
5. Identify different types of caste, class, social change and its influence on health and health practices.
6. Develop understanding about social organization and disorganization and social problems in India.
7. Integrate the knowledge of clinical sociology and its uses in crisis intervention.

COURSE OUTLINE
T – Theory

Unit	Time (hours)	Learning outcomes	Content	Teaching/ learning activities	Assessment methods
I	1 (T)	Describe the scope and significance of sociology in nursing	**Introduction** • Definition, nature and scope of sociology • Significance of sociology in nursing	• Lecture • Discussion	• Essay • Short answer

Unit	Time (hours)	Learning outcomes	Content	Teaching/ learning activities	Assessment methods
II	15 (T)	Describe the individualization, groups, processes of socialization, social change and its importance	**Social structure** • Basic concept of society, community, association and institution • Individual and society • Personal disorganization • Social group—meaning, characteristics, and classification • Social processes—definition and forms, cooperation, competition, conflict, accommodation, assimilation, isolation • Socialization—characteristics, process, agencies of socialization • Social change—nature, process, and role of nurse • Structure and characteristics of urban, rural and tribal community • Major health problems in urban, rural and tribal communities • Importance of social structure in nursing profession	• Lecture-cum discussion	• Essay • Short answer • Objective type

Unit	Time (hours)	Learning outcomes	Content	Teaching/ learning activities	Assessment methods
III	8 (T)	Describe culture and its impact on health and disease	**Culture** • Nature, characteristic and evolution of culture • Diversity and uniformity of culture • Difference between culture and civilization • Culture and socialization • Transcultural society • Culture, modernization and its impact on health and disease	• Lecture • Panel discussion	• Essay • Short answer
IV	8 (T)	Explain family, marriage and legislation related to marriage	**Family and marriage** • Family—characteristics, basic needs, types and functions of family • Marriage—forms of marriage, social custom relating to marriage and importance of marriage • Legislation on Indian marriage and family • Influence of marriage and family on health and health practices	Lecture	• Essay • Short answer • Case study report

INC Syllabus

Unit	Time (hours)	Learning outcomes	Content	Teaching/ learning activities	Assessment methods
V	8 (T)	Explain different types of caste and classes in society and its influence on health	**Social stratification** • Introduction—characteristics and forms of stratification • Function of stratification • Indian caste system—origin and characteristics • Positive and negative impact of caste in society • Class system and status • Social mobility—meaning and types • Race—concept, criteria of racial classification • Influence of class, caste and race system on health	• Lecture • Panel discussion	• Essay • Short answer • Objective type
VI	15 (T)	Explain social organization, disorganization, social problems and role of nurse in reducing social problems	**Social organization and disorganization** • Social organization—meaning, elements and types • Voluntary associations • Social system—definition, types, role and status as structural element of social system • Interrelationship of institutions • Social control—meaning, aims and process of social control • Social norms, moral and values	• Lecture • Group discussion • Observational visit	• Essay • Short answer • Objective type • Visit report

Unit	Time (hours)	Learning outcomes	Content	Teaching/ learning activities	Assessment methods
			• Social disorganization—definition, causes, control and planning • Major social problems—poverty, housing, food supplies, illiteracy, prostitution, dowry, child labor, child abuse, delinquency, crime, substance abuse, HIV/AIDS, COVID-19 • Vulnerable group—elderly, handicapped, minority and other marginal group • Fundamental rights of individual, women and children • Role of nurse in reducing social problem and enhance coping • Social welfare programs in India		
VII	5 (T)	Explain clinical sociology and its application in the hospital and community	**Clinical sociology** • Introduction to clinical sociology • Sociological strategies for developing services for the abused • Use of clinical sociology in crisis intervention	• Lecture, • Group discussion • Role play	• Essay • Short answer

UNIT 1

Introduction to Sociology

 CHAPTER OUTLINE

- Introduction
- Definition of sociology
- Nature of sociology
- Scope of sociology
- Significance of sociology in nursing

 Learning Objectives

After reading this chapter, students will be able to:
- Define sociology
- Explain the nature of sociology
- Discuss its scope
- Learn about its importance and application in nursing

 Key Terms

- **Sociology:** Study of society
- **Formalistic school:** The subject matter of sociology consists of forms of social relationships
- **Synthetic school:** The school of thought of the scope of sociology

Unit 1: Introduction to Sociology

INTRODUCTION

The term Sociology was coined by Auguste Comte, a French philosopher in 1839. Auguste Comte is the father of sociology.

The word sociology is derived from the Latin word 'Societus' which means 'society' and 'logos' meaning study or science. It is the science of human society. All individuals have to interact with other individual, socialize with others in order to survive.

Sociology is the modern science that uses various methods of empirical investigations and critical analysis of the society.

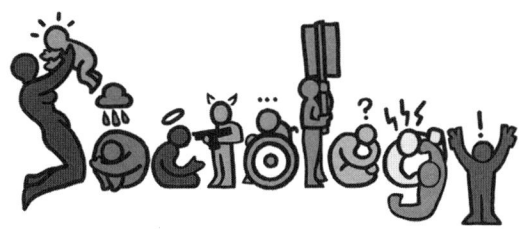

DEFINITION OF SOCIOLOGY

'Sociology is a systematic study of human society and their social life.'

'Sociology can also be defined as the scientific study of the interaction among different organized groups of human beings.'

'Sociology is the study of human interactions and interrelations, their conditions, and consequences.'
—**H Ginsberg**

'Sociology in its broadest sense may be said to be the study of interactions arising from the association of living beings.' —**Gillin and Gillin**

'Sociology is the science that deals with social groups, that is, their internal forms of organization, the process that tends to maintain, or change these forms of organization, and the relation between groups.'
—**Johnson**

'Sociology may be defined as a body of scientific knowledge about human relationships.' —**JF Cuber**

'Sociology is the science of collective behavior.'
—**RS Park and FW Burgess**

'Sociology deals with the behavior or men in groups.'
—**Kimball Young**

'Sociology is the science of social institution.' —**Durkheim**

Unit 1: Introduction to Sociology

'Sociology is the science of social relationships.' —MacIver

'Sociology is the science of society or social phenomena.' —LF Ward

'The subject matter of sociology is the inter-action of human minds.' —LT Hobhouse

From the above definitions we can summarize as follows:
- Sociology is the science of society. Sociology is a study of social relationships.
- Sociology is the study of human behavior in groups.
- Sociology is the study of social groups or social systems.

The main task of sociologists is to determine the nature and character of human societies and social institutions. They attempts to discover the evolution of man and society, its system and structures, development, and functions of social institutions.

Sociologists also investigate the connections between family structure and societal economic structures, between forms of government and wealth distribution, between religion and capitalism, and so forth. Knowledge of all these relationships is essential if we are to comprehend the workings and design of society.

NATURE OF SOCIOLOGY

There are different views expressed about the nature of the sociology as science. Some critics do not consider sociology as a science, but some considers:

a. Sociology cannot be regarded as science

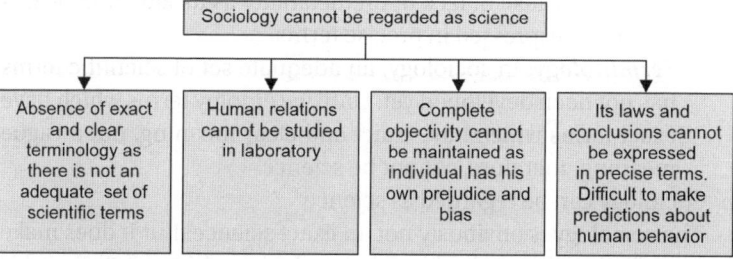

- **Validity:** The subject matter of science such as physics/chemistry include the process of experiment or validating the findings whereas sociology is the study of human relationship in group which cannot be studied in laboratory.

- **Generality:** The scientific laws are universally applicable. The generality of a finding refers to the degree to which a functional relationship obtained in one situation is able to predict the obtained relationship in a new situation. In sociology, the universal applicability is rarely achieved because of the heterogeneous nature of the society.
- **Predictability:** Predictability describes the likelihood at which an event is going to occur. In physical sciences, experiments can be done in laboratory to predict the melting point of an element whereas in sociology we do not use any laboratory for experiments as no prediction is possible.
- **Objectivity:** When a phenomenon is observed in its true form without being affected by observer's own views, it may be termed as objective observation. All the observers must come at the same opinion about the phenomena, e.g., coal is black, full moon is round. In social sciences, it means that conclusions arrived at as the result of inquiry and investigation are independent of the race, color, creed, occupation, nationality, religion, etc. If the research is truly objective, it is independent of any subjective element, any personal desire that he may have. This kind of objectivity is difficult to achieve in social science. Because factors of many varieties distort the process of inquiry (Francis Bacon 1561-1626). Social phenomena are to last and human motivation are too complex.
- **Exactivity:** The exactness of science depends on its subject matter. Science should be able to frame certain laws enable us to predict accurately. So, sociology cannot be considered as a science because of lack of predictability as its laws and results cannot be expressed in precise terms.
- **Terminology:** In sociology, an adequate set of scientific terms has not been developed yet. Until we employ terms which have exact terms which have exact and clear meaning, not a vague meaning, therefore, cannot be science.

b. Sociology can be regarded as science

The sociology is obviously not an exact science. But it does make use of scientific methods in the study, its subject matter and is therefore entitled to be called a science, the social science.

The concept was first developed by Emile Durkheim. It uses scientific methods, investigation, and uses different bodies of knowledge.

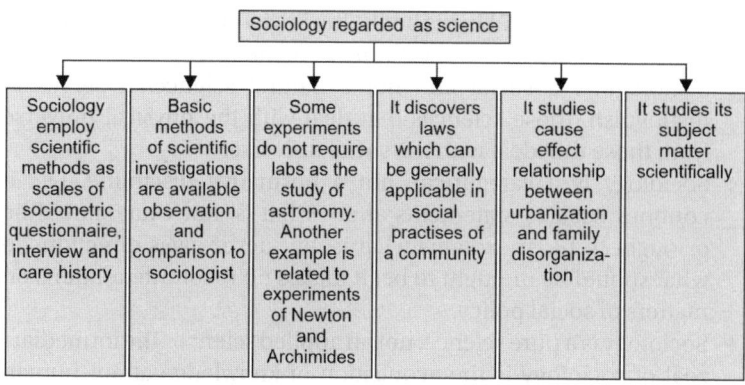

- **Experimentation**: Sociology is not a science because it cannot make experimentation. Sociology deals with human relationships which cannot be put to laboratory test. We can't see or weigh human relationship because it is abstract in nature. We can't do experiment with abstract things.
- **Scientific method**: Sociology also employs methods such as schedule, interview, and observations for data collection, sociometry, projective techniques and case history to quantity the social phenomena which are comparable to the method of experimentation.
- **Factual**: It deals with only facts, uses scientific principles involved to solve the problems.
- **Predictability**: Like natural sciences sociology can not make prediction accurately. Natural Sciences make prediction on the basis of certain data. But Sociology deals with social relationships and human behavior which are so uncertain and peculiar that we can't make any accurate prediction about it. We can't predict what will be one's behavior at a certain point of time nor we can predict about the trends or speed of social change. Hence sociology is not a science.
- **Universal**: The laws of sociology prove to be true at all times and places, as long as the conditions do not vary. The laws are devoid of any exceptions.
- **Cause and effect relationship**: It structures for the cause-and-effect relationship in its subject matter and in this connection, it provides universal and valid laws.
- **Generalization**: It gives generalization about the social behavior of human beings.

Robert Bierstedt (1957) in his book 'The Social Order' mentioned the following characteristic of the nature of sociology.

- Sociology is a social and not a natural science. It serves to distinguish, those sciences that deal with the physical universe from those that deal with the social universe.
- Sociology is a categorical, not a normative discipline, i.e., it confines itself to statements about what is, not what should be or ought to be. It explains what is, but never gives directions to what should be or ought to be. It makes no recommendations on matters of social policy.
- Sociology is a pure science, not an applied science. The immediate zeal of sociology is the acquisition of knowledge about human society not the utilization of that knowledge sociologist does not determine questions of public policy, do not tell legislators what laws should passed or repeated and do not dispense relief to the ill, the lame, the blind or the poor. Sociology as a pure science is engaged in the acquisition of knowledge that will be useful to the administrator, legislator, and the diplomats.
- Sociology is relatively an abstract science and not concrete one. This does not mean that it is unnecessarily complicated or unduly different. It is not merely interested in the concrete manifestations of human event but rather in the form that they take and the patterns they assume.
- Sociology is a generalizing and not a particular being or individualizing science. It seeks general laws or principles about human interaction and association, about nature form, content, and structure of human groups and societies and not in the case of history, complete and comprehensive descriptions of particular societies or particular events.
- Sociology is both a rational and spherical science.

SCOPE OF SOCIOLOGY

There are many differences of opinions about the scope of sociology. It is said by some that sociology studies everything and anything under the sun. This is too vague and vast view about the scope of sociology. As a matter of fact, sociology has a limited field of enquiry and deals with these problems which are not dealt with by other social sciences.

Sociology does not investigate the moral principles that should govern society, sociologists, like common man who spreads information to improve things. Acting politically, and attempting to make things right are both similar actions. Most of them are committed to some direction of social reform.

In order to limit and demarcate the field of sociology, there are two schools of thoughts among sociologists which are the following:

Specialistic or Formalistic School

According to formalistic school, the subject matter of sociology consists of forms of social relationships. **Simmel, Small, Vier Kanalt-Max Weber, Tonnie, Von Wiser** are the main advocates of formalistic school.

Simmel, a German sociologist demarcates socially clearly from other branches of social study and confine it to the enquiry into certain defined aspect of human relationship.

According to **Simmel**, the distinction between sociology and other social sciences is that sociology deals with the same topics as they put a different angle, from the angle of the different modes of social relationships. It should confine its study of formal behavior instead of studying actual behavior. Thus, according to **Simmel**, sociology is a specific social science, which describes, classifies, analyzes and delineates the forms of social relationships and study them in abstraction.

In **Small's** view, sociology is the study of generic form of social relationship, behavior and activities.

Vier kandt's view, sociology is concerned with the mental and psychic relationship by which people are related to one another in society. While dealing with culture, sociology should not concern itself with the actual contents of cultural evaluations, but it should confine itself to the discovery of the fundamental forces of change and persistence. It should abstain from a historical study of concrete societies.

According to **Max Weber** (1864–1920), the aim of sociology is to interpret or understand social behavior. According to him, sociology is concerned with the analysis and classification of types of social relationships.

Von Wiese and **Tonnie's** also limit the scope of sociology to one special aspect of social relationships and behavior. **Von** has given his view that sociology is the study of forms of social relationship. **Tonnie** has interpreted the social processes quantitatively and has given mathematical formula as given below-

$$P \quad A \quad X \quad S$$
Social Process Attitude Situation

Criticism of Formalistic School

- It has limited scope of sociology.
- It is difficult to study abstract forms separated from concrete relations.
- The conception of pure sociology is impractical.
- Sociology alone does not study social relationships. Thus, the fields of sociology are narrowed and confined to the limited field.

Synthetic School

According to synthetic school, sociology synthesis of social sciences of a general science. It says that all aspect of social life is interrelated, and it is an encyclopaedic and synoptic.

Ginsberg, **Durkheim**, **Hobhouse**, **Sorokin** and **Karl Mannheim** are the main advocates of the synthetic school.

Ginsberg's opinion is that the study of social relationships in abstraction as suggested by **Simmel** is not correct. According to him, sociology should not be limited the study of social relationship in general, but it should be widened by the addition of study of the relationships embodied.

In the different spheres of culture under special sociologies like the sociology of religion, of arts, of laws and of knowledge, etc. Ginsberg divided the subject matter of sociology into four parts: (1) Social morphology, (2) Social control, (3) Social processes and Social pathology.

Ginsberg has summed up chief functions of sociology as follows:
- Sociology seeks to provide a classification of types and forms of social relationships into institutions and association.
- It determines the relationship between parts of social life. For example, economical, political, moral, and legal, etc.
- It discusses the conditions of social change and persistence and to discover sociological principles governing social life.

Durkheim (1858-1917) accepts the scope of sociology as suggested by Ginsberg. According to him, the subject matter of sociology is broadly divided into three branches namely:

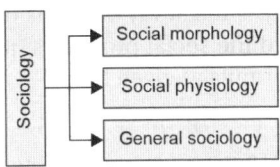

Social Morphology

Social morphology is concerned with geographical or territorial basis of the life of people and its relation to types of social organization, and the problems of population as well as its volume and density, logical distribution, etc.

Social Physiology

Social physiology is divided into a number of branches such as sociology of religion, morals, laws of economic life, language, etc., which deal with the social facts, i.e., activities related to the various social groups.

General Sociology

General sociology deals with the general principles of the society. It discovers the general principles of the society, general characters of social facts.

According to **Hobhouse**, sociology is a synthesis of numerous social studies, but the task of the sociologist is threefold.
- As a sociologist, he must pursue his studies in his particular social field.
- Sociologist should try to study the interconnections of social relations.
- Sociologist should interpret social life as a whole

According to **Sorokin**, the subject matter of sociology includes:
- The study of general features of social phenomena, e.g., marriage, family, culture, etc.
- The study of relationships behavior of the different aspects of social phenomena, e.g., family, marriage, religion, economic organization, etc.
- The study of relationship between the non-social, man and environment.

According to **Karl Mannheim**, the sociology can be divided into two main sections:

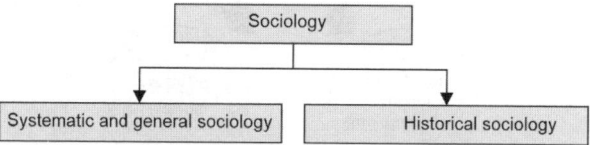

1. **Systematic and general sociology** describes all the important sections living together that is sound in every society.
2. **Historical sociology** deals with the historical variety and actuality of the general form of society. Historical sociology falls into two main sections:
   a. **Comparative sociology** focuses on how the same social phenomenon has changed historically and attempts to make conclusions by contrasting general features with industrial features.
   b. **Social dynamic** deals with the inter-relations between the various social factors and institutions in a given society.

Thus, the scope of sociology is very wider. It is a general science, but it is also a special science. The subject matter of all social sciences in society. What distinguishes them from one another is their viewpoint. Thus, economics studies social relationships and society itself.

Sociology studies all the various aspects of society such as social traditions, social processes, social morphology, social control, social pathology, etc. It deals with the general principles underlying all social phenomena. It is the science which deals with human social groups, classifies them, and analyses the nature of their structures.

Importance of Sociology

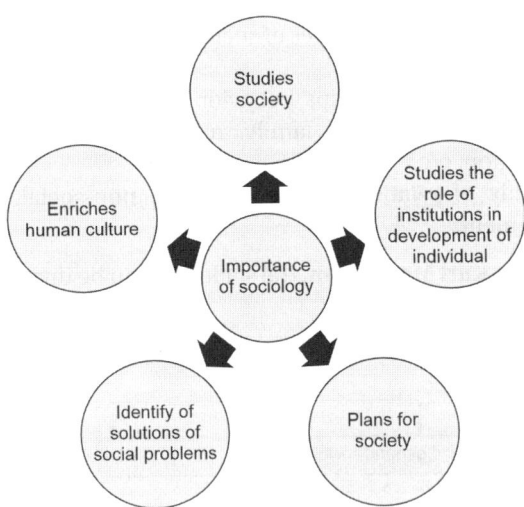

Sociology is important to study because:

- **Studies Society**: Sociology studies society in true scientific manner. If an individual has knowledge of society, he can use that knowledge in improvement of human affairs.
- **Studies the role of institutions in development of individuals**: The study of social institutions and relation to individuals has been made in sociological studies. Sociology studies, how the institutions are helpful in development of an individual and studies the weak point and support restrengthening them in order to have better individual.
- **Planning of society**: It is possible to mend society through adequate and proper planning. It is necessary to have knowledge about the society, before social policies are framed and carried out which later on will be helpful in shaping the society.
- **Identify solutions of social problems**: Sociology study the cause of social problems through the methods of scientific research and tries to identify solution for these social problems. This helps in controlling the social problems and also in improvement of social life. In India there are no. of problems like waving of bond of marriage, increased broken homes, disintegration of joint family, urbanisation, unemployment, etc. Sociology studies these problems, find out the cause, plan for society to improve or eliminate these problems.
- **Enriches human culture**: It enables a man to have better understanding of culture. It stimulates an individual to provide services for common good.

Importance and Application of Sociology in Nursing

Sociology is a very useful science especially for the nursing profession. Sociology helps nurses and doctors to understand the culture and social life of the patient.

In this world every society group has its own culture. All the causes of the diseases are not merely pathological disorder. For many diseases cultural, behaviors, habitual, environmental, and psychological causes are responsible. STDs, oral cancer, lung cancers are concerned with cultural causes, for hypertension, diabetes, mental stress, the psychological depression is the main causes. Therefore, the medical personnel should know the culture of the groups.

Nursing plays a vital role in health care profession. Nurses are the key persons who have significant influence over the group member within the society. Nurses have to work for maintenance of healthy lifestyles and high standards of living.

Knowing the community resources and facilities that are available is essential for being an effective health promotion agent. Sociology, often known as the science of human society, can play an important role in this process which is understanding and improving the community lives.

Technological progress has successfully eliminated many diseases, but it has brought new problems, and challenges to the nurses. The problems of the aged patient suffering from AIDS or persons due to industrial or other types of accidents are examples. The ability to handle such situations effectively requires a deep understanding of human behavior, relationship, and psychology.

Sociology Helps the Nurses

- To understand the problems of clients.
- To provide total patient care in a comprehensive manner.
- To suggest the individuals the ways, work with families and communities.
- To understand the emotional reaction patterns of the patient and other individuals in groups.
- To make diagnosis of people beliefs and practices to various diseases.
- To study the social interactions and social relationships in society, in social environment and in the community.
- To study the social problems related to behavior and suggest preventive medical approaches effectively.
- To understand the cause and meaning of many kinds of patient's behavior to make them comfortable and treat them alike for improvement of client care, in relation to society.
- To understand the problems of clients.
- To suggest the ways to work with families, community agencies and group of persons to provide health counselling in planning for continuity of care.
- To gain greater insight into human problems as related to the illness.
- To develop emotional soundness, maturity in dealing with situations and effectivity.
- To make diagnosis of people's belief and practices to various diseases.

Contd...

Contd...

- To identify some of the sociocultural barriers and promotes the activities related to treatment, prevention of diseases and promotion of health.
- To select suitable healthy education methods.
- To understand the client and anticipate in order to meet the emotional needs of the clients.
- To plan social interactions and to establish good interpersonal relationship with superiors, subordinates, class IV employees, clients, students, visitors, and community.
- To study the social problems related to behavior and suggest preventive remedial approach to tackle the problematic situations in the community in efficient manner.
- To identify and analyse different social situations which are responsible for the incidence and prevention of morbidity and mortality.
- To act as an effective liaison between client and the health team members.

- Auguste Comte, a French philosopher coined the term 'Sociology' in 1839. Auguste Comte is known as the father of sociology.
- The word sociology is derived from the Latin word 'Societus' which means 'society' and 'logos' meaning study or science. It is the science of human society. Various authors have defined sociology from their own perspective.
- The nature of sociology is a controversy, whether it is a science or not.
- In scope of sociology, two schools of thought- formalistic school and synthetic school have discussed. Formalistic school have been criticised due to its limited scope.
- Study of sociology is important as it studies society, studies the role of institutions in development of individuals, plans for society, identifying the solutions of social problems, enriches human culture.
- It is important to study sociology in nursing. Sociology helps the nurses to know about society, existing interpersonal relationships, culture, lifestyle of human beings, etc.

Review Questions

Multiple Choice Questions

1. Sociology is derived from which two words?
   a. Society and logy
   b. Societus and logus <ANS>
   c. Society and logus
   d. Societus and study
2. Social psychology deals with which of the following?
   a. Importance of religion, superstitions
   b. Human behavior <ANS>
   c. Different Culture
   d. Study of origin, growth, and function

Short Answer Questions

1. Define sociology.
2. Sociology is a science. Justify the statement.
3. Sociology cannot be regarded as science. Comment.
4. Discuss the importance of sociology.

Long Answer Questions

1. Define sociology. Explain the scope of sociology.
2. Discuss the nature and scope of sociology.
3. Write down the importance of sociology. Explain its importance in nursing.

2 UNIT

Social Structure

Chapter Outline

- Basic concept of society, community, association, and institution
- Individual and society
- Personal disorganization
- Social group – meaning, characteristics, and classification.
- Social processes – definition and forms, Cooperation, competition, conflict, accommodation, assimilation, isolation
- Socialization – characteristics, process, agencies of socialization
- Social change – nature, process, and role of nurse
- Structure and characteristics of urban, rural, and regional community.
- Major health problems in urban, rural, and regional communities

Learning Objectives

After reading this chapter, students will be able to:
- Develop good knowledge on social structure
- Learn the basic concept of society, community, association, and institution
- Explain the nature and theories of society
- Differentiate between the community and society
- Understand personal disorganization
- Learn about the social group and social processes
- Discuss about socialization
- Explain the structure and characteristics of urban, rural and regional community.

Key Terms

- **Society:** Web of social relations, complex of organised associations and institutions within community
- **Community:** Human population living within a limited geographic area
- **Social organization:** Interdependence of different aspects of society
- **Social structure:** Pattern of interrelations between individuals
- **Social group:** Two or more, who interact with each other and recognise as a distinct social unit.
- **Status:** Rank or hierarchical position
- **Caste:** A group bearing common name and traditional occupation.
- **Socialization:** Process of learning group norms, habits, ideas and working together.
- **Social change:** Difference in the social phenomenon over a period of time.

BASIC CONCEPT OF SOCIETY, COMMUNITY, ASSOCIATION, AND INSTITUTION

There are various words that people use on a daily basis that have particular meanings in sociology. It is vital that you all comprehend the significance and definitions of each to have better comprehension of the vocabulary you may encounter when working in the community or in any health setting.

Society

Society is defined not merely as an aggregate of individuals and groups living together, but is explained as a concept in sociology, where a system of set pattern mechanism exists comprising a complex web of norms, interactions and interrelations of individuals and groups that keep them bound together with a common purpose of co-inhabitation from generations together within a given territorial dimension.

The word society is usually used to designate the members of a specific group, persons other than social relationships of these persons. Society is the subject matter of the study of sociology. Thus, we say that sociology is the scientific study of the society. In society, we have groups, associations, and institutions

Community

Although family as a social entity sometimes are self-sufficient, but families do not live by themselves. For some reasons ranging from economic interdependence to shared cultural values, families normally bond together to form communities. The community, rather than the family, then becomes the social setting for most everyday economic, political, religious, educational, recreational, and similar activities. In brief, a community is a social organization that is territorially localized and through which its members satisfy most of their daily needs and deal with most of their common problems.

Institution

A social institution is a procedure, practice and an instrument, combination of variety of customs and habits accumulated over a period of time. Institutions are instruments and tools of human transactions. An institution is thus a stable cluster of norms, values and roles.

A social institution is an organized complex pattern of behavior in which a number of persons participate in order to further group interest. The family, the school, the church, the club, the hospital, the political parties, professional associations are all social institutions. Within each institution, the rights and duties of the members are defined.

Social Organization

The term 'social organization' refers to interdependence of different aspects of society and this is an essential characteristic of all enduring social entities.

Herbert Spencer used the term 'social organization' to refer to the interrelations of the economic, political, and other divisions of society.

Social organization is a process of merging social factors into ordered social relationships, which become infused with cultural ideas.

Social Structure

Social structure refers to the pattern of interrelations between individuals. Every society has a social structure, a complex of major institutions, groups, and arrangements, relating to status and power. Social structure is an arrangement of social activities that is seen to exist over some period of time and that is believed to depict underlying pattern of social order.

Association

As social life is becoming increasingly complex, with social actors pursuing a widening variety of goals through collective action, they create various kinds of specialised organization. Each of these organizations is limited in its range of activities, focuses on only one or a few aspects of social life. The generic name for such specialised organization is association.

An association is a social organization that is more or less purposefully created for attainment of relatively specific and limited goals, for example a Trained Nurses Association of India, Teachers Association.

INDIVIDUAL AND SOCIETY

Society

Man is a social animal as he cannot live alone and needs society. In sociology, the term 'Society' refers not only to a group of people but to the complex pattern of norms of interaction that arise among them.

Individual

Individual is a unit of society. He lives in society after having been born in it. In short, individual is a such unit of the society that he or she cannot live without society.

Definition of Society

'Society is a system of usages and produce authority and mutual aid, of many groupings and divisions of control of human behavior and liberties.'
— **MacIver**

'A society is a collection of individuals, united by certain relations or modes of behavior which mark them off from others who do not enter into these relations or who differ from them in behavior.'
— **Ginsberg**

It must be noted here that social order is often stable but never static, that is the basic feature of a particular arrangement of social relationships may persist for some time, but these patterns exist among ongoing relationships, which in one way or another always varying.

'Society is an abstract term that connects the complex inter-relation that exist between and among the members of the group.'
—**LB Reuter**

'Society is the union itself, the organization, the sum of formal relations in which associating individuals are bound together.'
—**Giddings**

'Society means men in interdependence.' —**Timashaff**

Society: This term is used to designate institutions when we speak of Arya Samaj society or Brahma Samaj. Man is a social animal. In this context society plays an important role. Society is the study of social process, social group, individual and other social organizations. A number of theories have been put forward to explain about society. Society is creation of God. Just as God created all animals, and inanimate objects in this world, so he created the society as well.

According to **Green** *'A Society is the larger group to which only individual belongs.'* It means all the individuals are directly/indirectly belongs or connect with other individuals.

Elements of Society

- Mutual interactions of individuals.
- Mutual interrelationship between individuals.
- A pattern of system.
- Reciprocal awareness is an essential ingredient of social relationship.
- We feeling / common propensity.
- Like-mindedness.
- Society also implies difference / diverse / variations.
- Interdependence.
- Cooperation.

Man, lives in the society for his mental and intellectual development. Society safeguards our culture and transmits to future generations. The mind of man without society remains the mind of an infant at the age of adulthood. The cultural heritage directs our personality.

Though the individual is a product of society, sometimes there may be a conflict between them. Sometimes the individual may develop a personality, which is incompatible with the environment, in which he is placed.

Deterioration of the societal system may also cause opposition between the individual and society. Therefore, individual and society are interdependent. The relationship between them is one sided. Individual and society interact with each other and depend on one another. They are complementary and supplementary to each other.

Nature of Society

Man is a social animal, in this context, society plays an important role. Society is the study of social process, social group, individual and other social organizations. A number of theories have been put forward to explain about society. These are:

a. **Social contract theory**

According to this theory all individuals are born free and equal. Society is created by mutual agreements of individuals. There are various authors like **Hobbes, Locke** and **JJ Rousseau** has given their views under social contract theory.

- ♦ **According to Hobbes**

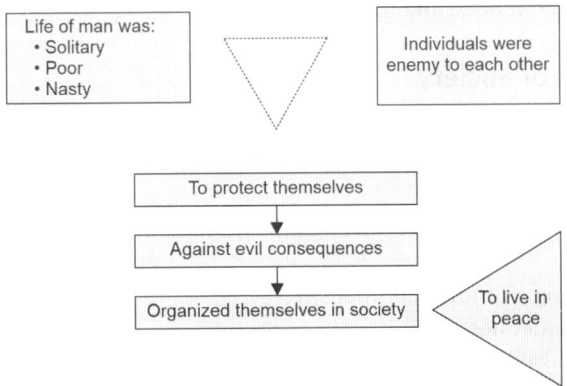

- ♦ **According to Locke**

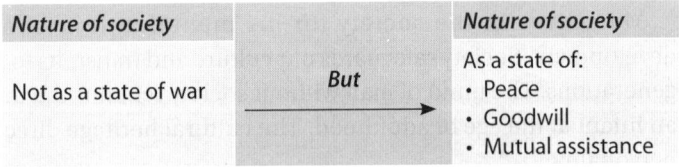

♦ **According to JJ Rosseau**

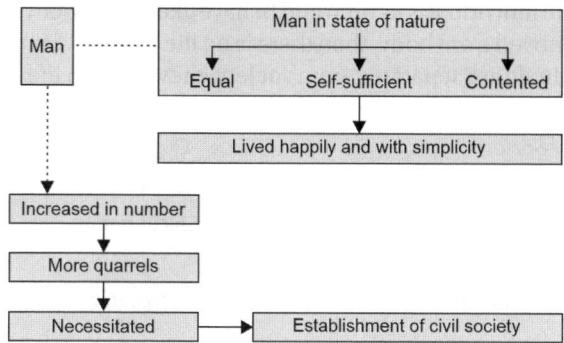

Thus, Society is creation of God. Just God created all animals and inanimate objects in this world, so he created society as well. Man is not born human, nor is he born social, but he becomes both through interaction and intercommunication between the members of the primary groups. Social relationships are characterized by a balance between likeness and cooperation, conflict, etc.

Limitations of this theory
- It does not provide adequate explanation.
- Society has emerged gradually, did not came into existence on a particular day.
- Force is an important factor in evolution of society but can not be regarded as single cause for origin of society, even other factors were also responsible.

b. **The organic theory of society**

This is an ancient theory. **Plato** divided the society into three classes based on the three faculties of human soul.

Society into classes	Human soul
The rules	Wisdom
The warriors	Courage
The artisan	Desire

According to **Aristotle**, the symmetry of state is same as of individual and individual is an intrinsic part of society.

Murray has summed up the points of resemblance as stated by **Herpert Spencer** that society is small aggregate of individuals. Individual and society grow in size. The various parts of society are interdependent with the growth, the simplicity is replaced by complexity. On this basis, it can be concluded that society is an organism. The individual is its limb and behave like cells of body. If the limbs are removed from body, then there is no life in limbs. Similarly, when individuals are separated from society, they have no life.

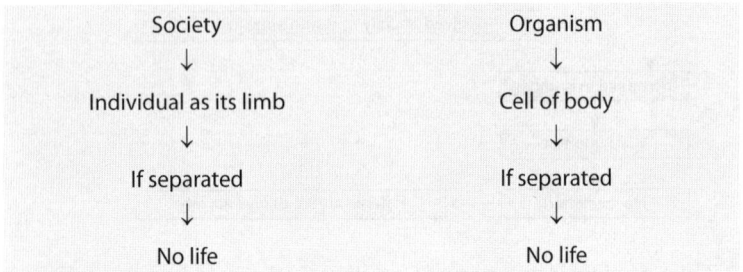

Limitations of Organic Theory

- The union of individuals in society is not in the same way as of two cells
- Society does not die in a similar way as individual dies.
- Society cannot be an organism as it has no body.

Types of Society

The type of society has not been the same everywhere on this planet nor has it been similar throughout the course of human history. Three main types of society are:
1. Tribal society
2. Agrarian society
3. Industrial society.

For example: African society is tribal, the Indian society is agrarian society and American society is industrial society.

Tribal Society

It is a social group in which there are many clans, nomadic bands, villages, or other subgroups which usually have definite geographical area, separate language, singular and distinct culture and either common political organization or at least a feeling of common determination, common name united by blood relationship, speaking a common dialect, occupying or profession to occupy common territory and is usually not too endogamous.

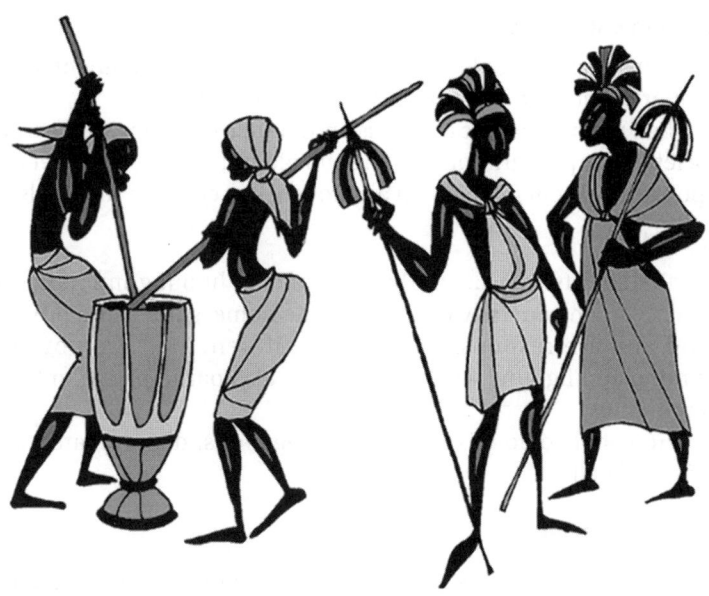

Characteristics of tribe

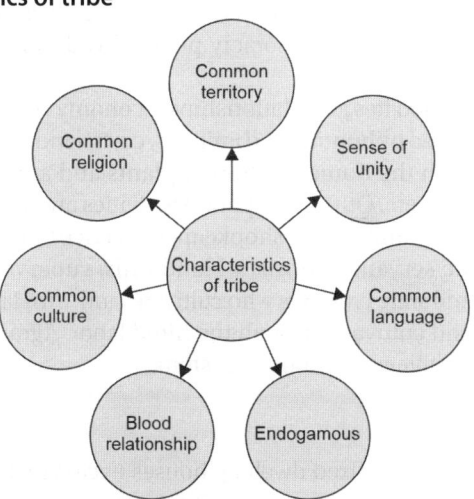

Structure and features of tribal society

Tribal society is a type of primitive society, which existed in the early period of human history, though it can be found in the backward regions of Asia, Africa, and Europe.

Economic structure

The tribal society people live close to the physical environment which supports them and determines the economic activity.

Their main economic activity is hunting and gathering. Some tribal societies rely primarily on hunting and plant gathering. They depend upon animals not for food but also for shelter, clothing, and tools.

Social life

In tribal society, men are the bread winner by hunting and gathering food. Women generally take care of the home, gather, and prepare food and are responsible for the children. Men are not only hunting and fighting with enemies but also participating in tribal ceremonies.

The tribal society is simple, homogenous, disintegrated and differentiated.

Agrarian Society

The title indicates it is agricultural economic activity. Agrarian society is called as peasant society. The development of agriculture greatly influenced in past century. The families' economic activity is agriculture. The agrarian society people lived in relatively small bands.

Basically, blood ties are relationships. Economy consisted of seeds and root gathered by hunting and animals, cows, land, and cultivation. Associated with the domestication of plants and animals like cow, goat, and sheep, etc. Other occupation activities are weavers, potters, watchman, blacksmith, petty shopkeepers, service holders, sweepers, and domestic servants, consist of landlords, supervisory farmers, cultivators, and stare croppers who cultivate land, own land, supervise cultivation and cultivate through the hired labor. Agrarian society is popular by its village community system.

Village

Village is made up of fixed dwelling houses necessary for living close together for protection and cooperation. Living nearer to the land gave birth to agricultural villages. The village is not only the residential place of farmers, but also the social integration. It serves as the nucleus of the society. Life operates almost completely within the village. In the village life pattern of the people are fixed. Their habits, attitudes and ideas are sharply marked off from those of the people living in the industrial society.

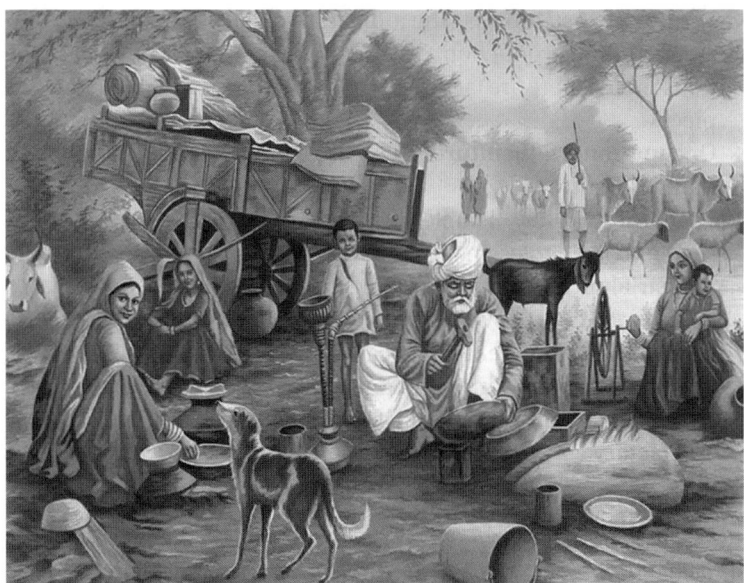

- The agrarian society is homogenous society whose people are engaged in the same economic pursuit. The people tend to be more much alike in body build as well as cultural patterns.
- In agrarian society family plays an important role not only for the reproduction and child rearing agency but as economic unit.
- The members of agrarian society exhibit a strong in a group feeling. In the name of the village glory, the people are ready to sacrifice their lives.
- In agrarian society any outsider violating the village norms and customs is heavily punished.
- In agrarian society neighbourhood is one of the important units which has disappeared from the industrial society.

Industrial Society

A very important factor in the history of society which has brought about far-reaching consequences in the structure of societies. The social structure began to change with the beginning of industrial revolution. An entrepreneur, an industrialist, capitalist come in and took over some operations.

Features of industrial society

- **Emergence of modern family:** The family in industrial society has move from an institution to companionship.

- **Economic institutions:** The industrial society is marked by a new system of the production, distribution, and exchange. In place of households there are factories where the work is divided into little pieces.
- **Occupational subculture:** These are extreme division of labor in industrial society.
- **Segmental roles:** People in industrial societies have been segmentalized roles. In personality of relationships is exhibited in industrial society.
- **Social mobility:** Movement of persons within a class system has been increased rather than in caste system.
- Position of women in industrial society is diverse. The women have many opportunities and have brought women to workshops and factory.

COMMUNITY

'A social group with the 'we feeling' and 'living in a given area.'
—**Bogardus**

'The smallest territorial group that can embrace all aspects of social life.'
—**Kingsley Davis**

'An area of social living marked by some degree of social coherence.'
—**RM MacIver**

'A group or collection of groups that inhibits a locality.'
—**Ogburn and Nimkoff**

'Group of people who live and belong together and share whole set of interests.' —**Manneheim**

'A human population living within a limited geographic area and carrying in a common independent life.' —**Lundberg**

'The community may be described as the entire population keeping a certain territory or in case of nomads, habitually moving, in association hold together, by a common system of rules regulating the intercourse of life.' —**Ginsberg**

'A community is the smallest territory group that can embrace all aspects of social life.' —**Davis**

'Community is a group living in one locality or a region under the same culture and having some common geographical focus for their major activities.' —**Kimball Young**

'By community is meant a unit of territory within which is distributed population which possess the basic institutions in their simple and specialized forms by means of which common life is possible.'
—**Dawson Gattys**

From the above definitions of community, the meaning of community is a group of people inhabiting in a given geographic area sharing a common way of life, working together for certain ends, aware that they belong to the community as well as the larger society.

Features of Community

The following are the elements or features on the basis of which we can decide whether a particular group is a community or not.

- **Locality**: A community is a territorial group. It occupies defined geographical area. They reside in that locality. Community is locally limited. People will develop social contacts, to get safety, security, and protection. Community promotes the people to fulfil their common interests and needs.

    People possess a strong bond of social solidarity. Locality is basic factor for community. Transport and communication facilities will be concentrated for a specific community.

    The community includes the physical factors like fertile soil, minerals, forest, fisheries, vegetation, resources, climate, etc. Community provides peace, protection, common culture, and social system.

- **Community sentiment**: A feeling of belonging together/we feeling. People will stay together, have their common interests and be conscious of their unity.

    People will be identified by their own group, which promotes sense of awareness, living and sharing, developing bondage among the members.

    In modern times, this community sentiment is slowly going down as people may not have common interest and a common look. Hence, attachment among the members is gradually changing as they belong to complex nature of society.

- **Group of people**: Groups of people share the basic conditions of common life. Group members can act collectively in an organized manner.

- **Permanency**: Includes permanent group life in definite place. Community is relatively stable.

- **Neutrality**: Community is established in a normal and natural way, they are not created or made by act of will or by planned

efforts. Individuals become members of the group by birth. The community life is comprehensive.
- **Likeness**: Language, practices, customs, traditions, folkways, mores are common. People share the common way of life and works through customs and traditions.
- **Wider ends**: People associate not for the fulfilment of a particular end. They are natural and wider but not artificial. The membership of community is of wide significance.
- **Particular name**: Each community will have its own specified name indicating the reality in individuality and describes the personalities.
- **Size of community**: There are bigger or wider communities, which includes small community like village, towns, cities, tribes, etc.
- **Regulation of relations**: A bundles of rules, regulations, customs, traditions, institutions, defines and shapes the members. In the rural community informal means of social control is observed like customs, folkways, rituals, mores, and beliefs. Whereas in urban community formal means of social control, e.g., law, police, court, armed forces are observed.
- **Dependency**: An individual is physically dependent on community for fulfilment and satisfaction of physical needs. Psychologically also he is dependent on community as it saves from isolation and solitude.

Basic Elements of Community

Although members of the community lead similar life, but the community does not have only one end. Community has various ends and for the achievement of these ends several institutions and associations are formed. It is so because these ends are more comprehensive than element.

- **Community and neighbourhood**: Sometimes community and neighbourhood are confused as one. There is no doubt that usually a person belonging to a community live in neighbourhood. But neighbourhood is not synonymous with community. It is quite possible that in the neighbourhood of a member of the community, member of another community may be living. No doubt, neighbourhood is helpful in the development of community feeling.
- **Community is extensive while neighbourhood is limited**: In the community circle personal acquaintance is wide but it is not so in regard to neighbourhood.

Importance of Role of Community in Social Life

Community has been playing vital role in our social life all these years. Integrity of society has been very much influenced by the community feeling. In the modern world the community is diminished because the feeling of universal brotherhood or the concept of the world society is gaining strength. In spite of it, it cannot be denied that community plays a very vital role in society and in our social life.

Benefits of Community Life

- Provides the individual needed security and protection.
- It strengthens the unity among people.
- Provides cooperation among the members. It encourages collective forces and efforts for the fulfilment of community needs.
- Depends on community system among the members.
- Provides individual the opportunities for the expression of his/her talents, abilities, and personality's development.
- Provides sense of belongingness.
- Community life has its own conflicts and contradictions

Difference between the Community and Society

Characteristics	Community	Society
Definition	Community refers to a group of individual living within a definite locality with some degree of we-feeling.	Society refers to a system or network of relationships that exists among these individuals
Locality	A community always associated with a definite locality	Society has no definite locality or boundary because it refers to a system of social relationships. Hence, it is universal or pervasive
Nature	Concrete	Abstract
Scope	A community is narrower concept. Hence, community is smaller than society	Society is a broader concept. Because there exists more than one community within a society
Interest	Particular or specific interests prevail in a community.	Common and diverse interests are present in society

Contd...

Contd...

Characteristics	Community	Society
Relations	May or may not have conscious relations	Conscious relations are more important than mere population in society
Communities	In community, there cannot be societies	In society, there can be many community
Community sentiments	There can be no community without community sentiments	Community sentiments are not present in society
Self-sufficiency	Cannot be self sufficient due to its limited scope	Self sufficient
Objectives	Less extensive and loosely coordinated	More extensive and closely coordinated
Development	An individual cannot have fullest expression of personal self and has to obey the commands of community	Individuals have wider scope to develop themselves and giving expression of their personality
Likeness	Likeness is more important than differences in community	Society involves both likeness and differences
Norms	It exhibits and creates certain norms and values, and social institutions.	It can exert pressure on the individual to confirm to norms
Regulation	Informal means of regulation are more important in community	Society involves both formal and informal means of social regulations.
Communication	People in community communicate involuntarily. Therefore, it is not necessary to interact	Communication and interactions are important in a society which builds social relationship

PERSONAL DISORGANIZATION

Definition

'All personal disorganisation represents behaviour upon the part of individual which deviates from the culturally approved norm to such an extent as to arouse social disapproval.' —**Mowrer**

According to **Prof. Ralph Kramer**, 'The individuals are actors in the drama of society and their relationships are ties that bind them together. Each person is only as strong as his social relationships, for no man lies upto himself alone. Hence, although social disorganization properly refers only to the failure and dissolution of relationship between individuals, the actors themselves are inevitably involved in the process.'

Concept

- Personal disorganization represents the behavior of the individual which deviates from the social norms. It results in social disapproval which may express itself in a wide variety of degree.
- The individual may also react in different ways. Social reality presents an endless confusion of social disapproval from time to time. It may be mild or violent. Individuals may respond either positively or negatively to social disapproval. This kind of personal disorganization does not deeply disturb the social order.
- The social disorganization is that in which there is violent social disapproval and yet the individual responds positively.
- In this the individual's response to social disapproval is subjective, the person retreats into an individually defined inner world. His innovations lose their social character.

Classification of Personal Disorganization

- **Physical disorganizations:** The genetic defects like low IQ and congenital abnormalities, cancer, AIDS, alcoholism, and drug addiction are the examples of physical disorganization.
- **Mental disorganizations:** Mental health is the basement of physical health. The problems like stressful situations, frustrating moments will change the emotional status of the individual. It leads to mental illness.
- **Social disorganizations:** Social disorganization consists of the incoordination of individual responses as a result of the operation of consensus and control.

Personal organization refers to the coordination and integration of the attitude systems within the personality. A change in the cultural context which destroys the functioning of coordination that constitutes the social order represents social disorganization. Similarly, any variant behavior which disturbs the integration of the attitude systems within the personality represents personal disorganization.

Causes of Personal Disorganization

- Mental deficiency
- Physical deficiency
- Lack of personal resources
- Biological Inheritance
- Cultural level
- Uncertainly of roles

Forms of Personal Disorganization

- Juvenile delinquency
- Crime
- Drink
- Sex
- Mental deficiency
- Insanity
- Suicide

SOCIAL GROUP

In sociological terms, a group is any number of people with similar norms, values and expectations who regularly and consciously interact. College sororities, dance companies, tenants' associations, and chess clubs are the examples of groups.

It is important to emphasize that member of a group share some sense of belonging. This characteristic distinguishes groups from mere aggregate of people, such as passengers who happen to be together on an airplane or train or from categories who share a common feature, but otherwise do not act together.

Social group is a basic unit when two or more persons interacting with each other interpersonal relationships are directed towards fulfilment of certain common goals or purpose.

A social group consists of two or more people who interact with one another and who recognize themselves as a distinct social unit. Frequent interaction needs people to share values and beliefs. This similarity and interaction cause them to identify with one another. Identifications and attachment in turn stimulating more frequent and intense interaction each maintains solidarity with all to other groups and other types of social system.

Meaning

Social group is a collection of human beings in its elementary sense. A group is a number of units of anything in close proximity to one another. Thus, we may speak of a group of houses on a field by group we mean 'any collection of human beings who are brought into social relationships with one another.' Individuals in group are connected to each other by social relationships.

A true group exhibits some degree of social cohesion and is more than a simple collection or aggregate of individuals such as people waiting at a bus stop. Characteristics shared by members of a group may include interests, values, representations, and kinship ties. It regards the defining characteristic of a group as social interaction.

Definition

According to **Ogburn** and **Nimkoff**, *'Two or more individuals come together and influence one another.'*

According to **Bogardus**, *' Two or more individuals who have common objects of attention, stimulating to each other who have common loyalty and participate in similar activities.'*

According to **Eldredge** and **Merrill**, *'A social group may be defined as two or more persons who are in communications over an appreciable period of time and who act in accordance with a common functions or purposes.'*

According to **Gillin** and **Gillin**, *'A social group grows out of and requires a situation which permits meaningful inter-stimulation and meaningful responses between the individuals, focusing of attention on common situations or interests and the developments of certain common drives, motivations, or emotions.'*

According to **MacIver** and **Page**, *'Group is any collections of social beings who enter into distinction of social relationships with one another.'*

According to **HM Johnson**, *'It is system of social interaction.'*

According to **Horton** and **Hunt**, *'Group are aggregates or categories of people who have a consciousness of membership and of interaction.'*

According **WG Green** *'Groups are aggregate of individuals which persist in time, which has one or more interests and activities in common which are organized.'*

According to **Williams** *'A social group is given aggregate people playing inter-related roles and recognized by themselves or others as a unit of interaction'*

Characteristics of Social Group

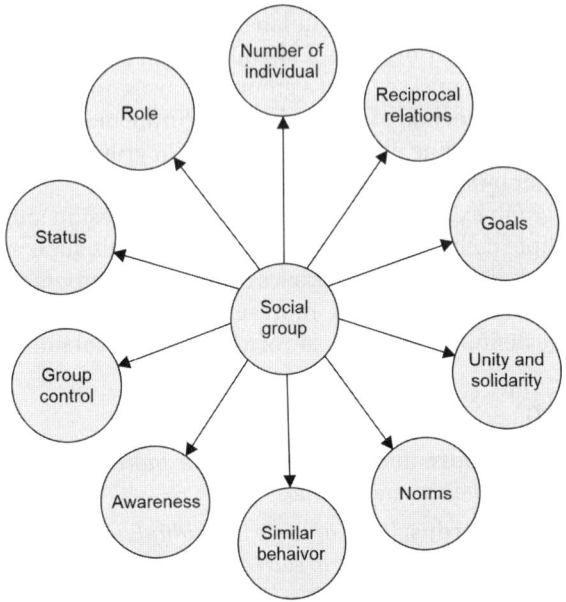

- **Number of individuals:** A social group consists of two or more number of individuals. These individuals belong to the group as members of the group and are considered as a unit of the group.
- **Reciprocal relations:** Among group, member's reciprocity is more. These reciprocal relations among the members are the basis or foundation of social group without which social group cannot be formed. The members must interact or interrelated with one another.
- **Goals:** It is another important characteristic of social group. The aims, objectives and ideals of the members are common. For the fulfilment of these common goals social groups are formed. Here individuals' interest is sacrificed for group interests.
- **Unity and solidarity:** Members of social group are always tied by sense of unity and bond of solidarity; members of a social group are characterised by a strong sense of we-feeling. This we-feeling fosters cooperation among members. Because of this we-feeling the members identify themselves with the group and consider others as outsiders.
- **Norms:** Every social group has its own regulations and norms which the members are supposed to follow. With the help of these rules and norms the group exercises control over its members. These norms may be written or unwritten. Any violation of group

norms is followed by punishment. The group norms maintain unity and integrity in the group.
- **Similar behaviors:** Members of a social group show similar behavior. As their interests, ideals and values of a group are common hence its members behave in a similar manner. This similar behavior helps in the achievement of common goals.
- **Awareness:** Members of a social group are aware about the members about their membership which distinguishes them from others. This is due to the consciousness of kind as opined by **Giddings**.
- **Group Control:** Social group exercises some sort of control over its members and over their activities. This control may be direct or indirect. The group exercises control on over non-conformists or deviants.
- **Status:** Status within the group, which determine the rank or hierarchical position which an individual occupy in the group.
- **Role:** The people have status in the group. Based on this they perform the activities.

Social groups dynamic is nature. The nature of change may be slow or rapid, but it is bound to happen.

Groups may be permanent or temporary in nature. There are permanent groups likes family and temporary groups like crowd, mob, etc.

Importance of Social Group

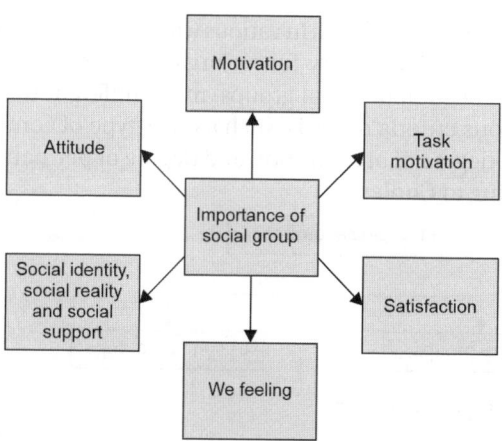

- **Motivation:** The group members influence and motivate each other. For example- In family, parents motivate children for higher education and status.

- **Task motivation:** The members gather together to achieve the goal of mutual activity. For example: In case of disaster management programmes, nurses gather to participate to manage the cases of disaster victims and provide efficient care. Other groups such as disaster relief group etc are formed to help the individuals.
- **Satisfaction:** Combined activities of social group brings rewards of achieving goal, which provides net satisfaction and greater identification within the group.
- **'We' feeling:** Social group bring cohesiveness
- **Social identity, social reality, and social support:** Social identity means individuals become involved with one another and aware of each other as members of the same social unit. In hospitals, orientation programmes are being organised by nursing group to orient the newcomers and to provide identity to them in nursing field. The newcomers are also informed of norms which inform them about the social reality. They are introduced to seniors and about the help, which they can seek during the problem while on job from them, there by acting as social support.
- **Attitude:** Social group through influential and motivational behavior change the attitude of members of groups, who don't behave according to expected one.

Classification of Group

Groups have been categorised in various ways by different sociologists. A classification is necessary for an organised analysis of groups. For the classification of social groups, many different thinkers have chosen various criteria or basis, such as size, type of contact, nature or interests, degree of organization and degree of permanence, etc.

1. According to **Cooley**

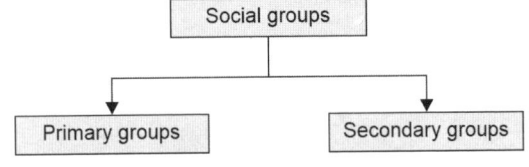

2. According to **Summer**

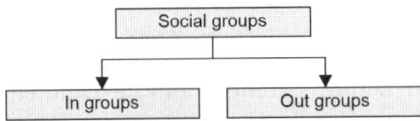

Unit 2: Social Structure

3. According to **FH Giddings**

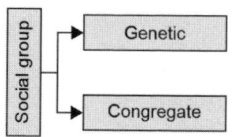

4. According to **Miller**

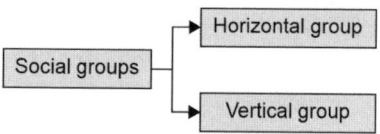

5. According to **Leopold**

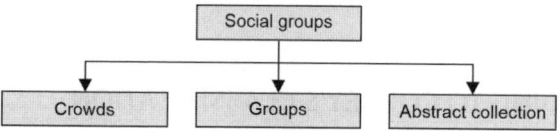

6. According to **Dwight Sanderson**

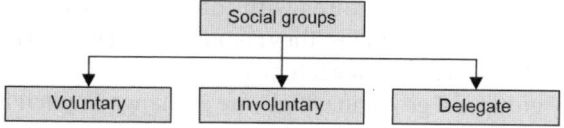

7. According to **Charles A Ellwood**

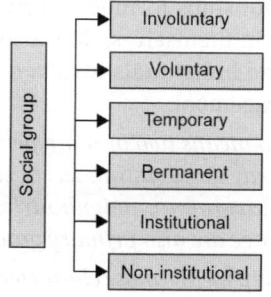

8. Acccording to **Tonnies**

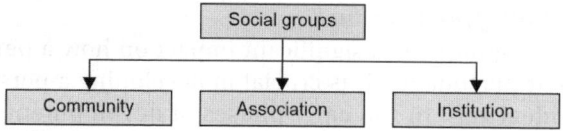

9. According to **Park and Burger**

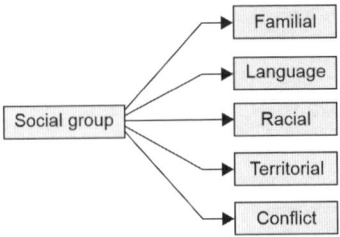

10. **Others**

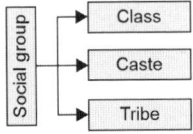

ACCORDING TO COOLEY'S CLASSIFICATION

Primary Group

Primary groups are small groups with intimate, kinship-based relationship, for example, families. They commonly last for years. They are small and display face to face interaction.

A primary group is a group in which one exchange implicit items such as love, caring, concern, animosity, support, and such examples of these would be family groups, love relationship, crisis support groups, church groups and such relationships formed in primary groups are often long lasting and goals in themselves, they also are often psychologically comforting to the individuals involved and provide a source of support and encouragement.

According to **Lundberg**, *'Primary group means two or more persons behaving interaction to each other in a way that is intimate, cohesive, and personal. For example, family, playground, neighbourhood, friend's group, work team and small village are also primary groups.'*

According to **CH Cooley** *'By primary group means those characterized by intimate face to face association and cooperation. They are primary in several senses, but chiefly they are fundamental informing social-nature and ideals of the individual.'*

The primary group has a significant impact on how a person develops their personality. It is crucial in developing a person's social and ideal self. In the early phases of development, the person adopts the views of others through identifying with them.

In the family, child gets training in meeting his friends, learning cooperation, competition, and struggle. The agent of socialization is the family.

The primary group not only satisfies the human needs but also provides a stimulus to each of its members in the pursuit of interest. Primary group not only offers members security but also manages their behavior and controls their relationships. The family transmit culture and, in this respect, and make him to acquire basic attitudes towards people, social institutions and the world around him. 'We' feeling is more in primary group. In this way primary groups run the society smoothly and maintain its solidarity. It creates sympathy and mutual understanding among members.

Characteristics of Primary Group

The characteristics of primary groups may be classified into.
- **Physical conditions:**
  - **Proximity**: The members should be is close proximity which develops intimate relationships and have face to face interactions. This close contact provides an opportunity to the members to express their views, ideas, opinions and even it is possible to visualise the facial expressions and gestures while having communication.
  - **Small size**: Primary group should be small, approximately it consists of 50 to 60 people to develop intimate relationships between groups.
  - **Durable relationship**: In primary group, the relationship is permanent and must exist for a long time or lifelong e.g., family. All the members of the primary group try to fulfil the condition of continuity or durability of relationship.
  - **Stability**: It is required for primary group which will promote the intimacy of relationship among the members of group.
  - **Cooperation**: All the members of group gather together in a spirit to participate co-operatively to study a common subject or to remove the grievances. This common feeling provides satisfaction among members of group.
  - **Common interest**: Group members share the common interest because of devotion and energy of all of the members of group in achieving goal. It not only sustains the common interest but sustains the interest of living itself.

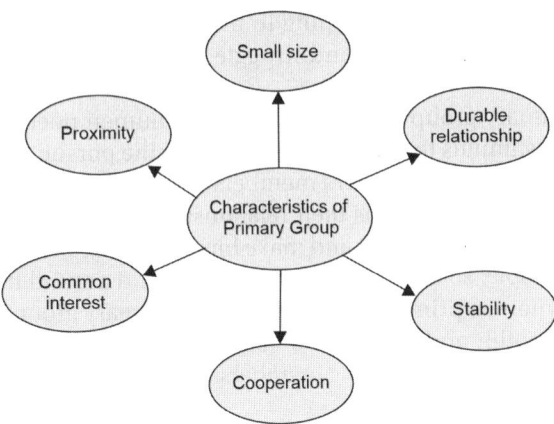

- **Internal characteristics:**
  - In primary group, the aims, objective, and ambitions of the members are identical.
  - The relationship is for the sake of love and affection not to attaining any particular end. The relationship is personal that is in between parents, friends or parent and child.
  - Relationship in primary group possesses power to control the individual and it is voluntary.

Family is the primary group, has less number of members, stable and exist for longer time period. All the members of family live under one roof which shows that they live in close contact having verbal communication. Non- verbal communication specially gestures can be seen during exchange of views and ideas face to face. This helps in better understanding between each other. All members cooperate with each other as they have close identification and do the same thing together with desires and attitudes. They work together in cooperation with each other to achieve their common interest.

From the above points for primary group, it can be concluded that the primary groups are important for individuals as well as for society.

Importance of the Primary Groups

The primary groups are important for individual and society because of these following reasons:

For individual	For society
An individual learns about cultures	Maintains social control over its members
Shapes the personality of the individual	Helps in process of socialization
Associates the individuals together	
Let the members express their aspirations and resentment	Teaches its member to work according to rules in society
Provides stimulus to each of its members in the pursuit of interest	Develops the basic attitudes towards social institutions
Encourages its members towards the achievement of objective	Provide cementing force to social structure and prevent social disintegration. So, the primary groups are important for individual as well as for society. Within the group, consensus is achieved because of authority, compromise, enumeration and integration
Boosts the morale of its members	
Creates 'we feeling' and brings cooperation among members and also unity for achievement of objectives	

Functions of Primary Group

- As family a primary group, which fulfil very vital functions for the members of the society.
- As family is a primary group where individuals are born and brought up.
- As society is a primary group where socialization of the individual takes place.
- It teaches high deals to individuals like freedom, love, sacrifice, justice, loyalty, patriotism, etc.
- Important functions of society like sex satisfaction reproductions, emotional security and social control are fulfilled in primary group itself.
- Primary groups are responsible for social order

Secondary Groups

Secondary group may be defined as those associations which are characterized by impersonal or secondary relations and specialization of function. They are also called as special interest groups of self-interest groups. Secondary groups are large and human contacts are superficial.

For example, a city, nation, a political party, corporation, labor union, an army, a large crowd, etc.

According to **Cooley**, *'Secondary groups are wholly lacking in intimacy of association and usually in most of the other primary and quasi-primary characteristics.*

According to **Mazumdar H.T.**, *'When face to face contacts is not present in the relations of members, we have secondary group.'*

According to **Ogburn**, *'The secondary groups are the groups that provide experience lacking in intimacy.'*

Therefore, it can be concluded that the secondary groups lack in intimacy and do not have face to face contact in the relation of its members.

Secondary groups, in contrast to primary groups are large groups in-volving formal and institutional relationships. They may last for years or may disband after a short time. The formations of primary groups happen within secondary groups.

Secondary groups, characterized by anonymous impersonal and instrumental relationships, have become much more numerous people move frequently often from one sections of the country to another and they change from established relationship and promoting widespread loneliness.

People in a secondary group interact on less personal level than in primary group and their relationship are temporary rather than long lasting. Since secondary groups are established to perform functions, people's roles are more interchangeable. Secondary groups are based on interests and activities. They are where many people can meet close friends or people. They would just call acquaintances. Secondary groups are groups in which an exchange explicit commodity such as labor for wages, services for payments and such examples of these would be employment vendor to client relationship.

The new range of the interests demands a complex origin station especially selected persons act on behalf of all and hence arises hierarchy of official called bureaucracy. These features characterize the rise of modern state the great corporation, the factory, labor union, university for nationwide political party and so on. These are secondary groups. **Cooley** mentioned the second type of social group of groups.

Characteristics of Secondary Group

- ❖ **Large:** Secondary groups are relatively large in size. For example, a political party, trade union, international associations, such as rotary club, the Red-cross society which consists of thousands of members scattered all over the world.

- **Formality:** The relations of members in a secondary group are of a formal type. Secondary group exert influence on the members indirectly. They are controlled by formal rules are regulations. Formal control such as law, legislation, police, court, etc. are very much important for the members.
- **Impersonality:** Secondary relations are impersonal in nature. In the large-scale organization, there are contacts, and they may be face-to-face and impersonal.
- **Indirect cooperation:** It is another characteristic of secondary groups. In its members do different things interdependently. In the large-scale organization where division of labor is complex, the members have not only different functions but different degree of participation, different rights and obligations.
- **Voluntary membership:** The membership is most of the secondary groups is not compulsory but voluntary. Individuals are at liberty to join or to away from the groups. It is not essential to become the member of Rotary international or Red Cross Society. However, there are some secondary groups like nation or the state whose membership is almost involuntary.
- **No Physical Proximity:** Secondary groups are not characterized by physical proximity. Many secondary groups are not limited to any definite area. These are some secondary groups like the rotary club and lions club which are international in character. The members of such groups are scattered over a vast area.
- **Specific Ends or Interest:** Secondary groups are formed the realization of some specific interests or ends. They are called special interest groups. Members are interested in the groups because they have specific ends to aim at. Indirect communication contacts and communication in the case of secondary groups are mostly indirect. Mass media of communication such as radio, telephone television, newspaper, movies, magazines and post and telegraph are resorted to by the members to have communication.
- **Communication:** Communication may not be quick and effective. Impersonal nature of social relationships in secondary groups is both the cause and the effect of indirect communication.
- **Group Structure:** The secondary group has a formal structure. A formal authority is setup with designated powers and a clear-cut division of labor in which the function of each is specified in relation to the function of all. Secondary groups are mostly

organized groups. Different statuses and roles that the members assume are specified. Distinctions based on caste, color, religion, class, language, etc. are less rigid and there is greater tolerance towards other people or groups.

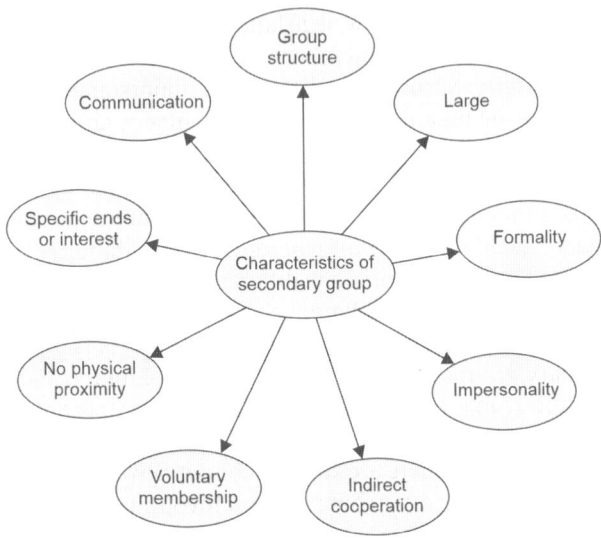

Importance of Secondary Groups

Due to the shift in modern society from small to larger communities, man is increasingly more dependent on secondary groups for his needs.

For example: Earlier, childbirth delivery used to be done at home, baby was born in the family (primary group) but now a days due to advancement and to reduce the mortality and morbidity institutionalised (hospital) delivery is preferred, now babies are born in hospital (secondary group). The secondary groups are considered important because:

* The secondary groups occupy dominant place in modern civilized and industrial societies. The small communities have now given way to large communities. The place of cottage industry we have now grant corporations employing thousands of people. The changing trends of modern society have swept away primary groups. The efficiency is improved in specific field of activity and in consciousness, they become experts. A formal authority is set up with the responsibility of managing the organization efficiency.

- The secondary group broadens the outlook of its members. It accommodates more individuals and localities which widens the outlook of its members. It is more universal in its judgement than the primary group. Many professional and occupations are opening the way for specialized careers.
- Secondary groups provide a greater chance to develop individual talents. The talented individual may rise from an unknown background to the highest position in business, industry, civil and technical services.
- The functions of secondary groups are essential in present society. The people are becoming more and more dependent on those groups. The tremendous advances in material comfort and in life expectancy in modern world would be impossible without the rise or goal-directed secondary groups.
- Rules formed by the group, will increase the efficiency of the work
- It breaks the barriers of class, caste, and province.

Difference between the Primary and Secondary Group

Characteristics	Primary group	Secondary group
Meaning	Primary groups are those that are bound together by strong emotional bond and common interests. It provides the typical experience of social unity and harmony, to its members.	Secondary groups are the groups which are formal, segmental and utilitarian. The relationship between members exists due to contractual obligation or interest.
Size	Small both in size and area.	Relatively larger and widespread.
Durability	Long-lasting and permanent.	Short term or long term, depending on the condition.

Contd...

Contd...

Characteristics	Primary group	Secondary group
Interest of Members	Diffused	Specific
Found in	Family Setting	Educational and Employment Setting
Significance in the life of people	Greater significance	Little significance
Group focus	Relationship	Task
Relationship	Personal, Direct, and Intimate	Impersonal and goal-oriented
Principle	Particularism	Universalism
Structure	Informal	Formal
Communication	Direct, quick, and effective	Indirect
Member's Role	Stable	Interchangeable
Cooperation	Direct	Indirect

Reference of Groups

A reference group is a concept referring to a group to which are individual, or another group is compared.

Reference groups are used in order to evaluate and determine the nature of a given individual or other group's characteristics and sociological attributes. It is the group to which the individual relates or aspires to relate himself or herself psychologically. It becomes the individual's frame of reference and source for ordering his or her experiences, perceptions, cognitions, and ideas of self. It is important for determining a person's self-identity, attitudes, and social ties. It becomes the basis of reference in making comparisons or contrasts and in evaluating one's appearance and performance.

OTHER TYPES OF GROUPS

Peer Group

A peer group is a group with members of approximately the same age, social status, and interests. Generally, people are relatively equal in terms of power when they interact with pears.

Clique

An informal tight-knit group, often in high school/college setting that shares common interests. Most cliques exhibit an established yet shifting power structure.

Club

A club is a group, which usually requires one to apply to become a member. Such clubs may be dedicated to a particular activity, for example, sport's clubs.

Household

All individuals who live in the same home. Anglophone culture may include various models of household, including the family, blended families, share housing and group homes.

Community

A community is a group of people with a commonality or sometimes a complex net of overlapping commonalities, often-but not always in proximity with one another with some degree of continuity overtime.

Franchise

An organization which runs several instances of a business in many locations.

Gang

A gang is usually an urban group that in a particular area. It is a group of people that of ten hangs around each other. They can be line some clubs, but much less formal.

Mob

A mob is usually a group of people that has taken the law into their own hands. Mobs are usually groups which gather temporarily for a particular reason.

Posse

A posse was originally found in English common law. It is generally obsolete, and survives only in America, where it is the law enforcement equivalent of summoning the militia for military purposes.

Squad

This is usually a small group, of around 3 to 8 people, who work as a team to accomplish their goals.

Team

Similar to squad, though a team may consist of many more members. A teamwork in a similar way to a squad.

ACCORDING TO SUMMER'S CLASSIFICATION

In Groups

The group to which an individual belong is his 'in group'. The members of in group have respect for one another's right and show co-operation. People feel comfort and secure.

For example: Family, college, institution, hospital etc.

Characteristics of In Group

Similar attitude and reactions
Sense of belongingness
Considerable degree of sympathy among members
Cooperative relationship and respect towards each other
Feeling of brotherhood
Members ready to sacrifice themselves for the sake of group
Pleasure of one member provides pleasure to all its members
Members have unity within the group

Out Groups

Out group is defined as the group to which an individual does not belong or the group in relation to outside the boundaries of his in group. People are hostile and lack of contact with other groups. It may lead to misunderstanding and suspicion. Out-group is dehumanized. Intense competition and frustration present in out-groups. The attitude of individuals towards out group ranges from mild negative attitude to intense negative or a feeling of hatred.

Characteristics of Out Group

Exhibit dissimilar activity among members
Have 'they' emotion
The person shows antagonism or enmity against the other party.
Demonstrates or displays a negative attitude toward the outgroup
No ethnocentrism

Ethnocentrism: It is the view of things in which one's own group is centre of everything and other are sealed and rated with reference to it. It is an assumption that the values, the ways of life and attitude of ones' own group are superior to those of others. It is one characteristic of in group.

Difference between In Group and Out Group

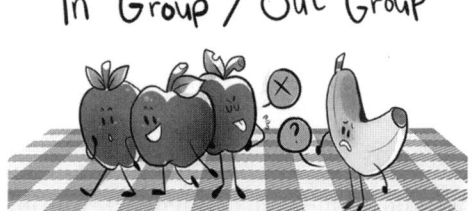

In group	Out group
The group with which an individual identifies himself/herself, has a sense of belonging with.	A group to which an individual feels individual has no sense of belonging/ identification
In groups sets the members of it apart from all other people	In out-groups the individuals belong to many groups, the membership of which is overlapping
It is a "we-group".	It is a "they group"
In a group their relationship displays cooperation, goodwill, mutual help and respect for one another rights	Although each group satisfies or other aspects of personality these groups are not necessarily complementary groups, indeed they are conflicting
There is a sense of attachment members of In-group	There is a sense of indifference and at times may be even hostility towards members of out-group

Contd...

Contd...

In group	Out group
We-feeling is seen, and organization is based on elements of inclusion and exclusion	They or other feeling exist, and the organization is undetermined
There are team efforts and sacrifices for the wellness of group no centrism is a character in group	Individual satisfaction is given priority and ethnocentrism is absent

ACCORDING TO FH GIDDING'S CLASSIFICATION

Genetic Group

The group in which individual is born i.e., family, involuntary in nature.

Congregate Group

The congregate group is the voluntary group into which one moves or joins voluntarily. For example- Union

ACCORDING TO MILLER'S CLASSIFICATION

Horizontal Groups

It refers to those group of individuals (members) who interact without any giving any importance to hierarchy. Ex- Group of friends

Vertical Groups

It refers to those group of individuals (members) who interact without a conscious sense of hierarchy. Ex- Person of different class, caste, and status.

ACCORDING TO LEOPOLD'S CLASSIFICATION

Crowds which are described as 'loose-textured and transitory'

Groups aggregations of long duration

Abstract collectivises such as a state or a church

ACCORDING TO DWIGHT SANDERSON'S CLASSIFICATION

Involuntary Group

It is based on kinship such as in the family. For example, a man has no choice to what family he will belong.

Voluntary Group

In this group a man joins his own will or volition. – He agrees to be a member, of it and is free to withdraw at any time from its membership.

Delegate Group

A delegate group is one which a man joins as a representative of a number of people either elected or nominated by some power, for example, parliament.

ACCORDING TO CHARLES A ELLWOOD'S CLASSIFICATION

Voluntary Group

Are those which members participate out of free will, e.g., clubs, trade unions.

Involuntary Group

These are those which person become members automatically, e.g., family, village, city or nation.

Temporary Groups

These are those which last for relatively short period, e.g., crowd and audience.

Permanent Groups

These last for long time, e.g., family, neighbourhood, and community.

ACCORDING TO TONNIE'S CLASSIFICATION

Community

Community is usually based on locality like village, city, or nation. A community is an inclusive group with three characteristics. Within the individual can have most of the experiences and conduct most of the activities that are important to him. It is bound together by a shared sense of belonging and by the sealing among the members that the group defines. The geographical area and sense of place set boundaries of common living and provide a basis for solidarity.

Example: Catholic community, Hindu community etc.

Associations

Associations are special purpose organizations such as trade unions, corporation, and political parties. Associations are usually based on limited utilization interests.

Example: Voluntary associations, clubs, veteran groups, factories, etc.

Institutions

The word 'institution' refers practices to 'established ways of doing things.' When an association serves public rather than merely private interests, and does so in an accepted, orderly, and enduring ways to called as 'institution'.

Example: Marriage, private enterprise, constitutional government, and thanksgiving, etc

Difference between Institution and Association

Institution	Association
Comprises of laws, customs, and systems	Comprises of human beings
Formless and abstract	Formal and concrete
It is evolved	It is constituted and formed
It is stable and permanent	Comparatively, it is less stable and permanent
It has procedure and method of working	It indicates membership
It has formed with the object of fulfilment of primary needs	It is formed with definite objectives
It depends on human activities and has a definite structure	It is based on mutual cooperation and no definite or specific structure
The discipline, rules and laws of institution are based on customs and traditions	The rules are formed after rational consideration

ACCORDING TO PARK AND BURGER'S CLASSIFICATION

Familial Group

Groups are based on blood relationships and kinships, e.g., family and lineage, etc.

Language Group

Those who speak the same language from a group, e.g., Tamilians, Punjabis, etc.

Racial Group

People of same race form one distinct group, e.g., Negroes, Mongoloids, etc.

Territorial Groups

People residing in the same geographical areas, e.g., state, nation, village, and city.

Conflict Groups

In this group there will be conflict with each other. Usually, the interest of one group is against that of the other, e.g., political parties, labor unions, etc.

CLASS (SOCIAL CLASS)

Class is a group of people who have particular position or status within the population as a whole. The class has its own social behavior. The occupation of people within one particular class is same. The class exhibits the standard of living. In social class, people have a feeling of equality in relation to member of its own class. A class is considered as a group of individuals having the following characteristics-

- Same occupation
- Common descent
- Similar mode of life
- Similar form of behavior
- Same level of education

Definition of Class

According to **Max Weber,** *'An aggregate of the individuals who have the same opportunities of acquiring goals the same exhibited standard of living.'*

According to **MacIver and Page,** *'A social class is a portion of community marked off from the rest by social status.'*

According to **Ogburn and Nimkoff,** *'A social class is the aggregate of persons having essentially the same social status in a given society.'*

According to **Cuber,** *'A social class or stratum of society is a major segment or category of population in which persons have about the same status or rank.'*

According to **Ginsberg,** *'A social class is a group of individuals who through common descent, similar occupation, wealth, and education have come to have a similar mode of life, a similar stock of those ideas, feeling, attitudes and forms of behavior and who on common or all of these grounds, made one another on equal terms and regard themselves, although with varying degrees of explicitness as belonging to one group.'*

According to **J.B. Gilter,** *'A social class may be defined as a category of persons with a set of privileges, responsibilities, power obtained through their position of a common degree of those qualities which are appraised as values in a particular culture.'*

According to **Capiere,** *'A social class is a culturally defined group that is accorded a particular position or status within the population as a whole.'*

Basis of Social Class

Different social thinkers have classified class on different basis. Economic difference as propounded by **Karl Marx** is said to be a most important basis of the class and class distinction. Given below is a list of the basis of the class:

- **Economic difference:** After the theory of **Karl Marx**, economic differences is considered to be most important basis of the class difference. **Karl Marx** in the 'communist manifesto' has said that history of all hitherto existing society is the history of the class struggle. Generally, those who oppose forward two arguments in this respect.
  - Many of classes are not based on economic distinction alone. In this respect Hindu society is quoted as an example. In this context, it is further contended that the classification of the Hindu society is based on 'karma' or 'deeds.
  - The second arguments advanced against the theory of class struggle is that classes have certain element of consciousness. In this respect **MacIver** has written, 'Economic division does not unite people and separate them from others unless they feel they are united or separated.
- **Occupation:** Occupation is also an important base of class division. Individuals in superior occupation are related as superiors while those in inferior occupation are considered as inferior.

- **Manual labor: Veblen** has put forward the view that labor is also the basis of class consciousness. According to this theory, those carrying on manual labor are considered inferior while those carrying on other jobs of labor are considered superior beings.
- **Various other factors in regard to basis of class distinction: Cattell** has enumerated other factors that are responsible for class distinction. According to him these factors are:
  - Intelligent quotient
  - Average income
  - Education
  - Birth restrictions

Types of Social Class

Authors **Merrill** and **Eldredge** have classified the class on the basis of various social factors under the following six heads:

Defined Class

Such classes are formed on the basis of pre-determined distinctions. Caste system in India is a case and example.

Cultural Classes

Different classes are formed on the basis of cultural influences. Those classes that are influenced by one culture before to one class, while those influenced by other culture are said to belong to other class.

Economic Classes

Classes formed on the basis of economic distinctions, and income groups. Capitalist's upper class, middle class, and labor, etc. are considered to be people belonging to different classes.

Political Classes

Sometimes classes are formed on the basis of political affiliations and membership of different political parties. Such classes are termed as political classes.

Self-identified Classes

Sometimes people because of their definite objectives join hands with others, because of this community objectives, feeling of oneness or we feeling develops in them, consequently a new class is formed. This class is termed as self-identified class.

Participation Classes

Sometimes classes are formed on the basis of eating together. People belonging to one class do not want to mix with people of other class or eat with them. Such classes are called participation class

The society has been classified into three distinct classes:
a. **Capitalist**: Capitalist own the means of production. They are the typically wealthy people who have a large amount of capital (money or other financial assets) invested in business, and who benefit from the system of capitalism by making increased profits and thereby adding to their wealth.
b. **Middle class**: It is a heterogenous group consisting not only of tradesman but also doctors, nurses, engineers, teacher, architect, lawyer etc. This class is superior to proletariat and inferior to capitalist. It is further divided into upper, middle, and lower middle class.
c. **Proletariat**: The proletariat is the social class of wage-earners, those members of a society whose only possession of significant economic value is their labour power.

Class and Caste

Sometimes caste and class are considered to be one, but fact is that these are two different institutions. Class is based on external as well as internal unity by caste is based move on internal unity and cultural factors. **Ogburn** and **Nimkoff** have said that 'a social classes are that aggregate of person having essentially the same social status in a given society'.

Influence of Class on Social Behavior

Class exercise vital influence on social behavior. This influence is open as well as closed

Open Class System

This type of class system influences the social behavior in the following manner:
- ❖ **Not based on birth:** Open class system is a system which is not based on birth. It is based on ability, capacity, and other qualities of merits. It means that people possessing certain merits and qualities can become members of open class system. In such a system there is every opportunity for progress.

- **Importance of individual achievement:** In this system, individual achievements are given a good deal of importance. In other words, it is the individual achievement that determine the social status of an individual.

Closed Class System

This class system is just the reverse of opened class system. In this system the individual behavior or social behavior is influenced in the following manner:
- **Based on births:** Closed class is based on birth. Status of an individual is determined according to birth and social descent. Individual achievements and merits have no place in this system.
- **Personal attainments:** In this type of class system, personal achievement, individual merits, and capabilities do not have any significance for recognition as a member of class. Stratification is already stated based on births and allied factors. This system, therefore, does not provide an opportunity to the individuals to improve their qualifications and make further headway.

TRIBE

The 'tribe' is largely used to describe non-white peoples. Tribe, viewed historically or developmentally, consists of a social group existing before the development of, or outside of states.

Many anthropologists use the term to refer to societies organized largely on the basis of kinship, especially corporate descent groups.

Tribe is a social group which have:
- Common territory
- Common religion
- Common language
- Common culture
- Common political organization
- Blood relations

Tribe has been defined as the social group which occupy the common territory, having ties of blood relationship and belong to common religion. Therefore, tribe is a group of people, often of related families, who live in the same area and share the same language, culture, and history.

According to **Imperial Gazette of India**, *'A tribe is a collection of families bearing a common name, speaking common dialect, occupying or professing to occupy a common territory and is usually not endogamous, though originally it might have been so.'*

Features of Tribal Society

- A tribe should least functional interdependence within the community.
- It should be economically backward.
- There should be a comparative geographical isolation of its people.
- They should have a common dialect.
- Tribes should be politically organized, and community panchayat should be influent.
- A tribe should have customary laws.

Schedule Tribe

The term 'Scheduled Tribes' first appeared in the Constitution of India. Article 366 (25) defined scheduled tribes as "such tribes or tribal communities or parts of or groups within such tribes or tribal communities as are deemed under Article 342 to be Scheduled Tribes for the purposes of this constitution".

They are socially and economically backward which was derived from their long-time habitation in geographically isolated areas with difficult terrain & practicing shifting cultivation. Lack of education and isolation from social mainstream made them vulnerable to exploitation by non-tribals and uprooting from traditional habitation and occupation so that they were relegated to lowest end of economic hierarchy.

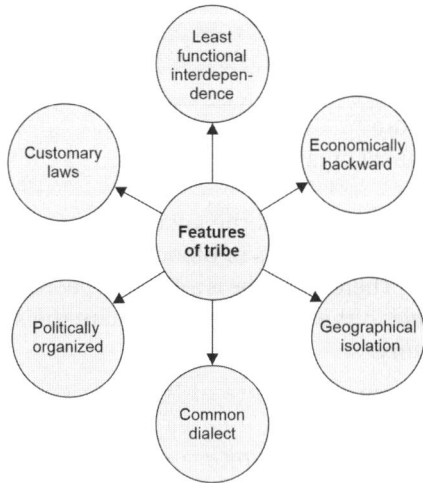

Problems of Tribal Community

The common problems that the tribes or tribal community faced are:

Land Alienation

The history of land alienation among the tribes began during British colonialism in India. The tribal property and lands were occupied by money lenders, zamindars and traders by advancing them loans.

Poverty and Indebtedness

Majority live under poverty line. The tribes follow many simple occupation based on simple technology.

Health and Nutrition

In many parts of India tribal population suffers from chronic infections and diseases out of which water borne diseases are life threatening. They also suffer from deficiency disorders.

Education

Most of the tribal areas are located in interior and remote areas, teacher would not like to go from outside and the children remain uneducated.

Cultural Problems

The tribal people are initiating Western culture in different aspect of their social life and leaving their own culture. It has led to degeneration of tribal life and tribal arts such as dance, music, and different types of craft.

CASTE

The Meaning of Caste: Origin of the Word

The word 'caste' owes its origin to the Portuguese word 'casta' which means breed, race, strain, or a complex of hereditary qualities.

The Portuguese applied this term to the classes of people in India known by the name **Jati**. The English word 'caste' is an adjustment of the original term. Caste means a group of people bearing a common name and having traditional occupation forming a homogenous community.

CH Cooley says, *'When a class is somewhat strictly hereditary, we call it caste.'*

According to **Green**, *'Caste system of stratification in which modality up and down the status ladder at least ideally does not occur.'*

According to **Megasyhanes**, *'Two elements of caste system are (i) there is no intermarriage and (ii) there can be no change of profession.'*

Kettar says, *'Caste is a group having two characteristics, membership is confined to those who are born of members and forbidden by inexorable social law to marry outside the group.'*

According to **Dharma shastra**, *'Caste means social exclusiveness with reference to diet and marriage; birth and ritual are necessary.'*

According to **Anderson & Parker**, *'Caste is that extreme form of social organisation in which position of individuals in the status hierarchy is determined by descend and birth.'*

Origin and Development of Caste System

Caste system is supposed to be sophisticated form of various dharma. In Rigveda, there is reference to three main classes—Brahmana, Kshatriya, and Vaishya. Sudra is considered to be a dasa, a class which is recognized in later period.

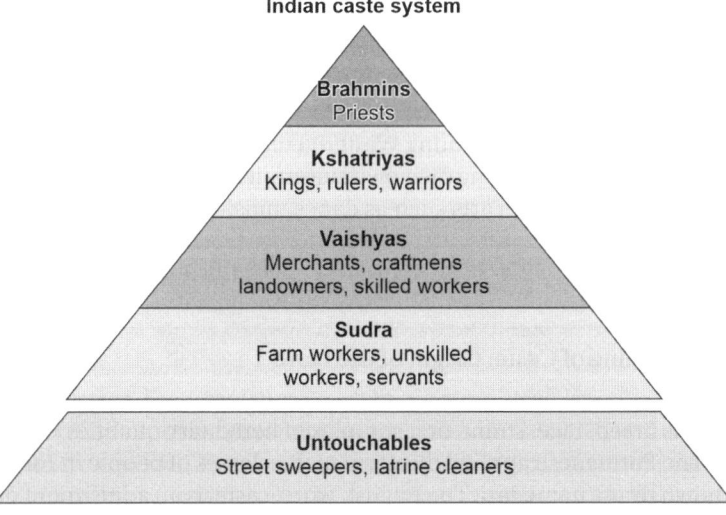

According to **GS Ghrye**, 'Caste in India must be regarded as a Brahmanic child of the Indo-Aryan culture, cradled in the land of Ganges, and then transferred to other parts of India by the Brahmin prospectors.

Rigveda mentions that Brahmin is created from the mouth of Purusha, Kshatriya from his arms and Vaishya from his thighs. It stresses the difference between Arya and Dasa not only in color but also in speech, physical features, and religious practice.

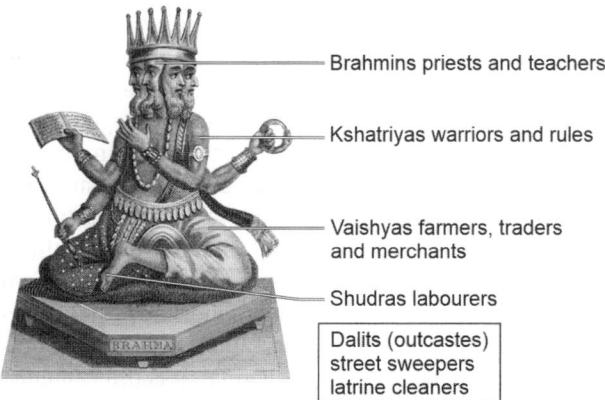

- Brahmins priests and teachers
- Kshatriyas warriors and rules
- Vaishyas farmers, traders and merchants
- Shudras labourers
- Dalits (outcastes) street sweepers latrine cleaners

The Dasa are mixed group born out of intermarriage of other three classes and considered as sudras or nishadas.

The classes mentioned in Rigveda are based on division of labor, viz, occupation adopted by the groups, but they were not stratified or rigid. They were open system of changing from group to group.

During the post Vedic period and medieval period, caste system developed into rigid and stratified institution based on birth, imposing severe restrictions on the relations between them. During the modern period, several changes have taken place in the structure and functions of caste.

An exact origin of caste cannot be easily traced as it is complex phenomenon prevailing since many ages. Several thinkers have attempted to explain its origin by formulating certain theories of caste system. The most important of these theories are traditional theory, occupational theory, religious theory, political theory, racial theory, and evolutionary theory.

Special Features of Caste System

Birth

The status of birth is an important characteristic feature of caste. It accounts for the hereditary tract of the individual. Every person born in his caste cannot alter his caste status till his death by any other means.

Differences in caste status have basically determined by birth. It is an unalterable hereditary disposition of the individual.

Hierarchical Division of Society

Among the four castes, the status is hierarchical. Brahmins at the top and Sudra at the bottom whereas Kshatriya and Vaishya are intermediary groups. The demarcation is high and lower is indicated in terms of birth and the individual remains in his caste status throughout of his life. The caste system has a caste council to regulate and guide the life of its members. It was known as caste. Panchayat to deal with offences committed by persons who violated caste regulations. Customs about birth, marriage and death varied among different caste groups. Castes are, therefore, small and complete units in themselves, definitely marked off from one another even though subsisting in a larger society. The doctrine of karma explains the birth of a person in a higher or lower caste. Caste is determined by ones past deeds and becomes at birth right for every individual. It is thus an eternal law that governs every person according to his karma. Restrictions on food drinks and social intercourse—caste regulations are stringent in respect of food, drink, and social intercourse. The sanctions and prohibits are peculiar and interesting. The notions of purity and impurity are the keynote of caste structure. Social intercourse between higher and lower caste is forbidden in terms of food, drink and even contacts. Food is classified into pakka and kacha. Pakka food is prepared by water, kacha food is considered polluted when prepared by a lower caste. Hindu members of lower castes may eat at the hands of a higher caste but not vice versa. Raw materials also other cooked food may be accepted by higher castes from lower groups. There is the idea of pollution by touch. Even wells are said to be polluted at the sight and the shadow of untouchables are considered as pollution by Brahmins. Ceremonial ablution of bathing and ritual are required to restore purity. All castes accept food and water from a Brahmin. Rigid restrictions of food, drink and social intercourse are more prominent between the highest and lowest caste groups. Civil and religious disabilities and privileges to certain caste groups: Segregation is an important feature of caste system. The untouchables like holeyas and madigas are segregated so as to live separately in the outskirts of the villages. They cause pollution by contacts and are forbidden to enter temples. Notions of purity and pollution are found even in different occupations. Dirty and repulsive work like washing and scavenging are regarded impure and persons who follow them are debarred. Brahmins are forbidden to officiate in cremation of lower castes.

Touch, drawing water from well, spitting on the street, wearing shoes, walking with umbrellas, entering temples, and moving in certain localities are forbidden to the lower caste groups. Brahmins who work on family priests for impure castes become polluted and regarded as inferior Brahmins.

Restrictions on Choice of Occupation

Each caste has a traditional occupation and is called functional caste by such occupation. Brahmins are called priests, kshatriyas as warriors, Vaishyas as traders and sudras as menials. There are restrictions on the choice of occupation among the different caste groups. It was not merely a moral restraint, but a restriction imposed by caste calling. Brahmin could not do the work of the toddy tapping or scavenging and in the same way, sudras cannot become a priest.

Restrictions on Marriage

Caste is an endogamous group imposing restrictions to marriage outside its own fold. Each caste or sub-caste forbids its members to marry outside its group. Endogamy is the essence of caste system. Those who violated the rules of endogamy were expelled from their caste group and deprived of caste privileges and condemned as out castes. Even the rights of inheritance were denied to children of persons, who married outside their own caste group. Inter-caste marriages are declared null and void by pandits and caste council.

Changing Trends in Caste System

Caste in India is supposed to be a rigid institution with many stratified groups in the form of sects and sub-sects. The emergence of a large number of jaties or sub-sects is due to violations of caste regulations in the original fourfold system. Caste rigidity is more stringent among sects and sub-sects than among the major four groups, man sub-castes have given up traditional occupations and dissociated from caste obligations. Buddhism, Jainism, Islam, Christianity, Sikhism, condemned the rigidity of hindu caste system but could not alter it. In the contrary, those religious groups were influenced by caste structure and its functions and many caste-like groups were introduced in those religion. Several reform movements like Arya samaj, Brahman samaj, Veerashaivism, Bhakti movement, Ramakrishna mission tried to denounce the institution of caste declaring that it has no religious sanction. Mahatma Gandhi struggled hard to eradicate the evil of untouchability in india and for promoting communal harmony between hindus and muslims in India. Changes in caste system may be analyzed under two periods: Preindependent days and postindependent period.

Changes in Caste System During Pre-Independent Period

During the preindependent period British administration had tremendous influence on the institution of caste. British rulers introduced several laws in order to bring about fundamental changes in traditional caste system. They applied equity in matters of administration and introduced certain legal norms to abolish the caste hierarchy. The lower caste groups become conscious of their legal rights and fought against higher groups to avoid exploitation. But the higher caste groups by their superior knowledge and economic resource thwarted their attempts.

- Western types of education in schools and colleges were liberal and secular to alter the traditional religious education of caste groups.
- Increasing opportunities of employment for both men and women and public offices and industries broke the barriers of caste.
- Occupations become pursuits of individual choice instead of being hereditary and traditional.
- Impact of new occupational patterns of caste created cultural diffusion and economic classes.
- Industrialization during the 19th century provided new uniform work styles and division of labor and several unions were started during 20th century.
- Migration of rural people from rural to industrial cities caused break of traditional caste ideas.
- Ascribed status of caste occupations changed to achieved status by performance of work.
- Family and kinship groups which were once the units of production were affected by new industrial system.
- Industrialization caused urbanization in which people of all caste groups mingled with new ideas of commercialisms, economic enterprise, leisure, and entertainment.
- The cumulative effects of industrialization and urbanization on traditional hindu caste society and envisaged in a gradual transformation ascribed status to dynamic achieved status of individuals.
- Modern education introduced by Britishers to some social reform movement like brahma samaj and arya samaj which attempted to ward off the evils of traditional caste system.

- The status of women changed with new concepts through education and employment opportunities.
- The concept of Sanskritization is a process of imitating the habits and cultural values of higher caste groups by lower caste.
- The word Brahminization interpret caste mobility of the lower caste groups by copying dress, food, and rituals of Brahmins.
- Brahminization to a wider concept of Sanskritization means a total change in the way of life applicable to all low caste groups and tribes. Sanskritization and Westernization affected the traditional caste system to a great extent.

There are various changes at different levels of new technology. Institutions of ideology and values rationalism, individualism, nationalism, humanitarianism, and secularism are the new concept of westernization, which led to a series of changes in institution and outlook of people. It led to various reforms cutting across the barriers of traditional caste system.

Changes in Caste System During Post Independent Period

- Indian constitution inaugurated on 26th January 1950 proclaimed India as a sovereign democratic republic with the main aim of creating a casteless and class less society.
- Hindu caste system based on inequalities of birth and social status was condemned by the fundamental rights incorporated in Indian constitution. India as a sovereign democratic republic establishes equality to all citizens irrespective of caste, creed, or religion.
- There are many restrictions in caste system on food drink, marriage, social movements, and religious practices. These setbacks are opposed to democratic principles.
- Hindu orthodoxy is considered as a great social evil and employment opportunities, recognizing inter-caste marriages, promoting civil control forms of marriage without traditional rituals, permitting remarriage of widows, providing facilities for social and economic betterment of lower caste groups are promulgated to eliminate the evils of caste system.
- Caste restrictions in respect of untouchables are most stringent, Mahatma Gandhi tried his best to ameliorate the conditions of harijans. Being downtrodden and depressed by higher caste groups the untouchables resorted to conversion to avoid ill treatment.
- Occupation patterns has changed. But associations among particular caste groups are formed for privileges and as a revolt against traditional restrictions.

- These have been anti-brahminical movements in Maharashtra, Tamil Nadu, and Karnataka.
- Gautama Buddha criticized Brahmin orthodoxy and many social reformers condemned Brahmins for their pre-eminent social positions. The rise of Mahars and Marathas as political groups in Maharashtra, Kammas and Reddys in Andhra Pradesh, DK and DMK movement in Tamil Nadu, Lingayat and Vokkaliga groups in Karnataka were anti-brahminical to wipe out Brahmins from power and pre-eminence.
- There has been a tendency towards formation of caste associations particularly among lower caste groups.
- Casteism has developed in a much narrower sense of group loyalty converted into politics. Caste consciousness has increased and rivalries between castes are intense and competitive in order to achieve power, privileges and status

Institutions of caste has secured new fields of activity in politics. Elections in many administrative bodies clearly reveal that caste element is a decisive factor. Caste is at present a political structure with a series of changes from its traditional imperatives.

POLITICAL GROUP

Max Weber defines the politics as a human community that successfully claims the monopoly of the legitimate use of physical force within a given territory.

Groups are formed to attain and maintain political power with specific goals. These political groups are of many types depending upon the type of political party. A person who belongs to a particular political party, it means that individual is a member of that political group.

Definition

A political group is a special interest group, which seeks to promote the interests of its members through external inducement political groups actively takes part in the formulation of government and trade unions.

A political party is an organised group of people having similar political aims and opinions. It is also defined as a political organization that seek to attain and maintain political power within government.

India has multi part system. Each political part has its own manifest. The number off political groups vary from state to state or country to country.

The main aim of the political group is to work for the welfare of the society. Political group plays a vital role in the election process. It includes nomination, canvassing and campaigning.

Political leaders are considered as the powerful personalities in the society. Entire political group is directed and guided by its leaders. There is always a risk of split. If the members are not satisfied with their leaders or policies, they may jump into another group, in India, lot of political groups are there. Even though the ultimate aim of political group is to do good for the public, many circumstances they said to satisfy the public

Types of Political Part System

1. **Nonpartisan**: It means there is no official political party exist.
2. **Single dominant party**: In this type of political system, one political party is legally allowed to hold executive power. Minor parties accept the leadership of dominant parties. Example- China
3. **Two-party system:** Only the two main parties have a serious chance of winning a majority of seats to form a government. The United States of America and the United Kingdom are examples of a two-party system.
4. **Multi-party system:** More than two parties have a reasonable chance of coming to power either on their own strength or in alliance with others. Thus, in India, we have a multiparty system.

Important Functions of Political Groups

- Bridges antagonism between different groups of the society
- Act as very effective mediator in setting disagreements in society in a peaceful and institutionalized manner.
- Ensure a two-way communication process between the government and the people as it is mainly through the parties that the government is constantly kept informed about the general demands of the society.
- Educate and instruct the people on public issues.
- Significant role in the process of political socialization in a country

RELIGIOUS GROUP

According to **Ogburn**, *'Religion is a belief in powers which control and direct the course of human life. Man believes in supernatural power which is higher to his own power and is governed by faith.'*

According to **Durkheim**. *'Religion is unified system of beliefs and practices relative to sacred things, things set apart and for bidden.'*

Tylor defines religion as a belief in spiritual beings.

In the modern world, there are thousands of religions, each religion has its own way of expressing the faith, religion always stresses the fellowship in development, teaching of religious insight and knowledge. It is a mixture of beliefs, problem of human existence. Religious groups are considered as society, important system of religious beliefs and practices, which are standardized, widely shared, and viewed as necessary and true.

According to **Anderson** and **Parker**, each religion has 4 components.

Belief in supernatural power	• Man believes that all human conditions are due to supernatural forces
Man's adjustment to supernatural power	• Man adjust himself to supernatural powers by doing some of outward acts according to religion such as prayer, kirtan, hymns, etc.
Acts defined as sinful	• When an individual is not performing the tasks or acts according to religion, then these acts are sinful • It is believed that the person performing sinful act has to suffer the wrath of God
Method of salvation	• Man adopted these method of salvation for removing the guilt • These are performed to keep an individual free from bondage of Karma

Important Functions of Religious Groups

❖ Each group has its own rituals and members are expected to follow.
❖ It defines the nature of relationship of human beings to one another and to God.
❖ It is service oriented, emphasize the service to poor, the needy and stock.
❖ Religious groups serve humanity through spreading education.
❖ Medical services are provided by many religious groups.
❖ Giving something in a charity is an important function of religious group
❖ It emphasizes on sacrifice and for heritance.
❖ All religious groups preach about nonviolence, encourage the sense of brotherhood.

By all these functions, we conclude religious groups light the human life by controlling and nurturing. Some religious groups misinterpret the preaching of their own religion and involve in antisocial activities. Each religious group is having their own beliefs and practices.

MOB

Mob is an aggressive crowd. It is the crowd of people, generally of criminal who act against the law. The mob gathers with a specific purpose for a temporary period of time.

The term mob can also be described sometimes to represent planned or organized form of crime. The mob behaves in extreme way often, we hear about crowd that get out of hand, people are trembled to death or about riots after a large spotting event which led to damage to property or injury to people.

Groups have incredible effects on individual's behavior and group behavior tends to be more extreme than typical behavior of its individual member. A mob is an influential force in changing people's behavior. Group encourage and brings a sense of anonymity in its members which results in antisocial behavior.

The term 'Mob' is derived from the Latin phrase 'mobile vulgus' which means easily moveable crowd. There is a term 'ochlocracy' which is a Latin word that means the government by mob or mass of people or intimidation of constitutional authorities.

Mob affect the policies. The crowd which causes violence on non-acceptance of decision of crowd, causes fear and frightens the large number of people and try to win the day.

Characteristics of Mob

- It affects individuals and group behavior toward extreme.
- It is influential force that change individual behavior.
- It encourages and brings a sense of anonymity in its members which results in anti-social behavior.
- Mob is the crowd that gone out of control.
- Mobs are usually involved in looting and grabbing power by means of fraud.
- Mobs are created by those individuals who exploit or cause violence.
- Policies and laws are affected by the mobs.
- Mobs are commonly manipulated by political leaders.
- Mob marches and shouts common demands if one is charged with uncomfortable task of refusing them.

CROWD

Crowd is a large and definable group of people. Crowd is 'gathering of a considerable number of persons around a centre of or point of common attention.' Crowd can also be called a mass.

Crowd is a physical compact of aggregation of individuals temporarily reacting to same stimuli in a similar way.

According to **Maclever**, *'A crowd is a physical compact aggregation of human beings brought into direct, temporary, and unorganised contact with one another.'*

According to **Contrill**, *'Crowd is a congregate group of individuals who have temporarily identified themselves with common values and who are expressing similar emotions.'*

According to **Thouless**, *'A crowd is a transitory contiguous group organized with completely permeable boundaries, spontaneously formed as a result of some common interests.'*

According to **McDougall**, *'Not every mass of human beings gather together in one place within sight and sound of one another constitutes a crowd in the psychological sense of the word.'*

Characteristics of Crowd

Generally, crowd is formed and is a part of social organization. The peculiar qualities of the crowd are in large. It arises only in the crevices of the social organization. Following are the characteristics of the crowd:

- Gathering or physical presence of individuals
- Temporary social group
- Unstable organization
- Polarization
- Transitory nature
- Anonymous
- Spatial distribution
- Sense of mass strength
- No sense of responsibility
- Does have any culture or own tradition
- Destructive in nature
- Unpredictable action

Apart from the general characteristics, crowd has certain psychological characteristics. These psychological characteristics are enumerated below:

- **Lack of intelligence**: In the crowd people do not apply intelligence. They behave like mass of people and guided more by emotions than intelligence. As individuals, many of the members of the crowd would not agree with their own behavior than they display as members of that crowd.
- **Lack of responsibility in a crowd**: In crowd people lack responsibility that is why crowd sometimes commits crime and resorts to violence.
- **Lack of volition**: Crowd lacks organization. It is formed for a transitory object. Once that object has vanished the crowd also disperses. The idea and the feelings of the members of the crowd are not permanent. They lack will power of volition.
- **Heightened susceptibility**: In a crowd suggestion acts very fast. Crowd is very suggestible and that is why people can use it as they like.
- **High emotionality**: In crowd every person is under influence of emotion. These high emotions trend is responsible for extraordinary behavior.
- **Credulity**: Members of the crowd accept anything that is told to them. This is due to their heightened suggestibility and emotional attitude.
- **Expression of unconscious impulses**: In a crowd people give vent to their suppressed desires as conscious impulses. According to Freud 'crowd provides an opportunity to the individuals to satisfy their suppressed desires and depressed feelings.
- **Instability of ideas**: In a crowd the ideas of people are unstable. They change very fast. This is lack of rationality and that is why the behavior of the members of the crowd is unstable and unpredictable.
- **Influence of leader**: Because of heightened suggestibility and emotionality, the influence of the leader acts fast on the members of the crowd. If the leader is successful, he is able to play upon the emotions of the members of the crowd.
- **Social facilitation:** Crowd is a collection of people at one place. Because of this collection their responses are very fast. Social facilitation or small social distances provide a good deal of motives and inspirations to individuals.
- **Immortality**: In a crowd people lack responsibility, they do not bother about moral values. They act as they think proper. That is why the behavior of the members of the crowd lacks all responsibility and morality.

Social Aspects of Crowds

Social aspects are concerned with the formation, management, and control of crowds, both from the point of view of individuals and groups. Often crowd control is designed to persuade a crowd to align with particular view, e.g., political rallies or to contain groups to prevent damages or mob behavior. Politically organized crowd control is usually conducted by law enforcement, but some occasion military forces are used for particularly large or dangerous crowds.

Classification of the Crowd

Crowd has been classified by various social thinkers in different ways.
1. According to **MacIver and Page**: MacIver and Page have classified the crowd on the basis of interests. They have classified it into two types:
   a. *Like interest crowd:* Such crowd is found when people because of their curiosity collect at one particular place around an object. They have a common interest, e.g., those interested in religion collect at particular place for worship or for some other reasons.
   b. *Common interest crowd:* Such a crowd collects, or such a crowd is formed because of some common object or interest. A very good example of such a crowd could be seen when the workers in a factory or students of an institution have gone on strike for the fulfillment of their demands.
2. According to **Kimball and Young**: Kimball Young has classified the crowd on the basis of relationship.
   a. *Attack rage crowd:* That crowd which is full of anger and is a mood to attack somebody or something is called attack rage crowd. Usually such a crowd is found when an accident has taken place due to negligence of somebody, then a crowd that has formed gets angry and takes the action of attacking the person, who has committed that negligent action causing accident.
   b. *Panic crowd:* When a crowd is formed because of fear and wants to run away to save itself, it is called panic crowd such a crowd is formed when some dangerous thing happened, of a communal riot has broken out or a bombardment has taken place, usually people collect together and afraid of the impending catastrophe, they not only collect together but also plan to run away, such a crowd is called panic crowd.
   c. *Passive crowd:* That crowd does not act and only remains passive spectator to the thing has happening is called a passive

crowd. Usually, it so happens when two persons or two bulls start fighting on the street, a crowd collects around the scene of the fighting but it does not take any action. It only remains as a passive spectator or a crowd onlooker.

3. According to **Roger W Brown**: The well-known social thinker Roger W Brown has categorized the crowd under the following heads:

   a. *Escape crowd or panicky crowd:* The crowd that collects because of some sudden fearful event and is full of panic is intending to run away is called panicky crowd, escape mob or crowd. It may be organized as well as unorganized.

   b. *Acquisitive crowd:* The crowd that collects at a place with the object of meeting some crisis or difficult situation about which it is acquired some knowledge in advance, the crowd that collects at the cinema counter for booking tickets in advance for a particular picture which is likely to attract huge crowds can be put under this class of the crowd.

   c. *Expressive crowd:* That crowd which lacks the qualities of the three types of crowds enumerated above is called the expressive crowd. As we have stated that this crowd aims at expressing or exhibiting some feeling or emotion. The crowd that forms itself into a procession at the time of 'Holi' rivalry is crowd of the category.

   d. *Audience:* This crowd is an organized crowd that has collected for a particular purpose we shall deal with this type of crowd at a separate place.

4. According to **Le Bon**: He categorise the crowd into-

   a. *Homogenous crowd:* Crowd formed from people of same caste, class etc

   b. *Heterogenous crowd:* Crowd may be anonymous like or not such as in case of street crowd and parliamentary assemblies respectively.

SOCIAL PROCESSES

The process by which people act and react in relation to others is called social interaction. The interaction process means the way in which partners agree on their goals, negotiate behavior, and distribute resources. Certain common forms of social interactions which are called as social processes exist all over the world. Social processes refer to respective forms of behaviors which are commonly found in social life.

The types of mode of interaction or social processes can broadly be divided into associative and dissociative types- cooperation, assimilation and accommodation are associative social processes, competition and conflict are dissociative social processes.

Those processes which link and connect individual either physically or mentally and brings them together are termed as associative process and those which disconnect people and sometimes develop antipathy seeing against each other are dissociative process.

Cooperation

Cooperation involves individuals or groups working together for the achievement of their individual or collective goals, in its simplest form, cooperation may involve only two people who work together towards a common goal.

For example: Two girls perform a dance jointly in cooperation towards achievement of a reward. The medical health team members work in cooperation to achieve the health of a patient.

There would have been no social life without cooperation. This is the most elementary process of society. Cooperation is possible in the form of social interaction where two or more persons work together to gain a common end. In the process of cooperation, it involves with two or more individuals or groups who have common goals. They have the sense of unity and work towards the common goal.

Definition

According to **Fairchild**: Cooperation is the process by which individuals or groups combine their efforts in more or less organized form for the attainment of common objective.

According to **AW Green**: Cooperation is the continuous and common endeavour of two or more persons to perform a task to reach a goal that is commonly cherished

Classification of Cooperation

According to **MacIver** and **Page**, it can be divided into five principal types:

Unit 2: Social Structure

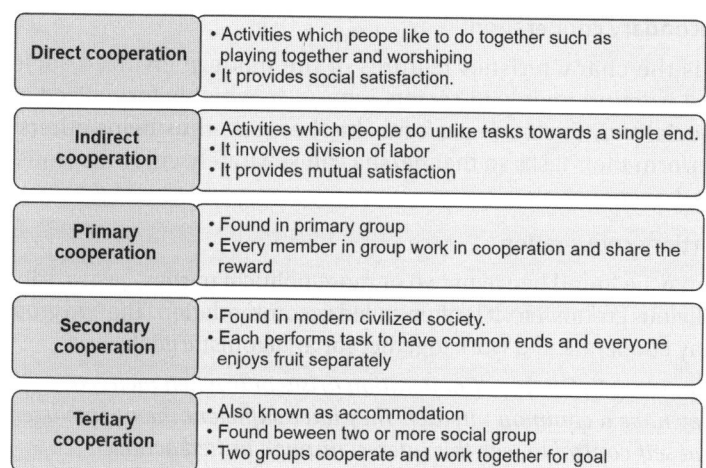

Direct cooperation

Those activities in which people do like things together, play together, worship together, labor together in myriad ways.

In the direct cooperation process, the cooperating individuals do like things together and perform identical functions they involve together either because of face-to-face relation while performing a task or because it brings them social satisfaction. All the activities, e.g., play together, worshiping together.

Indirect cooperation

Indirect cooperation includes the activities in which people do unlike tasks towards a similar end. Each member has his or her own specialized function. This is the special form of cooperation function of the principles of the division of labor. Indirect cooperation is playing a significant role in the modern society, e.g., doctors, nurses and all, health team members taking care of a patient.

Primary cooperation

It is found in primary groups such as family, neighbourhood, friend and so on. Here there is an identity end. The rewards for which everyone works are shared or meant to be shared with every other member in the group. Means and goals become one for cooperation itself is a highly priced value.

Secondary cooperation

It is the characteristics features of the modern civilized society and is found mainly in society groups. It is highly formalized and specialized. Each one performs his/her task, thus helps others to perform their tasks so that he/she can separately enjoy the fruits of his/her cooperation.

Tertiary cooperation

It may be found between two or more political parties, castes, tribes, religious groups, etc. It is often called accommodation. The two groups may cooperate and work together for antagonistic goals.

According to **Cooley**, *'Cooperation arises only when men realize that they have a common interact. They have sufficient theme intelligence and self-control to seek this interest through united action.'*

Cooperation and Social Life

- ❖ Cooperation is the fundamental unit of social life.
- ❖ Cooperation helps in the nurture and socialization of individuals.
- ❖ Cooperation is very much needed for the progress.
- ❖ Cooperation helps for the achievements of economical, political, religious, and educational institutions.
- ❖ Cooperation helps to face challenge arise in the social life.
- ❖ Cooperation is needed for both pleasure as well as survival.
- ❖ Cooperative in the basis of social progress and advancements.

Competition

Competition is modified form of struggle; competitive endeavour is a basic human drive manifested in procuring the needs of life. Men and women struggle by way of competition to secure social status.

Competition is neither free nor unrestricted. It is socially restricted. Some people think that competitive process is inherent in original human nature without any cultural holding. But cultural experience provides opportunities for competition and without cultural learning.

There is no social struggle or rivalry which induces competition. Competitive efforts, therefore patterned by culture. Competition is found not only within culture among its members but also between two or more different culture.

In modern society, competition is regarded as an ideal economic pattern. It is the life of trade and basis for modern economy, e.g., competitive business is found in modern economic life, very often it is hindered by monopoly through the cooperation of compelling businessman. Apparently free competition is not in place but remains ideal in modern democracy.

Competition is dynamic—stimulating aspirations and threatening failures. It may be cutthroat by bitter rivalries and monopolies.

Definitions

Mazumdar defines *'Competitions are the impersonalized struggle among assembling greatness for goods and services which are limited is quantity.'*

Bogardus defines, *'Competition is a contest to obtain something which does not exist in a quantity sufficient to meet the demand'*

According to **Park** and **Berger**, *'Competition is an interaction without social contact'*

Characteristics of Competition

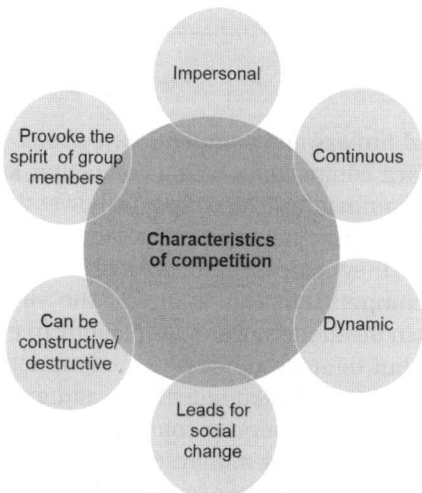

- Competition is mostly an impersonal process. The individuals may or may not be aware of but mostly he may not have personal contact with other competitions.
- Competition is an unconscious process. Mostly the individuals who are engaged in competition may become oblivious of the fact that they are in competitive race. Rarely they know about their competitions. It is universal and found in every country and every group.
- It is continuous process. There is no end for competition. It is found in every area of social interaction.

- Competition is a dynamic process. It stimulates achievements and contributes significantly to social change.
- Scarcity is the effect of competition.
- Competition leads for social change. It makes person to adopt new form of behavior to attain desired goals.
- Competitions may be constructive or destructive.
- Norms and rules are needed to control and regulate the competition.
- Competition provokes the spirit of the group members.
- Competitions aims at the attainment of the objective in orderly manner.
- Competition makes the society to become active otherwise the society would have remained static and becomes inactive.

Areas of Competition

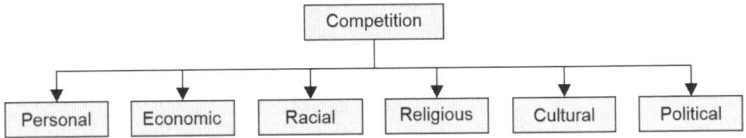

- **Personal and impersonal competition**: Personal competition is the face-to-face competition, or the competitor knows his rival. When people compete for leadership or for power, their competition is personal. In impersonal competition, the competitor does not know his rival. They compete as member of the group.
- **Economic competition**: This is one of the vigorous forms of competition in the modern world. Apparently free competition is not in place but remains an ideal in modern democracy. These competitions occur between individuals and groups to improve their standard of life, economic conflicts include conflicts arises for job, salary, promotions, money, wealth, and property, etc.
- **Racial competition**: This type of competition takes place between two racial groups. The clashes between Negros and Whites for power are the classical example.
- **Religious competition**: Religious competitions take place between two religious groups or two denominations in same religion. It can take place between Hindus and Muslims or protestant and catholic Christians.
- **Cultural competition**: Cultural competitions occur among people with different cultures or two groups with different cultural and ideological system.

- **Political competition**: Nowadays all the political groups want power. All the members in the political parties are struggling for that. Especially in the democratic set up the political competition is an unavoidable one.
- **Social competition**: Every individual wants to achieve something in his life. People always struggle to acquire higher status in the society. They compete to achieve the self-actualization. State in the Author **Maslow's** hierarchy of needs theory. This competition is known as social competition

Advantages of Competition

- Competition assigns individuals their respective place in the society.
- Competition always aims upward movement.
- It is a very good sources of motivation for the individual.
- Competition contributes to the socioeconomic progress.
- Competition provides the new and better opportunities to satisfy the individual's desire.
- Healthy competition helps the false development of personality of the members of the society.

Like cooperation, competition occurs at personal group and organizational levels, people competing for affections, promotion or public office all are example of personal competition. The competition is likely to know one another and to regard others defeat as essential to the attainment of their own goals.

Difference between Cooperation and Competition

Cooperation	Competition
Cooperation refers to a form of social interaction of two or more persons work together to gain a common reward Cooperation refers to a form of social interaction of two or more persons work together to gain a common reward	Competition is a form of sound interaction of individual to monopolize rewards by suppressing all the rivals
It is always based on joint errors of the people	It can take place either at group or individuals' levels
It normally brings positive results	It can bring either positive results or negative results

Contd...

Contd...

Cooperation	Competition
Cooperation requires qualities such as kindness, sympathy, concern for others mutual understanding to help	Competition requires qualities such as strong aspirations, self-confidence, the desire to earn name adventure, and the readiness to suffer and to struggle
It brings satisfactions and contentment	It may cause satisfactions as well as dissatisfactions, anxiety and uncertainty

Conflict

Conflict is a good oriented, just as cooperation and competition are, but there is a difference, in conflict one seeks deliberately to harm and/or destroy one's antagonists.

The rules of competition always include restrictions upon the injury that may be done to a foe. But in conflict these rules break down, one seeks to win at any cost, in talking about conflict, the notion of a continuum or scale is again useful.

It is useful in at least two ways, in differentiating conflict from competition and in differentiating personal form group and organizational conflict.

Conflict is one of the dissociative processes, conflict is just opposite to cooperation. This occurs when the interests are exclusive and in harmonious. In the conflict process two or more persons or groups try to prevent of the work. The attainment of certain objectives by other even to the extent of involving violence.

Definition

According to **Gillin** and **Gillin,** *'Conflict is the social process in which individuals or groups seek their and by directly challenging the antagonist by violence or threat of violence.'*

According to **AW Green**, *'The deliberate attempt to oppose, resist or coerce the will of another or others.'*

According to **Young** and **Young,** *'Conflict takes the form of emotionalised and violent opposition in which major concern is to overcome the component as a means of securing a given goal or reward.'*

Characteristics of Conflict

- Conflicts are universal
- They are personalised
- Conditioned by culture

Types of Conflict

George Simmel has classified the conflict into four types. They are:
- **War**: In war, conflicts develop between two or more groups or two nations for different reasons.
- **Fractional or feudal strike**: This conflict arises between the group members inside the groups. This is the Intra group conflict.
- **Litigation**: This is a judicial form of conflict; this conflict is made to assert own rights or claims.
- **Conflicts of impersonal ideals**: This is another form of small-scale conflict; this occurs because of different viewpoints and ideas clash between the individuals.

Other important forms of conflicts are:
- Direct conflict
- Indirect conflict
- Personal conflict
- Economic conflict
- Racial conflict
- Classic conflict
- Political conflict
- Group conflict
- Majority and minority conflict
- Religious conflict

Advantages of Conflict

- Conflict points issues in the group.
- Conflicts lead to find out the solutions for the problems.
- Conflicts increase the group cohesion.
- Conflicts make the group to be always alert.
- Conflicts promote unity in the group

Disadvantages of Conflict

- Conflicts create bitterness in the group.
- Conflicts lead to bloodshed, destruction, and other antisocial activities

- Conflicts develop intergroup tensions.
- Conflicts disrupts normal channel of cooperation.
- Conflicts divert attention of group members.

Effects of Conflicts

Effects of social conflicts according to Mazumdar:
- Conflicts increase two morals of the group.
- Conflicts promote solidarity of the group.
- Conflicts modify or alter the value pattern.
- Conflicts may help to find out the solutions for resolving the crises.
- Conflicts may lead to new consensus.
- Conflicts may bring changes in the status of the parties.

Conflict is an abnormal and universal form of social interaction as are any of the others. Analysis on conflict needs to describe both the ways in which it is harmful and destructive and the way which it is useful and socially integrative.

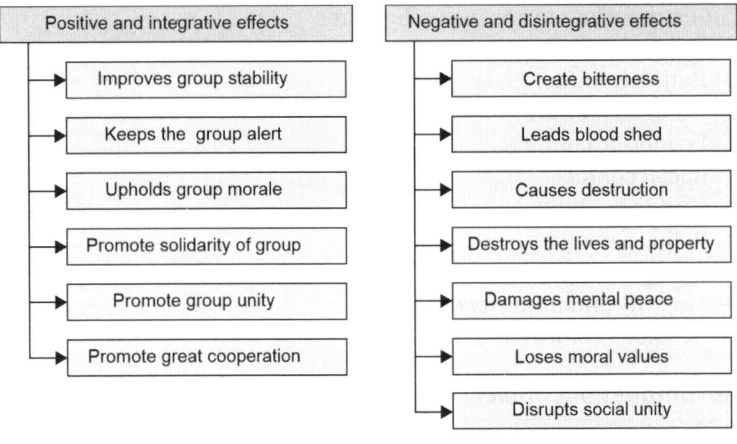

Difference between Competition and Conflict

Competition	Conflict
It is an unconscious process	It is a conscious process
Impersonal process	Personalized process
Continuous process	Intermittent process for a brief duration
It gives attention on the goal	Attention on the completion
It is non-violent	It may involve violence or threat of violence
Regard for the norms	No regard for any norms

Accommodation

This term 'accommodation' refers to several sorts of working agreements between rival groups that permit at least limited cooperation between them even though the issues dividing them remain unsettled. It does not technically end the conflict but holds in abeyance.

The accommodation may last for only short time and may be for the purpose of allowing the conflicting parties to consolidate their positions and to prepare for further conflict. It is more often their case, initial accommodation agreed upon by the parties may be part of the process of seeking solutions to the issues that divide them. If those solutions are not found, accommodation itself may become permanent.

Definition

According to **MacIver**, *'Accommodation refers particularly to the process in which man attains a sense of harmony with his environment.'*

According to **Ogburn and Nimkoff**, *'Accommodation is a term used by sociologist to describe the adjustment of hostile individuals or groups.'*

Accommodation is the first step in association process followed by cooperation. The term accommodation refers particularly to the process on which man attains a sense of harmony with his environment.

Characteristics of Accommodation

- Accommodation is impossible without a conflict.
- Accommodation is mostly an unconscious activity.
- It is universal.
- It is not stable one, continuous process.
- Accommodation process includes both love and hatred.

Different Forms of Accommodation

Summer refers accommodation as antagonistic cooperation. In the accommodation process the antagonism between conflicting elements is temporarily regulated.

Gillin and **Gillin** classified the different forms into the following:
- **Yielding to coercion or admitting one's defeat**: Meaning of coercion is used of force on there at by use of coercion conflicts can be terminated. It involves with the groups which are unequal

strength. The weaker groups yields because stronger group overpowered it.
- **Compromise**: When the conflict groups are utmost equal in power, they attain accommodation by means of compromise. In this process each group make some concessions and yields to some demand of the other, when the third groups or party involves in compromise that process is known as arbitration and conciliation.
- **Arbitration**: Arbitration is an effective device for bringing the compromise in which a third group or party tries to bring a solution to the conflict. The decision is binding on both parties.
- **Conciliation**: This is the form of arbitration. This attempt aims to find the solutions for the problems by developing friendship and understanding.
- **Toleration**: In this form of accommodation, there is neither settlement nor resolvement of the disputes, but only there is avoidance over the disputes, and conflict. This is based on live and let live policy. Both parties try to avoid each other or deliberately avoid conflict situation.
- **Conversation**: This form of accommodation involves a sudden reflection of one's own beliefs, convictions and loyalties and the adoption of other one group is convinced that they are wrong and tries to accept the viewpoint of the other group voluntarily.
- **Rationalization**: This form involves giving reasonable excuses or explanations for their behavior. Instead of accepting one's faults and shortcomings, the group tries to justify their own behavior. Americans had justified their attack towards Iraq that they want to destroy the nuclear threat.
- **Sublimation**: Sublimation involves the substitution of non-aggressive attitudes and activities for aggressive ones. This method is suggested by Jesus Christ to conquer violence and hatred by love and compassion.

Without accommodation social life is hardly possible. Accommodation checks and denies person and group to establish and maintain cooperation.

Assimilation

Assimilation is a social process of identification or integration of dissimilar individuals or group in terms of common interest attitude and outlook.

According to **Park**, *'Assimilation as a process of interpretation and fusion in which persons or groups acquire by memories, sentiments and attitudes of other persons or groups and by sharing their experience and history are incorporated with them in a culture life.'*

According to **Cuber**, *'Assimilation is a gradual process whereby cultural difference tend to disappear.'*

According to **Ogburn** and **Nimkoff**, *'Assimilation is the process whereby individuals or groups once dissimilar become similar and identified in their interest & outlook.'*

Assimilation generally referred to racial amalgamation. It represents a normative integration of dissimilar group in terms of similar standards, tastes, and interests. It denotes social acceptance. By assimilation a person or group acquires the values of another group.

Factors Contributing to Assimilation

- **Tolerance**: Without the human attitude of tolerance assimilation is not possible. It is a democratic virtue which fosters sympathy.
- **Intimacy**: Frequency and the nearness of human association is necessary for the start of assimilation process. Intimacy dissolves the walls of ultra-individualism which separates man from man.
- **Association**: Various association clubs and other places of public meeting are helpful. For the association only when people come together social process of all kinds including assimilatory set in and where there is still association of people there is likely to be no assimilation process.
- **Cultural similarity**: Often two persons, groups or cultures have many points in common. This mutual similarity creates mutual affinities which bring any of these two, i.e., individuals and groups are culture into better assimilation process.
- **Equal economical opportunity**: Modern age may be described as the age of money. Money is the supreme driving force, but to get favor of this money equal economical opportunities are required and any disparity in economical opportunity may mean diminished assimilation process.

Feeling of superiority and inferiority and exploration of weakness section of population by stronger one, contradictory to the assimilation process

Importance of Assimilation in Social Life

- Assimilation provides opportunity for close social contact.
- Assimilation process helps to overcome the economic difference among the members.
- Assimilation helps to adopt and adjust with the new culture.
- It promotes tolerance.
- It minimizes the ethnocentric feeling.
- It promotes harmony, unity, peace, and integration between the groups.

Difference between Accommodation and Assimilation

Accommodation	Assimilation
Accommodation may be a sudden process	Assimilation slow and gradual process
It may be temporary and provides only temporary solution	It is permanent method of adjustment of intergroup difference
Accommodation is deliberate and conscious effort	Assimilation is unconscious and it takes without any deliberate effort

Isolation

Isolation is another form of dissociative process. Interaction is the social behavior of all human beings. Every individual interacts with each other in the form of communication. Communication can be either in verbal or nonverbal. Without interaction an individual cannot meet his/her own needs and of others in the society effectively.

On some occasions, because of certain reasons, individuals are not allowed to communicate and interact with each other, and their communication measures are prohibited. In such type of condition, an individual remains alone, and he/she cannot perform his/her role properly. His productive life will be imposed. This situation is called as isolation.

Types of Isolation

Special isolation

This type of isolation is external. It happens due to external factors. The community to a person or group enforce it as an enforced deprivation of contacts when a person is put to solitary imprisonment. In such case, the individual is deprived of the production of the community. An individual subjected to special isolation become aggressive and in the risk of showing antisocial behavior special isolation may lead to develop metabolic conditions and antisocial activities.

Organic isolation

Organic isolation is an internal isolation. It is caused by certain defect like blindness and deafness. It is not enforced by any external factors. The physically defective individual cannot perform to duties like a normal person. He/She cannot communicate to everybody properly. As a result of that he/she may get very less chance to make friendship. He/She may become suspicious, irritable, distressful, and frustrated. Organic isolation is also considered as partial isolation.

Isolation and Social Life

- Most of the individuals do not like isolation because all the individuals are interdependent. They cannot satisfy their needs by themselves. Everybody needs the company of others.
- Without human interaction the personality will not develop as a person. Human personality is the product of social interaction. Isolation hides the personality in human beings.
- Complete isolation is not useful in one's life but on some occasion temporary isolation helps the individual to overcome certain problem.
- Isolated communities are maintaining poor standard of living compared to the communities which are interacting with each other.
- The new technological transportation and communication facilities decrease gap between the communities. Even the communities residing in the remote areas like hills and forest are reachable to other societies.
- Social change is very slow among isolated communities. They are setting less change in the exposure of other culture traditions and linguistic sectors.
- Isolation promote solidarity because there will not be any pressure from outside communities, but permanent isolation is hardly useful for the growth of the society.

SOCIALIZATION

The definitions and the study of socialization make it clear that socialization is a process. This process starts from the birth of the child. Human beings come into the world as biological organism with animal needs. He is gradually moulded into a social being and he learns the social ways of acting and feeling. Without this process of moulding, the society cannot continue itself, nor can culture exist and nor could the individual become a person. This process of moulding is called socialization.

Socialization is the process of establishing relationships with each other by social beings. It consists of complex processes of interaction through which individual learns the habits, skills, beliefs, and standards of judgement which are necessary for being a participant of social group and communities. In this process of socialization, one comes to acquire the quality of sociality.

Definition of Socialization

'Socialization is the process of working together, of developing group responsibility, of being guided by the welfare needs of others.'
—**Bogardus**

'Socialization is the process by which individual learns to conform to the norms of the group.'
—**Ogburn**

Process of Socialization

- ❖ **Rearing**: Bringing up the child plays a very important role in the process of socialization. The way, the parents shall rear a child, the way he shall grow and acquire the qualities and traits that are the result of that way of bringing up. That is why we find that child has not been properly brought up or his needs have not been fulfilled, acquires contain antisocial traits.
- ❖ **Sympathy**: Sympathy is very important part of socialization. It influences the social development of the child very much. In the childhood, a child needs help of many people, he/she is rebellious if the parents do not provide sympathy, he/she acquires self-confidence, also develops the attitude of identifying himself/herself with the family and the society.
- ❖ **Identification**: If a child gets sympathy from parents, family, and neighbourhood, he/she develops the feeling of identifying. himself with all of them. Consequently, the feeling of identifying develops with him/her and he/she imitates the language, the way of living with values, etc. of the society and the atmosphere in which he/she is living.
- ❖ **Imitation**: The child while living in the family and the society acquires the traits of other individuals. He/she imitates them

and tries to act accordingly. This imitation develops the social qualities of the child.

- **Social teaching**: In the family, the parents impart teaching to the child about behavior, ways of living and ways of behavior in the society. This training and education develop in the child, the imitation, belief, moral values, and ideals from the family by the child moves the school and there also he/she is imparted the social education or social teaching.

According to **Miller** and **Dollard**, this social teaching is based on the following four elements.
1. Drive
2. Cue
3. Response
4. Reward

In fact, the child has certain needs, and he tries to fulfil those needs and makes attempts for them. Sometimes he/she repeats those performances as result of which he learns certain things. The socialization process continues throughout all stages of human life.

- **Perceiving the situation:** A child has to change his or her behavior pattern according to the situation. He/she cannot behave similar manner in all circumstances. This process of perceiving the situation is very helpful in acquiring of social ideals.
- **New Responses:** When a person has perceived new situation, he/she acts accordingly. This acting according to the new situation is called new response. If he succeeds in it, he repeats it. But he fails he gives up.
- **Mutual behavior:** When an individual comes into contact with others, he/she is influenced by others and influenced by them also. He/She behaves with others according to the behavior which he/she receives from others.
- **Cooperation:** As a result of cooperation, the social qualities also develop in the individual. When he/she sees that cooperate with him/her and he/she develops certain qualities of cooperation. This is another way of developing social qualities and organizing the social personality.
- **Suggestions:** The child also tries to adjust himself/herself to the social needs according to the suggestions from others. Generally, these suggestions are received from the family, school and other agencies of education and socialization.
- **Reward and punishment or praise or punishment:** Generally, when a child acts according to social deals and values, he/she gets

rewards and praise consequently, he/she is encouraged to behave according to the needs of the society on the other hand when he/she acts against the interest of society, he/she gets punishment and insult. That is why he/she is discouraged to act against the interest of the society. Reward and punishment, therefore, help a lot in the process of socialization.

Stages of Socialization

The stages through which a child grows and acquires socialization can be divided into following four stages of socialization.
1. Oral stage
2. Anal stage
3. Latency stage
4. Adolescence

Oral Stage

This stage begins from the time of the birth and the main object of this stage is to be establishing the oral self-dependence or reliability. In this stage the child forms certain desires about eating. He learns the process of indicating his desire for the fulfilment of the wants. He establishes completed adjustment with the mother and in fact he or she becomes one with the mother. Through this stage a child learns the control of hunger drive.

Anal Stage

After oral stage anal stage begins. Oral stage ends at the end of one year and then anal stage begins, and it goes up the three years of age. Because of new desires certain crises develops, and the result the child learns to start some of his desires and wants. In this stage the child not only receives affection from the mother but also reciprocates. The oral stage, this is only one way traffic, and the child only gets affection from the mother.

Latency Stage

This stage begins at the age of 4 and continuous up to the age of 13 to 14. During this period the field of social atmosphere of the child becomes wide. Now he internalises all the four functions of the family, e.g., husband-father, wife-mother, son-brother, daughter-sister. At this stage the child starts going to the school where he learns stage gives him greater social equipment.

Adolescence

Adolescence begins at the age of 10 till 19 years. During this stage the child becomes still wider and so his social equipment becomes richer. During this period the child is anxious to get rid of the control of his parents, but he is not able to do it. He wants to keep out of the house as far as possible. There is desire to become free. Sometimes because of the control of the society and the family and the desire of the child to get rid of that control, there is also a clash, which is in fact a part of the social processor the process of socialization.

Factors of Process of Socialization

Socialization is the process of learning group norms, habits, and ideas. There are four factors of the process of learning which are imitation, suggestion, identification, language.

- **Imitation**: It is the copying the actions of another. It can be consciously or unconsciously. It has an important role in process of socialization. For example: A girl child imitates and do the same as her mother does. A boy attempts to walk, talk like his father through imitation.
- **Suggestion**: Suggestion is the way of communication information without logic or self-evident. The suggestions can be conveyed through language, pictures etc. It influences one's own and individual's behavior.
- **Identification**: With the growth of child by age, child become aware of nature of things which satisfy the needs. These things become the object of identification, through this identification, he becomes sociable. He starts playing with toys and enjoys it due to identification.
- **Language**: It is the way of transmitting the culture and moulds the personality of individual in accordance with society.

Agencies of Socialization

Socialization is the process which begins at birth and continues till death of an individual. The socialization process should not be left as it occur but should be controlled through institutional channels.

It makes the child a useful member of society. It gives social maturity and occurs by two sources.

First source include those who have authority over him. For example- teacher, parents, elderly persons

Second source include who are equal in authority. For example- friends, playmates, fellow on job in club.

Socialization involves the authoritarian mode as pattern of behaivour expected in the culture is innate whereas equalitarian mode is also important as child acquires something from his equals which he cannot acquire from persons in authority. Thus, both authoritarian and equalitarian relationships contribute to socialization.

The chief agencies are- family, school, playmates, religion and state.

- **Family**: Family has an extraordinary importance in the process of socialization. Family is the first who socialise the child. Children learn language, speech, and gesture from the family. Family environments influence the growth of child. Family teaches basic values to the individual.
- **School**: Educational institutions such as schools and colleges are important agencies of socialization. In these institutions, the children will come to contact with other children who come from different backgrounds and different ways of behavior. The children learn about the social system and conditions of other countries. The teachers also influence the process of socialization.
- **Peer group/friends**: In fact, neighbourhood and play group are not very distinct from each other. The children may learn social values and art of adjustment from neighbours. The neighbourhood reinforces the individual family as an agency of social control. In the neighbourhood group controls traditionally in the form of mores. They are kept alive and enforced by the elder members of the locality. Children learn cooperation, morality, fashion etc from friends which is also important from the social point of view.
- **Religion**: Religion is based on the systems of belief and faith. Religion provides the sense of identity of past and future. The religion beliefs also mould the personality of the individual to differentiate between.
- **State**: State makes law for people and lays down to mould the behavior of people. If anyone fails to adjust to the rules and regulations of the society, will be punished by the government to mould his behavior.

Elements of process of socialization
- **Heritage of individual**: Physical and psychological
- **Environment**: Family, community and society
- **Culture**: Child imbibes the culture of the family

SOCIAL CHANGE

Social change means the change or modification in ways of doing and thinking of people. It is the modification in the life pattern of people and involves changes in the structure and functioning of social forms.

Social change is a process through which social organizations, social relationships and forms of values and beliefs of the people in the society are altered. Every society undergoes change whenever new social, economic, or cultural forces of transformation undergo change. These changes may be endogenous (internal) or exogenous (external). Social change can also be conceived as a relatively extensive and enduring reordering and/or redefining of the process of social organization.

Definition

According to **Lundberg**, *'Social change refers to any modification in established patterns of inter human relationship and standards of conduct.'*

According to **Davis**, *'Social change is meant only such alterations as occur in social organisation, that is structure & functions of society.'*

According to **Gillin** and **Gillin**, *'Social changes are variations from the accepted modes of life; whether due to alteration in geographical conditions, in cultural equipment, composition of the population or ideologies and whether brought about by diffusion or inventions within the group.'*

According to **Anderson** and **Parker**, *'Social change involves alteration in the structure or functioning of social forms or process themselves.'*

According to **Jenson**, *'Social change may be defined as modification in ways of doing and thinking of people.'*

According to **HT Mazumdar**, *'Social change may be defined as a new fashion or mode, either modifying or replacing the old, in the life of a people or in the operations of a society.'*

According to **MD Jones**, *'Social change is a term used to describe variations in or modifications of any aspect of social processes, social patterns, social interactions, or social organization.'*

According to **S Koenig**, *'Social change refers to the modifications which occur in the life patterns of a people.'*

Nature of Social Change

Social change is a continuous process as the change in population, technology, values & ideologies keep on occurring. This change differs from society to society. This change occurs either naturally or as a result of planned efforts. The characteristics of nature of social change are the following:

- **Social Change is a Universal Phenomenon**: Society is web of social relationships undergoing constant social process. There is no society which is static. Social change occurs in all human societies, you find change in the social structure due to the diffusion, innovation, and evolution. But the speed of social change differs from society to society, place to place and time to time.
- **Social Change is a community**: Change Social change refers to the life of the entire community, it does not refer to an individual or group of individuals
- **Speed of Social Change is not Uniform**: The change that takes place in some society is not uniform. The rate of speed changes corresponding to the circumstances, example of the social change that has taken place in India before its independence is entirely different to that of its after independence. Further, the speed also differs from place to place. The social change in urban area is much faster than to the rural areas. Also, it differs from literate community to the illiterate community
- **The Definite Prediction of Social Change is not Possible** The amount and direction of social change cannot be predicted as it depends on several factors. The amount and direction of change that occurred is our society may differ in the other community through similar conditions prevailing.
- **Social Change Shows Chain Reaction Sequences** The change cause in one are leads to the change in the other area. This is a claim reaction causes in the society. For example, women education led the women to work in factories and offices which lead to the change in the role of the woman in the family which lead to the change in the economic progress of that family and society

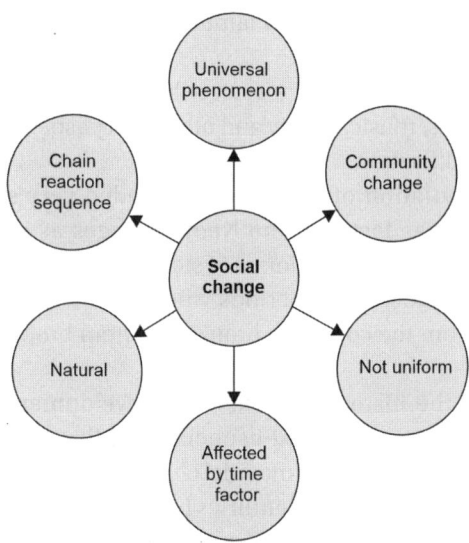

Forces of Social Change

Endogenous Forces (Internal to Society)	Exogenous Forces (External to Society)
Increase or decline in population growth due to factors like: • Migration --mainly rural to urban in Indian Society. • Practice of contraception. • Infant and child mortality rate. • Maternal mortality rate. • High rate of abortions • Introduction of government policies directed towards change. • Change of use of technology. • Social reform movements.	• French and Russian revolutions/ wars. • Breakdown of feudalism. • Agricultural and industrial revolutions. • Radical changes in lifestyle through scientific and technological innovations. • Nature of trade relations.

Process of Social Change

Social change, rapid in some cases slows in others has characterized all societies whether prehistoric, historic, or modern.

Increase in size of the group, alteration of diversities of economy, shift from normal to settled mode of life, modification of the social structure, new emphasis in religious beliefs and practice growth of science, new philosophies and famine are among the phenomena associated with such change.

The political structure of a society has altered in the course of history, customs, music, poetry and other every aspect of culture are subject to modification.

The accumulation of invention proceeded very slowly in the beginning. It was faster in the Neolithic ages as shown by the archaeological records, new forms of store and bone.

During the succeeding periods when the metal appeared the movements from the copper to bronze and from bronze to iron was faster still.

Finally, in the historical period, the development of material culture has been very rapid especially in the nineteenth and twentieth centuries. Not only material changes but since the outbreak of World War the numerous centuries have passed through changes in the political institutions, class structure, their economic systems, their mores, and modes of living. We also see social change going on continuously in society in the form of cooperation, competitions, conflicts, accommodation, and assimilation in various situations. The rate of change is different in different places and times. It is intermittent and continuous. It is in some cases sporadic in other cases it is continuous.

Sociologists hold the view that when the change is continuous it is known as social process. These processes take the form of cooperation, competitions, conflict, accommodation, assimilation, etc. There may also exists the feeling of subordination, super ordination of equality among the people. There are three components in which changes occurred, society, culture and civilization include in social change, changes only in social relationships or social structure and treat changes in other two components as cultural and civilization changes.

The sociologist **Dvias** who consider social change as a part of cultural change is stated by **Gillin** and **Gillin**, the mode of life includes not only social relationships but are generally accepted way of satisfying the needs of the group. The modes of life would include not only culture but also the cultural equipment.

Ideologies, religious beliefs, ceremonies, relations between in group and out group between the younger members of the group and the older, between males and females, the techniques employed in gaining a substance such as, methods of cultivation, hunting, fishing, building houses, protecting the crops and animals, and protecting the people themselves from and disease and other menaces. The modes of life also include the cultural equipment which people use for satisfying a change in social relationship and it is distinct thing from cultural and civilization change. The **contemporary world appears to behaviors more rapidly that at any time in human society.**

Theories of Social Change

Evolutionary Theory

It believes that every pattern of action, belief and interaction tends to generate an opposing reaction. It sees unequal distribution of power and authority as the fundamental source of conflict. It believes that societies are like organisms, which evolve in the same manner as **Darwin's** notion of biological evolution that societies go through series of stages based on increasing complexity towards higher and more advanced and developed state of existence.

Cyclical Theory

It is founded on the assumption that societies have pre-determined life cycle of birth, growth, maturity, and decline.

Functional Theory

It is based on the belief that societies change but they also tend to move towards equilibrium. Any disturbance in the system is easily accommodated within the existing structure.

Conflict Theory

It believes that every pattern of action, belief and interaction tends to generate an opposing reaction. It sees unequal distribution of power and authority as the fundamental source of conflict.

Terms Associated with Social Change

Social change suggests a difference through time in the object to which it is applied. The social change can be explained by the terms- evolution, progress, resolution, adaptation, growth, and accommodation.

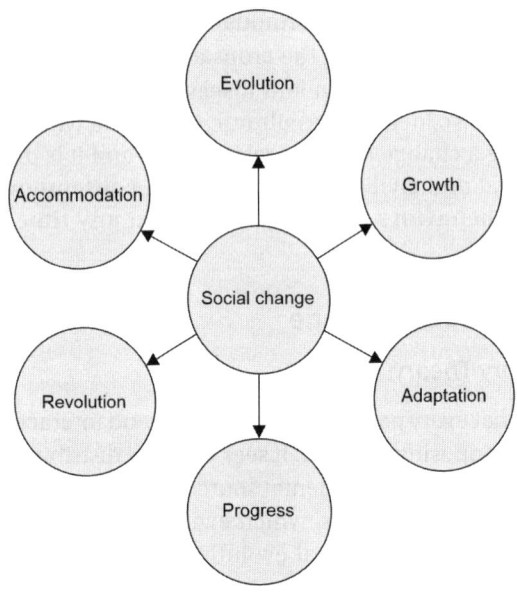

Evolution

The word evolution has been derived from Latin word 'Evolere' means 'to develop or to unfold'.

Evolution means change in size and structure. It is a process in which hidden or latent characters are revealed. Evolution is unfolding the variety of aspects belongings to the nature of changing object.

Von Baer, the German sociologist developed the concept of evolution as a process of differentiation-cum-integration. Societies show integration by increase in size and structure which can be seen that the number or population of societies has increased along with the structure.

Evolution also involves progress in coherence and multiformity. It is gradual, progressive and takes place in the way cosmic evolution occurs.

It is the process of detaching from an old group norm and ultimately achieving new norms. Social evolution is not an imaginary but is real according to **MacIver**. According to **Hob House**, 'Social evolution is developed, planned & unplanned of culture and forms of social relationship.

Growth

It means direction of change in quantitative character. For example, an increase in number of people in a society. Growth also shows that a social change has occurred in size.

Progress

It means development. According to **Ogburn**, 'Progress is a movement towards an objective, thought to be desirable by general group, for visible future.'

It means change for better which implies value judgement. It includes improvement in dignity, respect increasing freedom, promotion of liberty and aesthetic enjoyment of work of nature. Progress fulfils the desired aim. It is related to social system and require desire and volition.

According to **Mazumdar HT**, Progress contains at least following things:
- Enhancement of dignity of human beings
- Respect for each human personality
- Ever increasing freedom for spiritual quest
- Aesthetic enjoyment of works of nature
- Social order which promotes values
- Promote life and liberty

Revolution

Revolution means a sudden and great change. It brings social change. For example- The discovery of penicillin produces a revolution in medicine. Advancement in technology, computers have changed the life of human beings.

Adaptation

It means adjustment to different conditions. It is the change to meet different situations. With the advanced technology and techniques individuals adapt themselves to changing conditions.

Accommodation

It is adjusting oneself to the new environment. It may be physical or social environment. It is the social progress. It is the change in behavior of people which help them to adjust to the environment.

According to **MacIver**, 'accommodation refers particularly to the process which may attain a sense of harmony with his environment.'

Factor Influencing Social Change

Physical Environment

Major changes in the physical environment are very compelling when they happen. Climates change, soil erodes, and lakes gradually turn into swamps and finally plains. A culture is greatly affected by such changes although sometimes they come about so slowly that they are largely unnoticed. Human misused can bring very rapid changes in physical environment which in turn change the social and cultural life of a people. Deforestation brings land erosion and reduces rainfall. Much of the wasteland and desert land of the world is a testament to human ignorance and misuse. Environmental destruction has been at least a contributing factor in the fall of most great civilization. Many human groups throughout history have changed their physical environment through migration. In the primitive societies whose members are very directly dependent upon their physical environment migration to a different environment brings more changes in the culture. Civilization makes it easy to transit a culture and practice it in a new and different environment.

Population Changes

A population changes is itself a social change but also becomes a casual factor in their social and cultural changes:

When a thinly settled frontier fills up with people the hospitality pattern fades away, secondary group relations multiply, institutional structures grow more elaborate, and many other changes follow. A stable population may be able to resist change, but a rapidly growing population must migrate, improve the productivity, or starve. Great historic migrations and conquests of Huns, Vikings and many others have arisen from the pressure of a growing population upon limited resources. Migration encourages further change for it brings a group into a new environment subject it to new contacts and confronts it with new problems. No major population change leaves the culture unchanged.

Isolation and Contact

Societies located at world crossroads have always been centres of change. Since most new traits come through diffusion, those societies in closest contact with other societies are likely to change most rapidly. In ancient times of overload transport, the land bridge connecting Asia, Africa and Europe was the centre of civilizing change. Later sailing vessels shifted the centre of the fringes of the Mediterranean Sea and still later to the north-west coast of Europe. Areas if greatest intercultural contact are the centres of change. War and trade have always brought intercultural contact and today tourism is adding to the contacts between cultures. Conversely isolated areas are centres of stability, conservatism, and resistance to change. The most primitives' tribes have been those who were the most isolated like the polar Eskimos or the Aranda of central Australia.

Social Structure

The structure of a society affects its rate of change in subtle and not immediately apparent ways. A highly centralized bureaucracy is very favourable to the promotion and diffusion of change although bureaucracy has sometimes been used in attempt to suppress change usually with no more than temporary success. When a culture is very highly integrated so that each element is rightly interwoven with all the others in mutually interdependent system change is difficult and costly. But when the culture is less highly integrated so that work, play, family, religion, and other activities are less dependent upon one another change is easier and more frequent. A tightly structured society where in every person's role, duties, privileges, and obligations are precisely and rigidly defined is less given to changes than a more loosely structured society where in roles, lines of authority, privileges and obligations are more open to individual rearrangement.

Attitudes and Values

To people in developed nations and societies, change is normal. Children there are socialized to anticipate and appreciate change. Societies differ greatly in their general attitude toward change. People who reverse the past and preoccupied with traditions and rituals will change slowly and unwillingly. When a culture has been relatively static for a long time the people are likely to assume that it should remain so indefinitely. They are intensely and the consciously ethnocentric they assume that their customs and techniques are correct and everlasting. A possible change is unlikely even to be seriously considered. Any change in such society is likely to be too gradual to be noticed. A rapidly changing society has a different attitude toward change and this attitude is both cause and effect of the changes already taking place. Rapidly changing societies are aware of the social change. They are somewhat sceptical and critical of some parts of their traditional structure and will consider and experiment with innovations. Such attitudes powerfully stimulate the proposal and acceptance of changes by individuals within the society. Different groups within a locality or a society may show differing receptivity to change. Every changing society has its liberal and its conservatives. Liberals and educated people tend to accept changes more readily than the illiterate and uneducated. Attitudes and values effect both the amount and the direction of social change. No society has been equally dynamic in all aspects and its values determine in which area arts, music, warfare, technology, philosophy, or religion it will be innovative.

Cultural Factors

There is a connection between our values, our beliefs, and our social relationships. Culture helps us to understand individuals or groups of society. Culture again helps us to distinguish individual from individual group and society from society. Culture is the key that opens the door to an analysis of human beings. Any change in culture inevitably produces change certainly all cultural changes involve social change. Thus, both social changes and culture are closely interwoven.

Role of Culture and Social Change

Culture influences the direction and character of social change. Culture has become a determinant factor for any change, for instance the determinant school argued that culture is basic source of social changes. Though there is a relation between cultural change and social change, some sociologists do make a distinction between cultural change and social change. Cultural change denotes change in norms of a given society and social change means change in social structure and social behavior.

Technological Factors

The technological factors represent the condition created by a man which have a profound influence on his life. In an attempt to satisfy his wants, fulfil his needs and to make his life more comfortable man creates civilization. Technology is a by-product of civilization when the scientific knowledge is applied to the problems in life it becomes technology. Technology is a systematic knowledge which is put into practice that is to use tools and run machines to serve human purpose. Science and technology go together. In utilizing the products of technology man brings social change. The social effects of technology are far reaching. The loss of human freedom and the large-scale destruction of human beings are due to the increasing use of certain types of technology which has begun to thereafter the life support systems of the earth as whole.

Cultural Lag

The concept of cultural leg has become popular among sociologists. It is a concept that has been used when inventions discoveries and innovations are constantly disturbing the existing social order and the way of living. In short cultural lag means that one part of cultural lags the other part of culture and causes imbalance in society for example laws do not change quickly to meet social requirements. In contemporary society, the advancement in technology overtakes the non-material culture that is customs, beliefs, values, and laws. Since the material culture moves faster than the non-material culture the imbalance leads to the phenomenon of cultural lag. e.g., The presently educational system is lagging behind the requirement of society. It is, therefore, essential to meet growing demands of the society. Here, the educational system lags behind the social requirements. Social changes are very complicated matter and has several dimensions. Rarely whole society moves in one direction.

Theories of Social Change

Linear Theory

Some thinkers subscribe to the linear theory of social change. According to them, society gradually moves to an even higher state of civilization and that it advances in a linear fashion and in the direction of improvement. **Auguste Comte** postulated three stages of social change, the theological, the metaphysical and the positive. Man has passed through the first two they still prevail, believed that supernatural powers controlled and designed the world. He advanced in fetishes and deities to monotheism. This stage gave away to the metaphysical stage, during which man tries to explain phenomenon by resorting to abstractions. In the positive stage, man considers the search for be empirically observed. This implies progress which according to **Comte,** will be assured if man adopts a positive attitude in understanding of natural and social phenomenon. The factual evidence which is available to us can only lead as to remark that whatever direction social change takes in future that direction will be determined by himself.

Cyclical Theory

Cyclical theories contended that changes are not linear but cyclic (rise and fall). Societies are undergoing period of growth, maturity, and decline. Cultures pass through the same stage of birth, growth, maturity, decline and death like an individual. The civilization is the last stage of the culture (full maturity). The lifetime of a culture is approximately a thousand years. Culture can be characterized by senate culture and ideational culture. Senate culture means the value of sensory experiences, experiment. In contrast, ideational cultures stress the spiritual and religious factor. In the history of mankind either of this extreme culture dominates at one period, i.e., senate cultures dominate one period and ideational cultures dominate another period. As culture servings back and forth like pendulum, there are some periods where it reaches an idealistic point, a mixture of both senate and ideational value prevails.

Marxian Theory

Marxian perspectives provide a radical alternative to functionalist's views, they regard stratification as a divisive rather than an integrative structure. They said as a mechanism whereby some exploit others rather than a means of furthering collective goals. **Marx** used the term class refer the main strata in all stratification systems. In all stratified societies there are two major social groups or classes, a ruling class, and a subject class. The power of ruling class derives from its ownership and control of the forces of production. In capitalist society, there are two main classes, the bourgeoisie or capitalist class, which own the force of production and proletariat or working class whose members own only their labor which they hire to the capitalist in return of wages. **Marx** believed that all societies are divided into two major classes except primitive communism. Masters and slaves in ancient society, lords and serfs in feudal society and capitalist and wage laborers in capitalist society. Ruling class gains at the expense of the subject class and there is therefore a conflict of interest between them that is the capitalist want to extract maximum possible work from the laborer and laborers demand more wages and their due share in production. Political power derives from economic power. The power of the ruling class therefore stems from its ownership and control of the forces of production. Superstructure of society the major institutions, values and beliefs systems is seen to be largely shaped by the economic infrastructure. The political system and legal systems will reflect ruling class interests.

Functionalist Theory

Functionalists are primarily concerned with the function of social stratification with its contribution to the maintenance and well-being of society. Functionalist assumes that there are certain basic needs of functional prerequisites which must become, if society is to survive, social stratification also fulfils certain basic needs. They assume that parts of society form an integrated whole, and social stratification system is also integrated with other parts of society. They maintain that a certain degree of order and stability are essential for the operation of social system and social stratification systems help to maintain order and stability in society.

Role of Nurse in Social Change

All forms of social changes contributed very much for the improvement of health care delivery system. All sorts of advancement bring benefits for clients.

The improvement in the economy and the advance in the medical field resulted in more number of health care centres. More number of multi-specialty hospitals is established in the cities and other health care centres are established in the semi-urban areas. Nurses and health care workers also want to stay in the urban areas. As a result of technological changes, more number of devices are available to diagnose and to identify the exact nature of disease. Nurses should competent enough to handle the technological changes. Economical changes improve the status of the society, most of the people are affordable for the available treatment facilities. They have facilities like health insurances and medical coverage.

The latest advancement in the treatment facilities for the disease bring a new hope for the nurse and health care workers to face new challenges in the field of health. The development of information and communication field makes the public to become more aware about the health problems and health care facilities patients are having knowledge about the treatment modalities. Advancements make the student nurses in the field of health studies to gain more knowledge and help them to get wide exposure also. For example, various ownership rights of the capitalist class will be enshrined in and protected by the laws of the land. Thus, various parts of super structure can be seen as instruments of ruling class domination and as mechanism of for the oppression of the subject class. Ruling class ideology produces false class consciousness, a false picture of the nature of the relationships between social classes. Members of both classes tend to accept the status quo as normal and natural and largely unaware of the true nature of exploitation and oppression. In this way conflict interest between the classes is disguised and a degree of social stability produced but the basic contradictions and conflicts of class societies remain unresolved.

COMMUNITY

Community is a basic unit of social structure. The social life of people is affected by the kind of community in which they live. Community includes a group of people living in a geographic area with a common culture and the social system. In the community the members are conscious of their unity and act collectively, in an organized manner.

Definition

MacIver defined community as 'Whenever the members of a group small or large together in such a way that they share, not this or that particular interest, but the basic life, we call that group a community.'

According to **Lundberg**, *'Community is a human population living within a limited geographic area & carrying on a common inter dependent life.'*

The definition given by **WHO** Expert committee on community is as follows: "A community is a social group determined by geographical boundaries and/or common values and interests. Its members know and interact with each other. It functions within a particular social structure and exhibits and creates certain norms and values, and social institutions"

Characteristics of Community

- **Group of People**: Community is a group of people who share the basic conditions of common life.
- **Locality**: Community is a territorial group and occupies a geographical area. Locality is a basic element of a community. The area need not to be fixed forever. The people may change the area

of inhabitation from time to time, however some communities are well settled and developed strong bond.

- **Permanency**: A community includes permanent group life in a definite place, and it is stable.
- **Naturalism**: Communities are not created or made by will or act, but they are not natural. People who live in the community are the members of the group by birth itself.
- **Sentiment**: It means feeling of belonging or 'We' feeling. In community people stay together, share interests and ideas, maintain unity, and occupy a specific local area. Soundness of above all aspects increases the bond among members of the community. Therefore, sentiment plays an important role to create a community.
- **Wider Ends**: The ends of the community are wider and natural. The people associate in community not to fulfil a particular end.
- **Particular Name**: Each community has a particular name. For example, people living in India are called Indians, living in a state like Tamil Nadu are called Tamilians.
- **Legal Status**: A community has no legal status in the eyes of law. It has no particular rights or duties.
- **Dependency**: An individual in community is physically dependent on community for fulfilment and satisfaction of physical needs. Psychologically also he is dependent on community, as it saves from isolation and solitude.
- **Likeness**: In community, there is likeness to language, customs, traditions, practices, folkways, mores are common. People in community work through customs and traditions.

Types of Community

Types of community: Rural (village), Urban and tribal community

Rural/village community

Seventy percent of the Indian population lives in rural communities. Every village is self-sufficient unit. In each rural community nearly 2500 people lead their life, with face-to-face relations. Majority of rural people depend on agriculture.

Sanderson defined rural community as *'Consisting of people living on dispersed farm sheds and in hamlet or village which forms the centre of their common activities.'*

Rural community is a simple community of primary relations with low population based primarily on agricultural life. In rural life, where the family is relatively dominant and self-contained, a group responsibility prevails. The status of the individual is likely to be the status of his family. Property is likely to be thought of as a family possession.

The dominance of the family explains, in large measure, why social control in the rural community is exercised with minimum of formality and a maximum command. The group mores, reflecting a commonly shared system of values, are themselves effective as social pressure, in little need of support from specialized agencies.

Features of village community

- **Basis of social organization**: More than 500,000 people live in villages in India.
- **Group of people**: Members of the village community interact in person on a regular basis. They have similar customs and cultures.
- **Small in size**: Village communities are small in size. The census in India designates a place with 5000 inhabitants as a village community. Eighty percent of the Indian villages have less than 1000 population each.
- **A sense of unity**: Villagers have a sense of unity. All the families in the village are united and share sorrows and joys together. They also unite themselves to protect themselves from the invaders.
- **Importance of neighbourhood**: Community ties are yet another crucial aspect of village life. In a rural context, we-feeling, camaraderie, sympathy, and love are accessible to foster community ties in the village.
- **Community sentiment**: Community sentiment is the very essence of village community. The rural people express we-feeling with community sentiment. The members have a sense of dependence on the community for both physical and psychological satisfaction.
- **Intimate relation**: The villagers have intimate relations with each other, and they know each other personally.
- **Simplicity**: Simplicity and sincerity are the common characteristics of villagers. Kinship groups play a significant role in the village community's overall structure
- **Joint family system**: The villager communities give more value to the joint family system. All the members live together under the same roof, take food, hold property together, participate in common worship with the members in joint family.

- **Agriculture-the main occupation**: Agriculture is the main occupation in rural India. It is essentially a way of life for the rural people. A small section of the rural population depends upon non-agricultural occupations such as carpentry, pottery, basket making, etc. for their livelihood.
- **Caste system**: Caste system is a unique feature of the Indian village community. It determines the role, status, occupation, and marital relationships of the villagers.
- **Jajmani system**: The Jajmani relation binds the families of various castes into a hereditary, permanent, and multiple relationships. In the later days this system has been greatly weakened by socioeconomic and political changes in India.
- **Faith in religion**: Religion plays a major role in the village community. Religious influence is more on the activities like sowing, harvesting of crops, birth, marriage, illness, death, etc. On all such occasions, the villagers conduct religious ceremonies in the form of 'Puja', 'Mela' or 'Kirtan'. In this way, the faith in religion is very strong in villages.
- **Panchayat**: The functioning of the village as a political and social entity brought together members from different castes. The traditional village panchayat in the shape of village council performed a variety of tasks, including the maintenance of law and order, settling of disputes, celebration of festivals and construction of roads, bridges, and tanks, etc. On the other hand, matters relating to the caste rules, property and family disputes and other activities are judged by the caste panchayat.
- **Homogeneity in culture**: Homogeneity of population is another important feature of village communities. The members of a village exhibit similarities in their dress, speech, beliefs, values, attitudes, and behavior.
- **Informal social control**: In village communities, social control is informal and direct. The primary groups like the family, neighbourhood act as powerful agencies of social control in villages. The traditional village panchayat and the caste panchayat also exercise much control on the deviant members of the community.
- **Mobility**: Territorial, occupational and social mobility of the rural population is limited.
- **Status of women**: Generally, the women in villages are not much educated and their social status is lower than that of their counterparts in the towns. Factors like prevalence of child marriage, joint family system, traditional ideals, old values, and

lack of education among females are responsible for the low status of women.
- **Culture**: So far as village community is concerned, culture is more static than in towns. Greater importance is attached to religion and rituals.
- **Stability and continuity**: The village communities in India are relatively more stable. The reason is possibly attributed to the relative static character of villagers as a way of life the norms of behavior, customs of family relations, traditions of community life, etc. Life in the village is more stable and natural
- **Moral values**: The villagers have high mortality, and their life is being governed by norms.

Characteristics of Indian villages

Most of the characteristic features of Village Community in India are very similar to those elsewhere in the world, but there are certain peculiarities of Indian village. The peculiarities of Indian villages are:
- Joint family system
- Caste system
- Jajmani system – Under this system, members of caste or many castes offer their services to the members of other castes
- Agriculture is the main occupation
- Most simple Living
- Homogeneity in social life
- Stronghold of public opinion
- Lack of social mobility
- Importance of religion, customs, traditional mores

A large number of studies had been carried out with the assumption that the Indian village was not 'static', isolated' and 'homogeneous', but that it was changing, had connection with wider society. Migration, village exogamy, inter-village economic ties, dependence upon towns for market, division of labour and visits to religious places have also been basic feature of the Indian village.

The famous French sociologist **Louis Dumont** refers three meaning to the term "village community":
1. as a political society,
2. as a body of co-ownership of the soil, and
3. as the emblem of traditional society and polity. "a watchword of Indian patriotism".

Panchayat system

Article 40 of the constitution directs the government to establish Panchayats to serve as institution of local self-government. The panchayat in India generally refers to the system introduced by constitution amendment in 1952, although it is based upon traditional panchayat system in South Asia.

The modern Panchayati raj and its Gram panchayat are not to be confused with the extra constitutional caste panchayat found in northern India. The panchayat system was formalized in 1992 to implement decentralized administration.

Mahatma Gandhi advocated Panchayati raj as the foundation of political system, it would have been a decentralized form of government where each village would be responsible for its affairs. The term for such a vision was Gram Swaraj (Village Self-Government) is developed in India a highly centralized form of government. In Indian Panchayati raj now functions as a system of governance in which gram panchayats are the basic unit of local samiti (block level) and Zila Parishad (district level). It was formalized in 1992 by the 73rd amendment to the Indian Constitution.

The panchayat raj system is a three-tier system of decentralization. The elected members run this system. All the community development programs are implemented through this Panchayati Raj. The institutions of Panchayati Raj are:
- Panchayat at village level
- Panchayat Samiti at block level
- Zilla Parishad at district level

Various committees on panchayati raj
- Balwant Rai Mehta: Estabilshed 1957
- VT Krishnammachari: 1960
- Takhatmal Jain Study Group: 1966
- Ashok Mehta Committee: 1977
- GVK Rao committee: 1985
- Dr LM Singhvi Committee: 1986.

Panchayat system at village level
The Panchayat is a village level institution. It consists of:
- **Gram Sabha:** It is the assembly of all adult members of the village. It meets at least twice in a year. Gram Sabha discusses the proposals for taxation and elects the representatives for Gram Panchayat.
- **Gram Panchayat:** Grama Panchayat to executive organ of Gram Sabha. Its strength varies from 15 to 30 members. This is an agency for planning level. The elected Panchayat president is called as Sarpanch or Sabha Pati or Mukhiya, vice president and Panchayat secretary supports president. They take care of the socioeconomic development, civic administration, and public health.

- **Panchayat Samiti**: This is a block level institution. It consists of 100 villages. It covers the population about 80,000 to 1,20,000. It consists of all Sarpanches of village Panchayats, MLA's and MPs residing in the block area, representatives of women, schedule castes, schedule tribe members and co-operative societies. The important function of Panchayat Samiti is the execution of community development programs for the villages.
- **Zilla Parishad**: This is the district level institution. It is otherwise called zilla Panchayat. The members are all the heads of the Panchayat Samiti, MP, MLA's representatives of rural local self-government at the district level. The responsibility of Zilla Parishad is primarily supervisory and co-ordinating body. Their functions may vary from state to state.

Gram Sabha	Gram Panchayat	Panchayat Samiti	Zila Parishad
• All adults of village • Proposal of taxation, discusses annual programme • Elects members of gram panchayat.	• Executive members of gram sabha • Headed by sarpanch as president, assisted by vice president and panchayat secretary • Social and economic development of village	• Sarpanches of village panchayats • MLAs, MPs residing in block • Execution of community development programme in the block	• All heads of Panchayat samiti in the district • MPs and MLAs of district • Representation of women, SC and ST. • Two persons experienced in administration • Administrative functions • Health related activities.

Powers and responsibilities of panchayats at the appropriate level:
- Preparation of plan for economic development and social justice.
- Implementations of schemes for economic development and social justice in relation to 29 subjects given in eleventh schedule of the constitution.
- To levy, collect and appropriate taxes, duties, tolls, and fees.

The common department in the samiti are as follows:
- General administration
- Finance
- Public works
- Agriculture
- Health

- Education
- Social welfare
- Information technology and others

Functions
- Implement schemes for the development of agriculture.
- Establishment of primary health centres and primary schools.
- Supply of drinking water, drainage, construction/repair of roads.
- Development of cottage and small-scale industries and opening co-operative societies.
- Establishment of youth organizations.

Social dynamics
Social dynamics means the ability of a society to read inner and outer changes and deals with its regulation mechanism. Social dynamics is a mathematically inspired concept to analyse societies, building upon system theory and sociology. Sociologists, ethologists, criminologist anthropologists and biologists are utilizing it in their studies of systems and behavior.

Definition
Social dynamics is a comprehensive evaluation, performance measurement, social research and training firm creative, cost effective solutions that lead to improvements in programs, policies and operations.

Meaning of social dynamics
Culture and society are things that the human beings are emotionally bound to. They deal with ratings, with subjective needs. Different people have more or less different feelings, goals and opinions. This must be discussed as culture found upon least common denominator. Sociology sits on the fence, it is a mix of human and nature sciences, philosophy, and politics.

As this is stalled the progress of sociology, some people meant to bring new life into systemic to sociology. On a certain level, life and societies are nothing more than systems dealing with genes and culture. Therefore, system can be described by transmission functions.

Social dynamics in society
In small society, the individuals can come to a fine conscious in short time, which means, its attitude error is small, and its frequency broad width is high. But its absolute amplitude is small, so the society still depends on the big amplitude of nature, on the focus of nature. A big society can overcome hunger, disease, and poverty, but its political media are hogs, high but lagged and distorted output signal.

Modern societies rely on technology to invent and promote new technology. The problem with backpropagation is that it can complicate the system, make it dynamic hence hard to control. As mankind needs to align technology to human needs and needs to foresee the effects of its actions, social dynamics and its relatives are an important field.

Community development project and planning

Community development has been defined by **Barket Narain** as a process designed to create conditions of economic and social progress for the whole community with its active participation and the fullest possible reliance upon the community's initiative.

Community development project is aimed to improve the standards of the community. Community is the smallest part of a country. To improve the overall progress of the country, the community development project was established. Community development project is implemented at five levels. They are at the central levels, state level, district level, block level and village level.

Goals of community development project:

- Improving the available materials and human resources.
- Developing the community includes social, cultural, and economical aspects of people's life.
- Promote awareness on civil responsibility among the community people.
- Establishing cottage industries or local artifacts.
- Promoting co-operative effect.
- Improving the agriculture and animal husbandry.
- Concentrate on women and children welfare.
- Improving communication such as transportation, educational institution, housing, sanitation, and health.
- Developing human and natural resources.
- Development of initiative among members.

Important aspects of community development

- **Agriculture**: Agriculture is the occupation of almost all the villagers, community development programs in values in social improvement and conservation, development of irrigation facilities, distribution of high breed seeds, manure, and advance agricultural equipment. The farmer is benefiting in the form of subsidy and other facilities.
- **Transportation and Communication**: Community development program concentrate more on transportation and communication. Both facilities are determining the standard of a community. This

includes construction of new roads and repair of old one and establishing post offices in the villages.
- **Health and sanitation**: The department includes constructing a primary health centre in all sub castes in every block. Immunization programs are conducted regularly to prevent the communicable diseases.
- **Education**: In the education sectors, primary, middle, and secondary schooling are provided at free of cost. Textbooks, notebooks, and stationaries are also provided as free of cost. In most backward areas, free hostels are also provided.
- **Establishment of Cottage Industries**: Cottage industries are the important solutions for the unemployment. Assistance is provided for the establishment of cottage industries like poultry farming, carpentry, handicrafts, and loans are sanctioned for the establishment. Assistance is also given to sell their products.
- **Training**: Training centres are imparting knowledge to the villagers in modern techniques of agriculture, development of leadership quality and handicrafts production.
- **Housing**: Villagers are given loans to construct hygienic and standardized houses.
- **Social Welfare**: Social welfare programs includes establishment of recreational centres, organizing sport and games, arranging cultural programs, puppet shows, public television facilities and promotion of Mahila Mandals and youth clubs.

Changes in Indian rural life

Comparing to urban societies, the village is undergoing a slow change. But its change is unavoidable, and changes break some of traditions and long practices of the villages.

- **Caste system:** Previously the social system was mainly determined by one's caste. But nowadays the social status is determined by one's economic achievement. The restriction regarding selection of occupation loosened. The caste system in the village has lost its hold. The restrictions under caste system related to mode of living, dress up etc. are removed.
- **Changes in the Familial System:** The number of joint families in the village is rapidly decreasing. Nuclear families are increasing. Family is not considered an economic unit outside agencies are ready to perform the familial activities. The restrictions over food, dressing and marriage practices are weakened. As a result of girl's education, their status is also improved.
- **No Restriction on Occupational Choice:** Previously the village communities imposed hereditary and endogamous practices. It

is weakened nowadays. All are allowed to choose their education and occupation based on their preferences and qualifications. There is no differentiation in the payment of wages. Based on one's ability and his work the payment is made.

- **Flexibility in Marital System:** Marriage in the traditional village was arranged only by parents and other family members. But now the boy and girl are allowed to participate in their mate selection process. They are giving more preferences for education, occupations, economy, and external appearance. The child marriage is no more prevalent.
- **Changes in Rural Economy:** The Government Banks are established in rural areas. They relaxed their restrictions over sanctioning loans, on agriculture education. The cottage industries are increasing in the rural areas. The farmers are getting direct access to sell their products in the market.
- **Improving Standard of Living:** Day-by-day the standard of living in the villages are improving. No villages are isolated from other societies. Transport and communication facilities are improving. Most of the villages cannot be named as village such as they fall between the town and village category All forms of scientific advancement like TV, computer, mobile phones are available in villages. The housing pattern, the sanitary habits and drainage system are well planned. Youngsters are dressing almost like urban people. They are fashionable also. By external appearance one cannot make out whether the person is from village or town.

Availability of health facilities in rural community

In India major part of population is living in the rural areas. The status of India mainly depends on the development of rural areas. Keeping in mind Government of India, the Ministry of Rural Development implement many programs to improve the status of the villagers. These programs are as follows:

- **Integrated Rural Development Programme**: This program is implemented as part of new 20-point program. This program is meant for rural poor 3000 families per block, 1.5 million families are helped to bring their family income above poverty line. This program covers 30% families belonging to schedule caste and scheduled tribes.
- **National Rural Employment Programmes**: This program aims at improving the nutritional status of rural families. This also provides wages for the unemployed in the form of food grains
- **Rural and its Employment Guarantee Program**: This is also known as antipoverty programme. This program aims to provide

employment at least for one member of each landless labor household for a period of up to 100 days in a year.
- **Development of Women and Children in Rural Areas**: This program was started in the year 1982. This program enables the rural women, to participate more effectively in the rural development program in general and integrated rural development program in particular.
- **Special Livestock Production Programme**: This program was initiated in 1975-76. This program involves with livestock. This consists of two major parts. They are:
  - Cross breeding heifer rearing.
  - Setting up of sheep, poultry, and piggery production units.
- **Training of Rural Youth for Self-employment**: This program was initiated with effect from 15th august 1979. The main aim was of this program is to equip rural youth with 18-35 years age group with necessary skills and technology to enable them to take vacations of self-employment. This scheme is also an integral part of Integrated Rural Development Programme (IRDP).
- **Village Health Guides Scheme**: This scheme is implemented as part of primary health care. This was introduced on 2nd October 1977. The health guides are mostly women. They came from same community in which they work. They link community and governmental infrastructure. They provide the first contact between individual and health system.
- **Local Dais**: In remote villages, untrained dais conducts most of the deliveries. This program aims to train all local dais to improve their knowledge in the elementary concept of maternal and child health, sterilization aspects. The eighth Five Year Plan objective was to train all untrained dais practising in the rural areas.
- **Anganwadi Workers**: This Anganwadi workers scheme is implemented under Integrated Child Development scheme (ICDS). The Anganwadi worker is chosen from the community where she is expected to serve. She undergoes training in various aspects of health nutrition and child development for a period of four months. Along with the village guides, the Anganwadi workers are the community primary link with the health services and all other services for young children.

Other than these programs, Drought Prone Areas Programme (DPAP), Desert Development Programme (DDP) development of selected regulated markets, development of rural markets and establishing national grid of rural godowns are also established by Government of India to improve the status of the rural areas. Rural people are not ignorant. They are well aware of the Government schemes for their welfare. The poverty line has to come down because of the rural development schemes by the Government. They have work and payment and money throughout the year.

- **Education for children:** Villagers go to rural hospitals for illness no more depending on traditional medicine man. Integrated Child Development Scheme has improved under five children's health. Deficiency diseases among children have come to a standstill. Death due to diarrhea among children has reduced to a great extent due to rehydration therapy education for diarrhea affected children. Immunization program for vaccine preventable diseases among children has brought down morbidity and mortality among under fives. Villages voluntarily go and get immunization for their children. They seek trained dais for delivery conducting. Famine is averted by Government schemes. Villagers are happy and healthy accepting modern treatment. Balwadi Nutrition Programme started in 1970 for the benefit of children in the age group of 3-6 years in rural area. The Anganwadi workers looks after it. It provides preparatory education to these children.

Urban Community

The term 'urban' is derived from the latin word 'urbanus' meaning city or town. In the cities the relationships among individuals are in personal.

Urban community mean an area with a high density of population. In India, urban areas are the places which have a local authority like municipality, containment board, notified area committees. Urban people are gradually engaged in different occupational pursuits.

An urban community is a group of people having a certain minimum population and possessing certain specialized economic, political, and social structure.

Features of urban community

- **Large in size:** As a rule, in the same country and at the same period, the size of an urban community is much larger than that of a rural community.
- **Density of population:** Density of population in urban areas is greater than in rural communities.
- **Family:** Nuclear families are more popular in urban areas.
- **Marriage:** In urban community the family and marriage system is different compared to rural communities. There are love marriages and inter-caste marriages, divorce cases are more in towns. Sons

and daughters enjoy considerable freedom in choosing their life partners for marriage.
- **Occupation**: In the urban areas, the major occupation is employment. They will work in industries, administrative sectors and as professionals also. Divisions of labor and occupational specialization are very common in towns/cities/metropolises.
- **Class extremes**: In the words of Bogardus, 'Class extremes characterize the city.' A town and a city house the richest as well as the poorest of people. In a city, the slums of the poor exist and bungalows of the rich, the apartments of the middle-class members. The most civilized modes of behavior as well as the worst living conditions are found in the cities.
- **Social heterogeneity**: If villages are the symbol of cultural homogeneity, the cities symbolize cultural heterogeneity. The cities are characterized by diverse peoples, races, and cultures. There are great varieties regarding the food habits, dress habits, living conditions, religious beliefs, cultural outlook, customs, and traditions of the urbanites.
- **Social distance**: The urban people with less attachment, secondary group relations are more. In the urban community social responses are incomplete and half-hearted. There is no personal involvement in the affairs of others.
- **Mechanical attitude**: The attitude of urban community is mechanical as they show superficial manners of politeness and mutual convenience. They deal with strangers as animated machines rather than as human beings.
- **System of interaction**: Georg Simmel held that the social structure of urban communities is based on interest groups. The city life is characterized by the predominance of secondary contacts, impersonal, casual, and short-lived relations.
- **Mobility**: The most important feature of urban community is its social mobility. In urban areas the social status of an individual is determined not by heredity or birth but by his merit and intelligence.
- **Materialism**: In the urban community the social existence of man by wealth, status, and prestige. Status symbols are in the form of financial assets, salaries, costly home appliances count in urban nature. Once the contract is over, human relationship automatically ends in urban communities.
- **Rapid social and cultural change**: Rapid social and cultural change characterize the urban life. The importance attached to traditional or sacred elements has been relegated to the

background. The benefits of urban life have effected changes in respect of norms, ideologies, and behavior patterns.

- **Voluntary associations**: The urban community is characterized by impersonal, mechanical, and formal social contacts occurring among the people. Naturally they have a strong desire for developing genuine social relationships to satisfy their hunger for emotional warmth and sense of security. They form associations, clubs, societies, and other secondary groups.
- **Formal social control**: Social control in urban community is essentially formal in nature. Individual's behavior is regulated by such agencies as police, jails, law courts, etc.
- **Health and disease**: In urban community, overcrowding and pollution adversely affect the health of urban people. Sickness rate is higher in cities as compared to rural.

Growth of cities

In every great civilization there has been migration from the village to the city. In western Europe, the cities become more numerous and the growth of cities kept going on. The 19th century was a period of true urban revolution in advance.

The factors which led to the growth of cities are-

- **Surplus Resources**: In ancient times these resources were acquired through under dominate of man by man. (Slavery, forced labour and taxation by ruling). In modern times man has won over nature and extended his power. He has exploited the natural resources through technological improvements that now relatively few people can supply the basic needs of many.
- **Industrialization and commercialization**: Invention of machinery, development of steam power, application of huge capital led to the establishment of huge manufacturing plants which brought about the mobility of immobile groups of workers rushing their concentration around a factory area. While industrialization has stimulated city growth, trade and commerce also have played an important part in urban expansion. The development of modern marketing institutions (no need for face-to-face transactions) and of methods of exchange have greatly contributed to the growth of cities.
- **Development of transport and communication**: These facilities which are satisfying the urban dwellers desire. Industrialization depends upon transportation and communication so that raw material and manufactured goods can be transmitted to others. The local transport added to the population of the city by extending its boundaries.

- **Economic pull of the city**: City provide more opportunity for personal advancement than the rural areas. Modern business and commerce pull young men to the cities where they are paid liberal salaries. Employment opportunity are more in the city than in the village.
- **Educational and recreational facilities**: Until recently all high schools were in cities in India. Most training schools, examination centres, competitive examinations centres, colleges and technical schools are urban. Most big libraries are situated in cities. Amusement Park, theatres and musical drama are in urban city.

Urbanization and its impact on health and health practices

Urbanization is one of the unavoidable features of the modern society. Most of the semi-urban areas are becoming cities. Though there are many advantages and advancements, many disadvantages are also there in the process of urbanization.

Health hazards are more in cities, comparing to the villages. Some of the important problems are given below:

- The health care facilities are well advanced in the cities. All multispecialty and super specialty hospitals are situated in the cities. The patients can get high quality health care in cities.
- City is highly polluted. Both air and water pollution may cause some waterborne and airborne diseases among the citizens. It is too difficult to get pure air and water in cities.
- The level health awareness is very high in the cities. Most of the city citizens are employees and their standard of living is so high. For minor ailments also they go to the health care hospitals.
- The cost of health care is so high in city hospitals that the poor and middle-class members cannot afford for all the health needs.
- Slums are always in risky to develop communicable and other chronic diseases because of their negligence and their poor hygienic practices.
- In cities the citizens are leading a busy life. There is less time for them to interact with each other. The stress may lead them to develop emotional problems.
- Cities are overcrowded. There is no proper drainage and waste disposal system. As a result of that sanitation problem arise. Poor sanitation leads to develop waterborne and airborne disease.
- Most of the city workers are office job holders. The mental work is more than physical work. Because of less physical exercise, problems like obesity, diabetes and other health problems occurs.

Urban slums

The word slum was derived from the word 'slumberer', and now slums are the part of modern cities. They signify extremely complex phenomenon.

According to Webster dictionary *'slum is a fuel back street of a city with a slovenly vicious population characterized by a low qualified neighbourhood.'* A slum may be viewed as special type of disorganized area.

According to **Gist and Hibbert**, *'A slum is a building, group of buildings, or an area characterized by overcrowding with deterioration of civic amenities which endanger the health, safety, and morals of its inhabitants or the community.'*

Therefore, a slum is more than overcrowded and decrepit buildings, dirty and dark streets, the melancholic and poverty-stricken people, ill fed ill clad children, the diseased, the addicts, beggars, criminals, and prostitute's dwell. It is a social phenomenon in which the ideas, attitudes, practices, and way of behavior plays a major role. It represents a way of life

The urban expansion has led to expansion of urban slums. Slums are the colonies formed by the migrant labourer, who are economically weak to have houses to live in. The slum dwellers do not practice hygienic conditions because of shortage of resources. Not only this, but the social problems are also common among these, which affect the overall development of nation.

REGION

Problems and Impact on Health

Region is a large area of land, usually without exact limits or borders. Region combines urban and rural communities. In this world, many regions are there. Some of the familiar regions are arctic, tropical, and desert. The inhabitants belonging to a particular region has similar character.

Region is an integrated area of social life, which exhibits a balance state of dynamic equilibrium between various parts. The changes introduced into any part of the region will bring about changes in the entire region.

The community feeling within a region is known as regionalism. Regionalism promotes a feeling of oneness among the members with the land they share.

Definition

According to **Lundberg**, *'Region is an area within which the people and the different constitute communities are conspicuously more interdependent than they are with people of other areas.'*

Types of Region

Odam and **Moore** classified the regions into five kinds:
- **Physical region**: Physical region is demarcated by geographical factors. A mountain surrounded by a thick forest is one of the well-known types of physical region.
- **Metropolitan region**: It is a large city with its surroundings, which includes all trading, transport, communication, and other activities.
- **Sectional regions**: A particular set of folkways is prevailing.
- **Administrative region**: administrative region demarcated by political boundaries determined by convenience or political planning.
- **Group of states region**: The group of states region possesses the physical similarity, homogeneity, and cultural uniformities.

Regional Divisions in India

India is divided into different zones. Under the State's Reorganization Act 1956, India was divided into four zones. They are:
- **Northern zone**: North zone includes Jammu and Kashmir, Punjab, Rajasthan, Uttar Pradesh, and Delhi
- **Western Zone**: Western zone includes Maharashtra and Gujarat.
- **Eastern Zone**: Eastern zone covers Assam, Bihar, Odisha, and West Bengal.
- **Southern zone**: South zone covers Tamil Nadu, Karnataka, Andhra Pradesh, and Kerala.

Region and Health Problems

Health is a worldwide concern. All the nations are evolving many health programs to achieve the highest state of health. Even though everyone is in a risk of developing any sort of disease, certain diseases are more prevalent among a particular region.

Some of the facts regarding the important regional diseases and their influence in a particular region are as follows:

- Goiter and other iodine deficiency disorders (IDD) have been known to be highly endemic in sub-Himalayan regions. This region is called 'Goiter Belt'.
- Hookworm infection is more prevalent among tropical areas of America and Africa.
- Guinea worm cases are more in African regions specially Sudan, Nigeria and Ghana, India about 44 million population of tribal areas of Andhra Pradesh, Bihar, Odisha are affected by this disease.
- Filariasis cases are more reported at tropics and sub-tropics areas of Africa, Asia, and Western pacific regions of America.
- In India, union territory of Lakshadweep and Andaman Nicobar Islands are free of rabies disease.
- Most of yellow fever cases are reported from Bolivia, Brazil, Colombia, Peru and in the tropical forest regions of America.
- Japanese encephalitis cases are reported from western pacific countries and reminder occurs in Southeast Asia especially in India.
- Brucellosis or Malta fever exists in Mediterranean zone, Europe, Central Asia, Mexico.
- The incidence of trachoma, which leads to irreversible blindness, is very high in the regions of Africa and Asia.
- Leprosy is almost eradicated in the Western countries. The Northeast Asia region accounts for 80% of the global leprosy case load.

In India around 70% population is living in the village. But the 80% of the health care facilities are available in the urban areas. The quality of the available health facilities in rural areas is not satisfactory. This inequality leads to endless health problems. The inequality between urban and rural area persists not only in the health aspects but in the aspect of social life also. In India, there are disputes going on between many states. Best example is the Cauvery water dispute between Tamil Nadu and Karnataka. The growth of regional parties and political bargaining leads to instability, disintegrated and disharmony in a nation.

- Man is a social animal.
- Society is a web of social relationships. It refers to norms of interaction that arise among the individuals.
- Community and society differ based on community sentiments, definite locality, and concrete or abstract basis.
- Personal disorganization represents the behavior of the individual which deviates from the social norms. It results in social disapproval which may express itself in a wide variety of degree.
- A social group consists of two or more people who interact with one another and who recognize themselves as a distinct social unit.
- Groups are most stable and enduring social unit. The groups vary in size from two persons to large organization.
- The groups are important as they provide satisfaction, social identity, 'we feeling' affect the attitude and also motivate the human beings to achieve the goal
- Primary groups are small groups with intimate, kinship-based relationship, for example, families. They commonly last for years. They are small and display face to face interaction.
- Secondary group may be defined as those associations which are characterized by impersonal or secondary relations and specialization of function. They are also called as special interest groups of self-interest groups.
- The group to which an individual belong is his 'in group'. The members of in group have respect for one another's right and show co-operation. People feel comfort and secure. For example- Family, college, institution, hospital etc.
- Out group is defined as the group to which an individual does not belong or the group in relation to outside the boundaries of his in group.
- Mob is an aggressive crowd. It is the crowd of people, generally of criminal who act against the law. The mob gathers with a specific purpose for a temporary period of time.
- Crowd is a large and definable group of people. Crowd is 'gathering of a considerable number of persons around a centre of or point of common attention.' Crowd can also be called a mass.
- The process by which people act and react in relation to others is called social interaction. The interaction process means the way in which partners agree on their goals, negotiate behavior, and distribute resources.

Contd...

Contd...

- Competition is modified form of struggle; competitive endeavour is a basic human drive manifested in procuring the needs of life. Men and women struggle by way of competition to secure social status.
- Conflict is a good oriented, just as cooperation and competition are, but there is a difference, in conflict one seeks deliberately to harm and/or destroy one's antagonists.
- This term 'accommodation' refers to several sorts of working agreements between rival groups that permit at least limited cooperation between them even though the issues dividing them remain unsettled. It does not technically end the conflict but holds in abeyance.
- Assimilation means fusion of two distinct groups into one. It is a gradual process and occurs in all lasting interpersonal situation. It is concerned with absorption of culture by another and fusion into one.
- Isolation means keeping an individual away from personal contacts.
- Socialization is the process of working together, of developing group responsibility, of being guided by the welfare needs of others.
- Social change refers to any modification in established patterns of inter human relationship and standards of conduct.
- Cultural lag is a concept that has been used when inventions discoveries and innovations are constantly disturbing the existing social order and the way of living. In short cultural lag means that one part of cultural lags the other part of culture and causes imbalance in society for example laws do not change quickly to meet social requirements.
- Rural community is a simple community of primary relations with low population based primarily on agricultural life. In rural life, where the family is relatively dominant and self-contained, a group responsibility prevails. The status of the individual is likely to be the status of his family. Property is likely to be thought of as a family possession.
- Urban community mean an area with a high density of population. In India, urban areas are the places which have a local authority like municipality, containment board, notified area committees. Urban people are gradually engaged in different occupational pursuits.

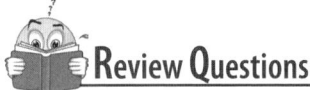

Review Questions

Short Answer Questions

1. Define society.
2. Define community.

3. Differentiate between community and society.
4. Discuss socialization.
5. What are the agencies of socialization?
6. Define personal disorganization.
7. Describe the features of group structure.
8. Discuss the importance of social group.
9. Discuss the panchayat system at village level.
10. Discuss community development project and planning.

Long Answer Questions

1. Define Society. Discuss its origin and explain its nature.
2. Discuss the various factors of process of socialization and agents of socialization.
3. Define social group and classify them.
4. Differentiate between Primary and secondary group and why these group are important.
5. Explain in detail about social processes.
6. Discuss the availability of health services in India.
7. Explain the theories of social change.

UNIT 3

Culture

Chapter Outline

- Nature, characteristic and evolution of culture
- Diversity and uniformity of culture
- Difference between culture and civilization
- Culture and socialization
- Transcultural society
- Culture, modernization and its impact on health and disease

Learning Objectives

After reading this chapter, students will be able to:
- Define culture
- Explain its nature and characteristics
- How culture is evolved
- Differentiate between culture and civilization
- Understand the concept of culture and socialization
- Discuss about the transcultural society
- Learn about the impact of culture on health and disease

Key Terms

- **Culture:** The way of life of a particular people shown in their behavior, habits and attitude towards each other.
- **Diversity:** The wide variety of something
- **Uniformity:** The quality or fact of being the same, or of not changing or being different in any way.

INTRODUCTION

Culture is derived from the English word 'Kulthra' and Sanskrit word 'Samskar' which denotes social channel and intellectual excellence. It means cultivating and refining a thing to such an extent that its end product evokes our admiration and respect. This is practically the same as 'Sanskriti' of the Sanskrit language. The term 'Sanskriti' has been derived from the root 'Kri (to do) of Sanskrit language. Three words came from this root 'Kri; prakriti' (basic matter or condition), 'Sanskriti' (refined matter or condition) and 'vikriti' (modified or decayed matter or condition) when 'prakriti' or a raw material is refined it becomes 'Sanskriti' and when broken or damaged it becomes 'vikriti'.

Culture is a way of life. Culture has an influence on social life. The food you eat, the clothes you wear, the language you speak and the God you worship, all are aspects of culture. In very simple terms, we can say that culture is the embodiment of the way in which we think and do things. It is also the things that we have inherited as members of society.

Culture can be used to describe all of humankind's accomplishments while living in social groups. Culture can be viewed as having elements like music, literature, architecture, sculpture, philosophy, religion, and science. But culture also refers to a person's outlook on different aspects of life as well as their conventions, traditions, festivals, ways of living life.

From place to place and country to country, cultures differ. Its growth is based on the historical process that is currently taking place at the local, regional, or national level. For instance, our greeting routines, attire, eating habits, and social and religious practises are different from those in the West. In other words, all nation's citizens are distinguished by their unique and distinctive cultural traditions.

MEANING OF CULTURE

The most commercially used meaning for culture is that when a person possess polished behavior, intelligence, refinement is said to be cultured and is generally conform to the accepted and recognized ways of society.

The person who does not conform to the ways of society considered that; the person is uncultured. But in anthropological sense, There is no such thing as an uncultured person because all humans have culture of their own which may be simple or complex. Culture is a design and plan for living in society. It is very difficult to live without the minimum of cultural elements for the sociologists, culture denotes acquired behaviors that are shared by and transmitted among the members of society and the same is also passed on from one generation to the other.

Many requirements of men are met by culture. It has the quality of being integrated. Culture is the special quality of men, and a reflection of their social heritage. The culture, what was created today combines with what has been first created by our ancestors. Thus, in every generation something new is added to the culture and thereby it is enlarged. Culture is sound only among the human beings who are the most highly evolved. By way of culture, we can distinguish the human society with that of animal society and by way of culture, the different human societies can be differentiated.

The only thing that constitutes culture is how man altered his environment to better support his way of life. The evolved and matured brain of man allows him to take advantage of his surroundings.

DEFINITION

According to **EB Tylor**, an English anthropologist, *'culture is that complex whole which includes knowledge, belief, art, morals, law, custom and any other capabilities and habits acquired by man as a member or society.'*

According to **EA Hoebel**, *'Culture is the sum total of integrated behaviour patterns which are characteristics of the members of a society, and which are therefore, not the result of biological inheritance.'*

According to **Ralph Piddington**, *'The culture of a people may be defined as the sum total of the material and intellectual equipment whereby they satisfy their biological and social needs and adopt themselves to their environment.'*

According to **Koening**, *'Culture is the sum total of man's efforts to adjust himself to his environment and to improve his modes of living.'*

According to **Malinowski**, *'Culture is the handwork of man and the medium through which he achieves his ends.'*

According to **Lundberg**, *'Culture refers to the social mechanism of behavior and to the physical and symbolic products of their behaviors'.*

According to **Lapiere**, *'Culture is the embodiment of customs, traditions, etc. of the learning of a social group over the generation.'*

According to **Herskovits**, *'Culture is manmade part of environment.'*

According to **AF Walter Paul**, *'Culture is the totality of group ways of thought and action duly accepted and followed by a group of people'.*

According to **Bierstedt**, *'Culture is complex whole that consists of everything we think and do and have as members of society.'*

According to **HT Naxumdar**, *'Culture is sum total of human achievements material as well as non-material, capable of transmission, sociologically, i.e., by tradition and communication, vertically as well as horizontally.'*

According to **Bogardus**, *'Culture is composed of integrated customs, traditions, and current behaviour pattern of human behaviour.'*

It can be concluded that the cultural behavior is learned behavior. It is essential to the concept of culture that instincts innate reflexes, and any other biologically predetermined forms of behavior be ruled out. Culture is, therefore, organized behavior.

Almost all aspects of culture come to be symbolically identified and symbolically transmitted from the old members of any society to its new members, so it is that every way in which the members of a society see and understand the world in which they live in shaped by the symbol system that makes up their culture.

As a result, there are many activities that people who lived in earlier eras of history are still capable of performing but that others who lived hundreds of years later are no longer able to. The recipe for creating the stained glass that adorned medieval buildings is unknown today. Culture may thus be conceived of as a kind of stream flowing down through the centuries from one generation to another.

NATURE OF CULTURE

The word culture is widely used in sociology.
- It is defined as the training and refinement of mind, tastes, and manners.
- Culture is the product of human society; a man is largely a product of his cultural environment.
- Culture is that it is acquired by man and persists through traditions.
- Culture regulates our lives at every turn from the moment we are born until we die there is culture, even we are conscious of it or not. Constant pressure upon is to follow certain types of behavior that other men have created for us.
- Culture represents a store house of readymade solutions to problems.
- Culture helps for insuring some stability in the functioning of the society as a whole.
- Culture refers to patterns of behavior developed because of membership in a society.

- Religion and family background can be used for cultural behavior.
- Cultural influences are probably more important than societies.

Culture is usually acquired through enculturation. It is the process through which an older generation induces and compels a younger generation to reproduce the established lifestyle. It is embedded in person's way of life. It tends to be so pervasive that it escapes everyday thought.

CHARACTERISTICS OF CULTURE

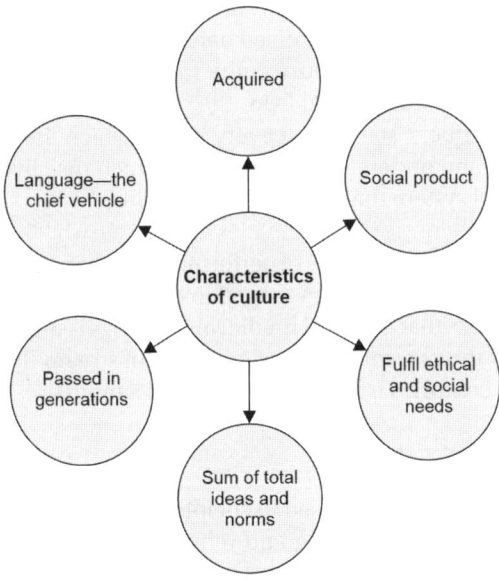

- Man is not born with culture. Culture is learned and acquired.
- Culture is based on some ideal and norms of behavior and each member of the society has to follow them.
- Culture provides socially acceptable patterns or regular ways of meeting biological needs (sex, procreation) and social needs, etc.
- Culture is human product of social interaction.
- Culture is learned by each person in the course of his development in a particular situation.
- Culture is always linked with past experiences and keeps on developing as it passes from one generation to another.
- Language is the chief vehicle of culture. Man lives not only in the present but also in the past.

- As man possesses language the knowledge that he learnt in the past is transmitted in present or future through the medium of language.
- The influence of culture is so great that it formulates the personality of an individual as well as community that he belongs to.
- Culture separates the individual from society to society.
- To each individual, his culture is great. This feeling of greatness and accepting the facts that his own culture is greater than other cultures make him non-cooperative to other cultures. This tendency is known as ethnocentrisms.
- Culture and society are interdependent. Culture possesses continuity and extends beyond the lifetime of those who possess, create, and utilize it.

ELEMENTS OF CULTURE

- Culture is a learned behavioral pattern. It is created by man for fulfilling some of the basic needs and necessities.
- Culture is a pattern of living or design for living. It is a way of life shared by all members of a group.
- Culture is than passed from generation to generation. Culture keeps on modifying as it passes from generation to generation to suit the passing of time and demands.

EVOLUTION OF CULTURE

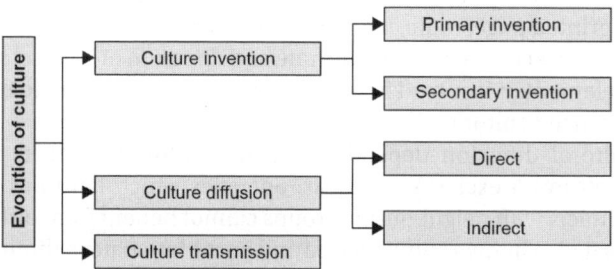

Cultural growth takes place in three ways. They are invention, diffusion, and transmission.

Cultural Invention

- Invention is the discovery of new material and non-material objects or ideas which serve as a stimulus to cultural growth. New materials or findings were discovered by accidents. Invention can be deliberate.

- Invention can be classified as either primary or secondary.
  - **Primary inventions** are those which make possible significant advances in humanity's struggle to shape the environment. They are the basic building blocks, upon which many other cultures developments rest, e.g., the wheel, the phonic alphabet is melting and atomic energy.
  - **Secondary invention** is those which represent improvement upon existing design, e.g., steering own at the year of sailing vessels, self-start or in an automobile.

Cultural Diffusion

- Diffusion takes place when societies borrow traits complexes or patterns from one another. Hence, it is popularly known as cultural borrowing. Influence of diffusion can be seen in the spread of the industrial revolution.
- One of the primary goals of modern third world nations is to borrow culture traits, complexes and patterns needed to create higher levels of industrialization.
- Diffusion can be direct or indirect.
  - The **direct** spread of culture takes place when members of different societies come face-to-face contact with one another, e.g., migration, trade, war, and missionary activities.
  - **Indirect** diffusion on the other hand does not involve personal contact. It depends upon communication media—such as printed page, radio, television, and films.
- Various factors affect both the rate and direction of cultural spread of element. It is spread from the more advanced culture to the less advanced culture.
- Cultural diffusion depends upon intercultural contacts which result in an exchange of ideas. Societies which fail to establish contacts with neighbouring groups cannot benefit from diffusion. It is tied to its own culture based and borne by whatever limitations that imposes. Cultural isolation is the result of geographical accident.

Cultural Transmission

Transmission is the process by which the accumulated knowledge of one generation is passed on the other generations, within societies that possess a written language, traits, complexes, and patterns can be transmitted in written form, within non-literate societies they are transmitted by word of mouth.

When the transmission of culture takes place imperfectly, certain aspects of culture are being lost. Such culture loss is especially apt to occur during the transmission of knowledge and skills which are exclusive prosperity of small groups or categories rather than entire societies, e.g., written language of Egypt.

The sociology of knowledge deals with the process by which knowledge arises in a particular culture. It also analyses how cultural knowledge is transmitted and controlled, and the effects that this has on behavior within the culture.

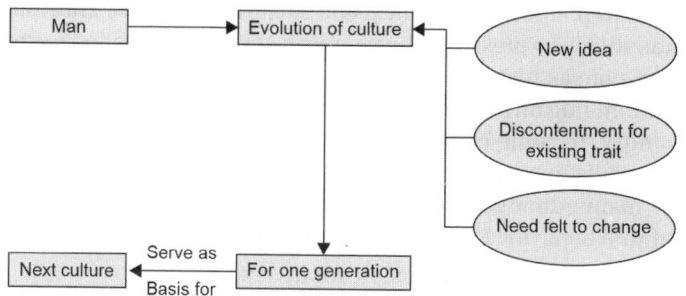

DIVERSITY AND UNIFORMITY OF CULTURE

Diversity of Culture

The biological drives influence human behavior in a significant way. For example, human beings have to eat and drink on a regular basis, optimally, a number of times each day. This means that hunting, gathering, fishing, and cultivating various forms of foods are essential activities in every human society. This satisfaction of biological drives through learned behavior not only permitted homo sapiens to survive but also accounts for human cultural diversity.

Culture is not innate, individuals create culture. It consists of set of principles and traditions transmitted from generation to generation. Human culture is linked to biological evolution of human beings. Human beings are creative by nature, so they have developed diverse or different ways of life.

Cultural diversity is the result of geographical location, religious beliefs, and lifestyles. It is found in heterogeneous society like India, where people belong to various religions, castes, subcastes, linguistic, etc. These variations subjects' people to differ in the way they live, eat, dress, work, etc. Hence, these emerges number of smaller groups within a larger group. The culture of particular smaller group (caste) in a larger whole (India) is termed as subculture. Hence, a subculture is a set of understandings behavior, practical and symbolic objects and vocabulary that distinguish a particular group from other members of their society. For a subculture to Geist individuals must identify with the others who identify with group and must interact with the group, both directly and indirectly. The existence of subculture indicates cultural variations in a society.

Some subcultures are not only different from, but also in opposition to, mainstream of society. Subcultures like those consisting of people who share the similar recreational interests, may have little impact on any group (political, economical and social or a society). These arise as the subculture pressures the people to commit for their own group.

There are as many as cultures as many groups. In some groups, we find monogamy while in other group we can find polygamy and polyandry. In some cultures, bride-groom goes to live at his wife's house, while in others, bride comes to live in husband's house. As a result, many ethnic groups throughout India exhibit distinct variances in cultural behavior, known as **diverse culture**.

The factors which are responsible for diverse culture are-

- ❖ **Geographical location**: Different civilizations have their roots in particular geographic regions. This is caused by the variety of materials that might be used. For example- flat grazing lands where there were large herds of cattle led to a nomadic culture.
- ❖ **Flexibility in behavior**: Human being is flexible and adjusts himself to his natural environment. This constant adjustment of cultural behavior has shown the diversity of culture.
- ❖ **Technological advancement**: Culture is diverse because one group may be backward technically than others. This can cause the change in culture from one to another.
- ❖ **Religious belief**: The group differ from one to another based on religious belief.
- ❖ **Lifestyle**: A group differs from another due to a change in lifestyle brought on by education.

Counter cultures are grouping whose members share values, norms and ways of life that contradict the fundamental beliefs and lifestyle of the larger, more dominant culture. These members reject some or all the core values and institution of society.

The most culturally diverse society in the world is India. In India, different culture exists due to change in level of education, lifestyle, technological advancements, and their beliefs of one group from another. It means diversity of culture is seen here.

- ❖ In India, there are 32 languages and each state with its different folk tales, songs, storytelling session show diversity of culture.

- India is composed of people from 3,000 castes (jaati) or subcastes, covers almost 200 languages and 630 regional dialects (Warsha, 1988).
- There are thousand of factories to produce specialised tasks for which management work, labour work and administrative work are divided. Each group has different types of behavioral pattern which has led to diverse culture based on different occupation.
- A number of religions are in India, the people of a particular religion have their way of living, beliefs and standard of living.
- Eating habits, dress up, differ from one culture to another depending upon state such as Punjabi culture, Haryanvi culture etc.

In India, Hindu majority (79%) has been at odds with people from different religious subcultures for hundreds of years. Since group identification and pride are so often rooted in language, religion, caste, and geographical residence. Societies with subcultural divisions along these lines are prone to conflict and violence

Cultural Uniformity

Uniformity of culture is far more complex than it seems. It means common culture or same type of culture prevailing all over the area. In India, uniformity of culture is based on belief that God in one, who is superior to all of us.

Globalisation affords the opportunity to internalise the universal culture and thus to become part of a whole. The cultural infrastructure, the global forces currently fabricating India, would pave the way for the internalisation of 'universal' culture.

Difference between Culture and Civilization

The term 'culture' is the way people live, reflected in the language they spoke, food they eat, clothes they wear and the Diet they follow or worship. It expresses the manner in which one thinks and do things.

Civilization is described as a process of civilizing or say developing the state of human society, to the extent that the culture, industry, technology, government, etc. reaches the maximum level. The term 'civilization' is derived from a Latin term 'civis' which indicates 'someone who resides in a town'.

Culture	Civilization
The term 'culture' refers to the embodiment of the manner in which we think, behave and act.	The improved stage of human society, where members have the considerable amount of social and political organization and development, is called civilization.
Our culture describes what we are	our civilization explains what we have or what we make use of.
Culture is an end; it has no measurement standards.	Civilization has precise measurement standards because it is a means
The culture of a particular region can be reflected in religion, art, dance, literature, customs, morals, music, philosophy, etc.	The civilization is exhibited in the law, administration, infrastructure, architecture, social arrangement, etc. of that area.
Culture denotes the greatest level of inner refinement, and so it is internal.	Civilization is external, i.e., it is the expression of state-of-the-art technology, product, devices, infrastructure and so forth.
Change in culture is observed with time, as in the old thoughts and traditions lost with the passage of time and new ones are added to it which are then transmitted from one generation to another.	Civilization is continuously advancing, i.e., the various elements of civilization like means of transportation, communication, etc. are developing day by day.
Culture can evolve and flourish, even if the civilization does not exist.	Civilization cannot grow and exist without culture

MacIver and **Page** have clearly stated the interrelationship between culture and civilization. They say that civilization is a ship "which can set sail to various ports. The port we sail to remains a cultural choice.

Without the ship we could not sail at all; according to the character of the ship we sail fast or slow, take longer or shorter voyages. But the direction in which we travel is not predestined by the design of the ship. The more efficient it is the more ports lie within the range of our choosing". In short, civilization is the driving force of society. Culture is its steering wheel.

CULTURE AND SOCIALIZATION

A certain group of people's shared beliefs, values, behaviors, and material possessions are referred to as their culture. Almost every element of our lives is influenced by our culture.

Our beliefs, attitudes, and behaviors are shaped and defined by the process of socialization, which also serves as a model for our behavior. As children become socialised, they learn how to fit into and to function as productive members of human society. Humans learn cultural values and standards through the process of socialization, which serves as a guide for daily living.

When an individual is born, he is helpless and depends upon others to fulfil the most basic physiological needs. As an individual grows, he experiences an outgoing process of social interaction which enables an individual to develop skills and also need to participate in human society. This ongoing process is called **socialization**. This process is important for human society as a whole because it is the means of teaching culture to each new generation.

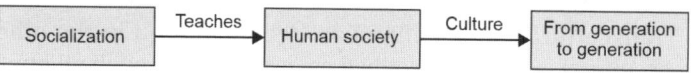

It means human infants are born without any culture. They must be transformed by the agents of socialization such as family, school, peers, and mass media into culturally and socially adept human beings. This general process of acquiring culture is referred as **socialization**. In socialization, language of culture is learned. We also learn about the occupational roles that their society has in store for them.

During socialization, we learn the cultural norms. It is also important in the process of personality formation. Much of human personality is the result of our genes, the socialization process can mould it in particular directions by encouraging specific beliefs and attitudes as well as selectively providing experiences.

Cultural learning directs the individual to get fit into the social group to which he belongs, and his drive areas also guided into approved channel of expression. An individual internalizes the cultural aspects with the mode of social learning. Hence, he/she becomes socialized in connection with the cultural learning. But it is noticeable that an individual does not learn the entire culture of their society.

Successful socialization can result in uniformity within a society. If all children receive the same socialization, it is likely that they will share the same beliefs and expectations on the basis of this national governments around the world standardize education and make it compulsory for all children. Education is the powerful tool for controlling people. Those, who internalise the norms of society, are less likely to break the law.

Socialization is the process by which we learn the fundamentals of our culture. The personality also develops, and we learn the appropriate roles to be performed in society.

TRANSCULTURAL SOCIETY

In the concise statement of the theme, a 'transcultural society' is presented as a multicultural society that employs consensual decision making. This should be read as correlation, rather than definition. Consideration should be given to the possibility of a transcultural society that does not employ consensual decision making. It is harder to imagine how a multicultural society that employed consensual decision-making (to a significant extent) could not transcultural it should be ruled out.

Transculturalism is defined as "seeing oneself in the other". Transcultural is in turn described as "extending through all human culture" or "involving, encompassing, or combining elements of more than one culture".

Transculturalism is characterized by the following:

- Transculturalism emphasizes on the problematic of contemporary culture in terms of relationships, meaning making, and power formation; and the transitory nature of culture as well as its power to transform.
- Transculturalism is interested in dissonance, tension, and instability as it is with the stabilizing effects of social conjunction, communalism, and organization; and in the destabilizing effects of non-meaning or meaning atrophy. It is interested in the disintegration of groups, cultures, and power.
- Transculturalism does not seek to privilege the semiotic over the material conditions of life, nor vice versa.
- Transculturalism accepts that language and materiality continually interact within an unstable locus of specific historical conditions.
- Transculturalism locates relationships of power in terms of language and history
- Transculturalism is deeply suspicious of itself and of all utterances. Its claim to knowledge is always redoubtable, self-reflexive, and self-critical.
- Transculturalism can never eschew the force of its own precepts and the dynamic that is culture.
- Transculturalism never sides with one moral perspective over another but endeavours to examine them without ruling out moral relativism or meta- ethical confluence.

- Transculturalism seeks to illuminate the various gradients of culture and the ways in which social groups create and distribute their meanings; and the ways in which social groups interact and experience tension.
- Transculturalism looks toward the ways in which language wars are historically shaped and conducted.

Transculture in Childhood

Of course, the children should not be isolated from other cultures. Every child should have at least one secondary culture and be exposed to a variety of cultures. The secondary culture serves as a counterpoint to the primary culture. The presentation of the other culture may resemble a buffet that is over-sampled over time as interest dictates.

Retaining Diversity

A more practical problem is the preservation of the distinctiveness of the root cultures given the overlaying transcendent culture. The danger is that the society would become more uniform and lose culture diversity. The loss of cultural diversity is considerable for many reasons including the loss of diversity invalidation perspectives for consensual decision-making.

Education for Diversity

One possible candidate to loss of diversity is to provide immersion schools during childhood. Every child can have a strong education within a root culture as a base from which to transcend cultural barriers. There is no reason that every child must be educated with the context of the same root culture. Thus, the transcultural society should foster the development of educational institutions representing different cultures.

INFLUENCE OF CULTURE ON HEALTH AND DISEASE

Culture and Health

Health beliefs and practices are a part of every culture. Most ancient and primitive societies had supernatural explanations for illness. The ancient people and even modern people believe that disease is due to wrath of supernatural power. Even today it is believed that a venereal disease leprosy is punishment from supernatural power.

Impact of Culture on Health and Disease (Illness)

Societies contain a variety of cultures. There are customs unique to each culture. These traditions begin even before birth and endure throughout life. All ceremonies are carried out in accordance with cultural traditions even after death. The goal of the numerous customs that may accompany pregnancy, childbirth, and weaning is successful reproduction as well as the protection of the mother and child's lives. However, when viewed from a contemporary, scientific perspective, not all of these traditions will be seen as beneficial. In fact, some of these might even be detrimental.

The cultural practices which have influence on health and disease are as follows:

- **Antenatal nutrition**: During pregnancy, the ladies are advised not to take healthy diet in some cultures. This is said with the aspect that childbirth will be easy, if the child is of small size. This unhealthy practice can cause low birth weight babies.
- **Breast feeding practices**: It has been observed that in some cultures, mother is not allowed to feed the baby for the first three days. But this is irrelevant practice affecting the health of a newborn baby.
- **No proper nutrition to girl child**: In some of culture, it is practiced that ladies or girls will eat the left-over food in family and they are even not provided with the adequate diet which can cause malnutrition, worm infestations and decreased immunity.
- **Handwashing**: Handwashing among the romans, Hebrews, and Egyptians was common before and after dinner. In early Greeks, it was considered ill mannered if the guests did not wash their hands before taking meal. Servants used to offer a vessel of water so as to carry out the custom of hand washing. This is a good custom as handwashing removes the germs from hands and prevents the ingestion of microorganisms with food.
- **Bathing**: There are occasions when the baths are fixed such as Vaisakhi, and woman have to take bath after menstruation for purifying themselves. According to religion, even priest advice ceremonial baths after childbirth. These baths are apart from regular baths. Bridal shower which is performed before marriage is an old tradition which is handed down to modern brides. It is a good tradition/custom of maintaining personal hygiene so as to prevent occurrence of certain diseases.

- **Hair care**: Woman kept their hair covered at all time and men get their beard shaved from barbers and even shave their heads. There were certain occasions when the men had to shave their head on the death of their parents. Traditionally, after the death of husband, even the woman's head were shaved. The barbers used the unsterilized blade, and one blade was used for shaving hairs of many people, so the chances of spread of infection were more as they were not having the idea of microorganisms.
- **Face care**: As women and men seldom washed their faces, so many men and women had developed unsightly acne scars by the time they had reached adulthood.
- **Nail care**: Nails were cut by men and women but on certain day only such as Monday, Wednesday, Friday & Sunday.

Customs Related to Food

- Food consumption and diet have been shaped by traditions and beliefs. People's dietary preferences are influenced by their religion or cultural practises. For example, non-vegetarian food is preferred in Muslim and Christian societies while vegetarianism is valued in Hindu culture. Even with a vegetarian diet, eating habits vary. Garlic and onions are forbidden in several religions. Timing of eating dinner before sunset is considered good in Jainism.
- Hot and cold foods concept is also prevalent. Some foods such as meat, fish, jaggery are considered as hot because they generate heat while foods such as curd, milk and lemon are cold foods
- Adulteration of milk with water is based on the belief that if pure milk is boiled, then the milk of donor animal will be reduced or dried up.
- Fasts have an effect on health and, in some cases, can worsen health, such as the Karva Chauth fast if kept by a pregnant woman or a diabetic woman. Muslims follow Ramadan, and Hindus maintain fasts on certain holidays like Janmashtami, Karva Chauth, Ram Navmi, etc. as well as on specific days like Monday (Shiv pooja), Tuesday (Hanuman pooja), etc. On their designated holy days, or "Pajusans," Jains observe fasting.
- In certain religions, customs related to eating are followed by women such as women eat left over food of husbands.

Customs Related to Marriage

- In tribal cultures, parents frequently planned marriages for their young daughters by setting up betrothals between them and their future husbands.

- In today's societies, it is normal for couples of opposite sexes to decide to get married based on their shared love (love marriage).
- In many cultures, a man must demonstrate his ability to protect his wife and their children from harm.
- In several societies, marriages are arranged, and parents select the partners for their son or daughter. Such type of marriages is commonly prevailing in India.
- Customs also dictates that the bride must always stand to the left of the groom during the ceremony.
- The compatibility of the prospective bride and groom is determined by consulting their horoscopes.
- The custom of newborn betrothals is still practised by traditional Hindus today.
- A Hindu priest will look at the couple's horoscopes to determine the best day to get married.
- Despite the legal age limit for male and female marriage, early marriage occur, which is still common in tribal and rural communities, is not deemed to be good.
- Certain religions are the most prone to consanguineous marriages, which might result in genetic illnesses among their marriages.
- Polyandry marriages, which are common in Todas of Nilgiri Hills, might lead to venereal illnesses in the population.
- Polygamy is still practised by religious groups who defend multiple marriages imposed by the deity they serve.
- Endogamy practises, including as marriages between family members, are still common, which has an impact on people's physical and emotional health. Even so, it discriminates against other castes.

Customs Related to Sexuality

- In several religions, it is customary to refrain from having sex during menstruation or periods.
- In some cultures, it is also taboo for men and women to engage in sexual activity before marriage.

Customs Related to Oral Hygiene

In order to have oral hygiene, twigs of neem and toothbrush is used. Use of ash and charcoal is not considered to be a good custom for maintaining oral hygiene.

Customs Related to Smoking

Customs related to smoking of bidi; pipe & cigar have dangerous effect on the health of human beings. Certain health problems such as tuberculosis, oral cancer, CAD, emphysema, angina pectoris, cancer of bladder can occur.

Customs Related to Purdah System

The purdah system (veils over head and face) in Muslims deprive the women of beneficial effect of sunrays and increases the incidence of ill health.

Customs Related to Sleeping Habits

Sleeping on grounds can cause insect bites according to customs, on certain occasions, the people have to sleep on ground.

Customs Related to Circumcision

It is a custom among Muslims in newborn babies.

Customs Related to Birth of Child

- It is considered bad custom to refrain the newborn from breastfeeding for three days and to keep the infant on water and sugar solution only.
- Prolonged feeding without weaning is considered not good.
- It is regarded as a good custom to combine prolonged feeding with weaning and exposure to sunlight for the infant.
- Conduction of deliveries by untrained dais is not appropriate as use of unsterile blade and improper cleaning can lead to infection.
- Branding of skin, which is a traditional custom among certain is not considered good, if unsterile blade or uncleaned technique is used.
- Applying of kajal in the eyes of newborn baby is sometimes harmful as it can cause eye infection and can transmit trachoma.
- Paste of turmeric on forehead is neither good nor bad custom.

Cultural Understanding and Awareness

To develop cultural understanding, you need to understand your own world view and that of your patient. At all costs you should avoid stereotyping. To have a deeper understanding of diverse cultures you need to inform yourself through education and research. A great way is to read about different religions, cultures, customs, and traditions if you have to develop appreciation for the richness of cultures of the world. What distinguishes Asian culture from European culture it helps to read history as well as educate yourself about societal and biological evolution to understand how we are all interconnected and how we all become 'different' because of events that shaped our culture and the environment that we live in.

Widening your prospective will not only help enrich your understanding of your patients from diverse background but it will enrich your understanding of life and yourself. In more practical terms, tolerance and flexibility are very important factors for cultural understanding. Respecting your patients (or all individuals for that matter) no matter what background is very important.

However, you should not make special privileges or overcompensate just because the patient is from a different cultural background. Respect should be given in the same accord as everyone what you have to do is give more understanding because it is not as easy compared to a patient that shares your world view.

- Culture is the way of life of a particular people shown in their behavior, habits, and attitude towards each other.
- The culture is acquired, a social product, fulfils the needs of group, total of ideas and norms of a group and also passed from first generation to generation.
- Culture can be acquired through enculturation. It is embedded in person's way of life. It tends to be so pervasive that it escapes everyday thought.
- Socialization process begins soon after birth. Through socialization, child learn language and fundamentals of culture.
- Culture influences the health and disease. The harmful activities of culture can cause morbidity and mortality among people whereas the good cultural practices maintain the health of people.

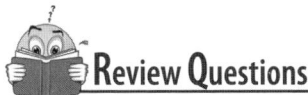
Review Questions

Short Answer Questions
1. Define culture.
2. Enlist the characteristics of culture.
3. Explain the nature of culture.

Long Answer Questions
1. Define culture. Discuss the evolution of culture. Write down the characteristics of culture.
2. 'Diversity and uniformity of Culture'. Comment.
3. How culture affects the health and disease?

UNIT 4

Family and Marriage

 CHAPTER OUTLINE

- Family – characteristics, basic need, types, and functions of family
- Marriage – forms of marriage, social custom relating to marriage and importance of marriage
- Legislation on Indian marriage and family.
- Influence of marriage and family on health and health practices

 Learning Objectives

After reading this chapter, students will be able to:
- Define family and marriage
- Explain the characteristics, basic needs, types, and functions of family
- Understand the forms of marriage and social custom relating to marriage
- Discuss the importance of marriage
- Understand the concept of legislation on Indian marriage and family
- How marriage and family influences health and health practices

 Key Terms

- **Family**: Biological social unit composed of husband, wife, and children
- **Marriage**: Approved social pattern whereby two or more establish a family

FAMILY

The family, a social institution, is the most fundamental of all social groups and it is universal in its distribution from time immemorial. It is fundamental and persistent social group, a basic social institution at the very care of society. The values institutionalized in the family have long been regarded as important enough to warrant strong measures against any behavior that violated them. Not only has the family been defined as fundamental to the existence of society, but it has been viewed as a source of morality and descent content. It has also been defined as a primary force for controlling behavior and civilizing the human animal.

Definition of Family

'Family is a group defined by sex relationship sufficiently pure and enduring to provide the procreation and upbringing of children.'
—**MacIver**

'Family is more or less durable association of husband and wife with or without children or of a man or woman alone with children.'
—**Nimkoff**

'Family is a biological social unit composed of husband, wife, and children.' —**Elliot and Merrill**

'Family is a group of persons united by the ties of marriage, blood or adoaption, constituting a single household, interacting, and intercommunicating with each other in their respective social roles of husband, wife, mother and father, son and daughter, brother and sister creating a common culture.' —**Burgess and Locke**

'Family is a group of persons whose relations to one another are based upon consanguinity and who are, therefore, kin to one another.'
—**Kingsley Davis**

'The family, in general, is a group based on marriage and marriage contact, including recognition of the rights and duties of parenthood, common residence for husband, wife and children and reciprocal economic obligations between husband and wife.'
—**William Newton Stephens**

Characteristics of Family

- ❖ **Mating relationship**: A family comes into existence when a man and woman establish mating relation between them. Mating relationship occur to meet the sexual desire of man and woman.

Unit 4: Family and Marriage

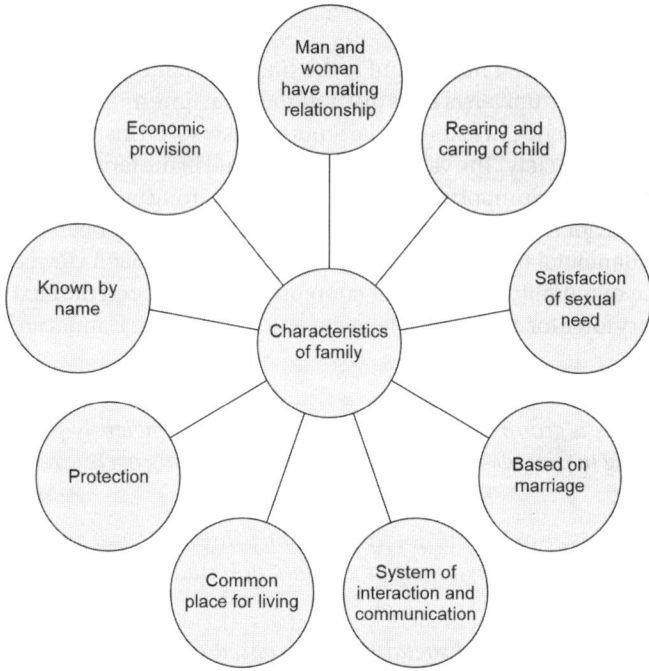

When the difference in opinion occurs, later on there can be break up leading to disintegration of family.

- ❖ **A form of marriage**: Mating relationship is established through the institution of marriage. The society regulates sexual behavior between opposite sexes through the institution of marriage. So family is a form of marriage.
- ❖ **A common place for living**: A family requires a home or household for its living. The members of a family have a common habitation or household. Some of the tasks such as childbearing and child rearing cannot be performed without having a common dwelling.
- ❖ **An economic provision**: Every family needs an economic provision to satisfy the economic needs. The head of the family carries on certain profession and earns to maintain the family. As per the current scenario, male and female members of the family being head of the family, collectively takes the responsibility to bear the burden of family in respect to economic needs.
- ❖ **System of interaction and communication**: The family is composed of persons who interact and communicate with each other in their social roles such as husband and wife, mother and father, son, and daughter, etc.

- **Protection**: Family provides protective services to its members by which they feel secure at home.
- **Satisfaction of sexual need**: The satisfaction of sex instinct makes for normal personality. If the sex instincts are suppressed, then it produces personality maladjustments and disrupts social relations. Satisfaction of sex instinct brings the desire for life-long partnership among men and women. It is important to mention that the family is composed of persons united by ties of marriage, blood, or adaption.
- **Known by name:** There is a system of reckoning descent which may be through either male or female line and ever family is known by a name i.e., in a family there exists a system of nomenclature.
- **Rearing and caring of child:** The family members i.e., father, mother, grandmother, rear and care the children. They take all the stress and tensions for caring the children.

Functions of Family

As a social institution the family has certain functions to perform for the society and the individual. It plays an important role for survival, protection and support, socialization, and societal identification of the individual. The Family serves the society as an instrument of sexual control and cultural transmission. Different sociologists have classified functions of the family in different ways:

Ogburn and **Nimkoff** have divided family functions into the six categories:
1. Affectional
2. Economic
3. Recreational
4. Protective
5. Religious
6. Educational

Groves has classified the functions of family in the following ways:
- Protection and care of the young
- Regulation and control of sex impulses
- Conservation and transmission of social heritage
- Provision of opportunity for the most intimate contacts

K Davis has mentioned four main functions of family:
1. Reproduction
2. Maintenance
3. Placement
4. Socialization of the young

According to **Lundberg** the following are the basic functions of family:
- Regulation of sexual behavior
- Care and training of the children
- Cooperation and division of labor
- Primary group satisfaction.

MacIver divides the functions of the family into two categories:
1. Essential functions
   - Satisfaction of sex needs
   - Reproduction
   - Provision of a home
   - Socialization.
2. Nonessential functions
   - Economic functions
   - Property transformations
   - Religious functions
   - Educative functions
   - Recreational functions
   - Wish fulfilment

Distinctive Features of the Family

Family is the smallest and the most intimate group of society. It is a universal institution found in every society. Family as the most important social institution possesses certain distinctive features. They are:

- **Universality**: The Family is a universal institution. Every human being is a member in the family.
- **Emotional basis**: Every family is based on human impulses of mating, procreation, motherly devotion and parental love and care. The members of a family have emotional attachment with each other. Love between husband and wife, parents and children make the family as an institution of self-sacrifice.
- **Limited size**: The family is very small in size. It is known as the smallest primary group. It is a small social institution. It includes husband and wife and the persons who are born in it or adopted. The relations among the members of family are direct, intimate, close, personal, and permanent.
- **Formative influence**: The personality of the individual is moulded in the family. The family's customs, traditions, mores, and norms have great influence in shaping the personality of its members during childhood. Family is the most effective agency of the process of socialization and social control.

- **Responsibility of the members**: The members of the family have responsibility and obligation for the family. All the members of the family have joint responsibility in maintaining duties to satisfy the needs of the family members. The children also learn about responsibility and cooperation from the parents.

Types of Family

- **On the basis of marriage**: Family has been classified into three major types—
  - **Polyandrous family**: This is a type of family formed where one woman marries many men and lives with all of them or with each other of them alternatively.
  - **Polygamous family**: The family formed where one man marries many women at one time.
  - **Monogamous family**-This type of family is prevailing all over world. In this, one man marries one woman.
- **On the basis of nature of residence**: Family can be classified into three main forms—
  - **Family of matrilocal residence**: In this type of family husband goes to live in house of wife.
  - **Family of Patrilocal residence**: This system of family is seen in many parts of India. In such type of family, wife goes and lives in the house of her husband.
- **On the basis of ancestor or descent**-Family can be classified into two main types—
  - **Matrilineal family**: In this type of family, ancestry continuous through mother. Mother is believed to be the ancestor of family. The rights of each member depend on the relation to mother.
  - **Patrilineal family**: This type of family is prevailing in most part of India. In this type, ancestry continues through the father.
- **On the basis of nature of relations among family members**- Family is classified into two main types—
  - **Conjugal family**: It consists of adult members, among whom exists sexual relationship
  - **Consanguineous family**: It consists of members among whom there exists blood relationship: brother & sister, father & son etc.
- **On the basis of authority**: Family is of two types—
  - **Patriarchal Family**: Under the patriarchal family the male head of the family possessed all powers. He is the owner and administrator of the family, property and right, to him all persons living in the family are subordinates. This type of family

was prevalent among the Hebrews, the Greeks, the Romans, and the Aryans of India.

The chief characteristics of patriarchal family are the following:
- The wife after marriage comes to live in the home of the husband.
- The father is the supreme lord of the family property.
- Descent is reckoned through the father. The children are known by the name of the family of their father.
- The children can inherit the property of their father only. They have no right over the property of the mother's family. With the passage of Hindu Code Bill, it has undergone a change.

- **Matriarchal Family**: In matriarchal family, the authority vests in the woman as head of the family with the males being subordinates. She is the owner of the property and rules over the family.

The chief characteristics of matriarchal family are the following:
- Descent is reckoned through the mother not the father because maternity is a fact while paternity is only an opinion. This is the matrilineal system.
- Marriage relations are transient. The husband is sometimes merely a casual visitor.
- The children are brought up in the home of the wife's relatives. Descent is not only matriarchal but also matrilocal.
- Property is transferred through the mother and only females succeed to it.

- The matriarchal family is said to prevail among the primitive people who led a wandering or hunting life. The matriarchal system has prevailed in many parts of the earth such as among the North American Indian, among people of Malabar (part of Kerala) and a few other parts of India. The Khasis have matrilocal residence and matrilineal descent.

❖ **On the basis of in-group and out-group affiliation**: Family may be classified into endogamous family and exogamous family.
- **Endogamous family**: It is one which sanctions marriage only among members of the in-group. Endogamy is the practice of marrying someone within a group to which one belongs. An endogamous family is one which consists of husband and wife who belong to same group such as caste or tribe. For example, in a caste-ridden society like India a member of a particular caste has to marry within his own caste. When a person marries within his caste group, it is called endogamous family.

- **Exogamous family:** It sanctions marriage of members of an in-group only with member of an out-group. In exogamy marriage with someone outside his group. For example, a Hindu must marry outside his Kinship group or Gotra. When a family is consisted of husband and wife of different groups such as Gotra is called exogamous family. In India marriage between same Gotra has been prohibited. Hence, one must marry outside his own Gotra.
- **On the basis of structure:** The family has been classified into nuclear and extended family.
  - **Nuclear family:** A nuclear family is one which consists of husband, wife, and their children. The children leave the parental household as soon as they are married. A nuclear family is an autonomous unit freedom from control of the elders.
  - **Extended family:** In an extended family all the brothers, their wives and sons and unmarried daughters live along with their parents in a common household and the father is succeeded by his eldest son. The Hindu family is an extended family.
  - **Joint family:** It is group of people belonging to the three or more generations who live under the same roof, eat food cooked from same hearth and participate in common activities.

Nuclear Family

A nuclear family is one which consists of husband, wife, and their children. The children leave the parental household as soon as they are married. A nuclear family is an autonomous unit freedom from control of the elders. It can be a nurturing environment in which to raise children, emotional support, low stress, and a stable economic environment.

Characteristics of Nuclear Family

- **Stable environment:** Children that grow up in a single parent household have higher chances of stability.
- **Behavioral stability:** Children get a sense of what is acceptable and unacceptable, as far as behavioral is concerned especially when both parents look after the nurturing the children.
- **A sense of consistency:** The children grown up in nuclear family, have a sense of consistency. This enables them to feel as a wider whole during get together of any family function.
- **Learning skills:** Children in nuclear family usually get far more extensive training in life skills. The mother teaches the children

about relationship skills and father about handiwork skills, sports skills as well as how to deal with outside world.
- **Sharing responsibility**: Children in nuclear family learn the sharing responsibility and roles are performed by expectations and example, rather than formal instructions.
- **Physical and emotional support**: Nuclear families have more physical and emotional resources with which they can reinforce the whole. Through observing their parents, they learn how to help in building the family.

Joint family

Joint families are made up of number of nuclear families, where all are related to each other. All people live in a common house, see blood relatives like grandparents, uncles, aunts, grandchildren, and other relatives live together. Usually more joint family's lives are found in villages of our India. Nowadays joint families are disappearing because of influence of modernization, institutionalism, industrialism, influence of urban society.

Generally, the joint family consists of three and four generations, joined together based on common ancestry and property. The members possess a set of reciprocal rights and obligations. Typically, they live in the same house and eat food prepared in the same kitchen. They work together, pool their income, expenditure, and property, and perform religious rituals as a family.

Characteristics of Joint Family

- **Authoritarian structure**: The power to take decisions regarding matters related to family and individual lie in the hands of head of family. His decision is taken as final, and everyone has to abide by it.
- **Family as an organization**: It implies the interest of the family as a whole is more important than individual's interest. One has to sacrifice one's personal wishes, likes and dislikes, which go against family norms or rules or traditions.
- **Status of member of family is determined by their age and relationship**: The status of a person higher in age is higher in joint family than person lower in age. Similarly, person is respected more because of the higher status in terms of marital or blood ties. A husband, an uncle, an aunt and in laws are respected because of higher status in relationship. A person's ability and achievement are not given importance in determining status.

- **Blood relationship**: Blood relationship gets preference over marital relationship. It implies that husband-wife relationship is subordinate to father-son or brother-brother relationship.
- **An ideal of joint responsibility**: Everyone shares the problems of other members of family and tries to help in whatever manner can.
- **Equal attention to all members**: The family income is pooled together and needs of the individual members are met according to their needs and not according to their contribution.

The joint family system is useful for agricultural and business-based families because both activities require manpower and pooling of economic resources such as land and money.

Merits of Joint Family

- It ensures economic progress as members of the family work collectively.
- Division of labor exists and therefore, the family runs smoothly.
- It is economical as members of the family purchase in bulk quantities for its consumption.
- The members of the family found leisure time as the members divided the work among themselves. The incapable and invalid people will fend social security as they are protected by the other members of the family.
- The fragmentation of landed property is avoided.

Demerits of Joint Family

- Laziness will develop among the members as the member think that the work will be done by the others, and they try to escape from doing work.
- The members will not develop individuality and personality as the head of the family controls the other members and suppress them in acting individually.
- There would be number of quarrels among the females of the family, they also develop jealous, hatred to each other. The children quarrel also creates conflict among the elderly people.
- Privacy for the young couple is denied.
- Uncontrolled procreation takes place as there would be competition among themselves.

Extended Family

An extended family is formed when two or more adults from different generations of a family, share a household. It consists of more than

parents and children. It may be a family that include parents, children, cousins, aunts, uncles, grandparents, and foster children etc. The extended family may live together due to many reasons such as:
- Help raise children
- Support for an ill relative
- Help with financial problem

The Modern Family

In the early historical period, family system was mainly patriarchal in which the father or oldest male member dominated the whole life of the family. The so-called matriarchal system meaning mother rule was not a common feature. Under feudal role, the position of women was more subordinated whereas that of male members was further strengthened. This was a necessary corollary of the authoritarian mores of feudalism.

Causes of the Decay of Patriarchal Family

After the renaissance and reformation came a new age of science and democracy which began to undermine the foundations of the patriarchal family. On the one hand, there were economic factors involving industrialism, urbanism and mobility which broke down the self-sufficiency of the patriarchal family on the ideals and the decline of religious orthodoxy, which were in less harmony with the prerogatives and attitudes of the patriarchal family.

Feature of Modern Family

Some of the salient features of modern family are as follows:
- **Decreased Control of Marriage Contract**: Marriage is the basis of family. In traditional family, the marriage was contracted by the parents. The marriage ceremony was based on the principles of male dominance and female obedience. In modern family, people are less subjected to the parental control concerning whom and when they shall marry. The marriage is now settled by the partners themselves. It is choice of mate by mate usually proceeded by courtship or falling in love.
- **Changes in the Relationship of Man and Woman**: In modern family, the woman is not the devotee of men but an equal partner in life with equal rights. The husband now does not dictate but only requests the wife to a task for him. She is now emancipated of man's slavery. She is no longer the drudge

and slave of olden days. She can divorce her husband as the husband can divorce her. She can sue the husband for her rights and likewise he sued.

- **Laxity in Sex Relationships**: The rigidity traditionally associated with sexual relationships no longer characterizes the modern family, cases of illegitimate sex relationship of the husband and wife too can be seen in modern family
- **Economic Independence**: Women in modern family have attained an increasing degree of economic independence. It is not only the husband who leaves the home for work but is also the wife who goes out of doors for work. The percentage of women employed outside the home is continually on the increase. In India, the number of women going for employment is steadily increasing. In upper classes women are property owners and in lower classes they are wage earners or professional workers. This economic independence has largely affected the attitude of modern woman. Formerly, she had no choice but to find a male partner who could marry her and support her economically. She is no longer helpless in the face of man, but rather resolves matters regarding her relationship with him. She is not a slave of the man who provides her with food, clothing, and shelter but now she can earn her own living. Such features did not mark the traditional family. In short, woman in the modern family has come as near achieving equality with men and children emancipation from parents.
- **Smaller Family**: The modern family is a smaller family. It is no longer a joint family. Moreover, the tendency is to have a smaller family and the contraceptives help in checking the birth.
- **Decline of Religious Control**: The modern family is secular in attitude. The religious rites of the traditional family such as early prayer, yagna, etc. are no longer performed, in modern family. Marriage also has become a civil contract rather than a religious sacrament. It can be broken at any hour. The authority of religion over the conditions of marriage and divorce has markedly declined. Divorce is frequent occurrence in modern family. In traditional family, it was a rare phenomenon.
- **Separation of Non-essential Functions**: The modern family has given up many functions which were performed by the traditional family. These functions have now been taken over by specialized

agencies. Thus, the hospital offers room for the birth of child, in the nursing home he is brought up, in the kindergarten he is educated and in the playground he recreates. Not only this much but many of the traditional talks of the household such as cooking and baking, cleaning, and washing are also performed outside the household by specialized agencies. The process advances still further as more and more families rely upon prepared and manufactured goods consumed by the family.

- **Filo-centric Family**: In the modern family the trend is towards the filo-centric family. A filo-centric family is one wherein the children tend to dominate the scene and their wishes determine the policy of the family. In modern family, physical punishment is rarely awarded to the children. The children now choose which school they will attend and what clothes they will wear, what will they eat, and where will they go to see a movie? The individuation of family members has reached a point beyond which it cannot go. The size and functions of the family have been reduced. It has suffered a change in regard to both its structure and functions. It now consists of the married couple and two or three children. Even this smallest family unit has shown a tendency towards instability. Its function has been taken over by several specialized agencies. The modern family is more individualized and democratic where woman enjoy a high prestige and position. From an institution, it has moved towards companionship.

- **Instability of Modern Family**: The striking problem that confronts the modern family is its instability. The control of the family over its members has decreased. The younger generation does not like any interference by their elders. There is lack of unity among the family members. The problems of working women have hindered the development of the children and increased conflicts between husband and wife. There is lack of mutual trust. The marriage bonds have weakened. There is sexual disharmony between husband and wife. The members of the same family are engaged in different pursuits, one in service, and the other in business, a third in politics. The modern family has shrunk both structurally and functionally and is gradually losing its primary characters. The state has undertaken to provide prenatal attention and infant schools, expensive medical facilities are available. Factory and office provide the place of work and women clubs and bars provide recreation. If people find their education, their work, and their recreation outside the family and if women can get jobs which make them independent, surely the chance of a broken home can be laid at the door of a modern family. The modern family is more individualized and democratic where women enjoy high prestige and position.

Dowry System

Dowry is a major problem of marriage in India, especially in certain communities with increasing importance of money, the amount of dowry is also increasing. Even the spread of modern education and enlighten, has not been able to diminish this problem.

Further, dowry has resulted in violence towards women. There are cases where the brides have been burnt as they were not able to satisfy more dowry.

In many communities throughout India, a dowry has traditionally been given by a bride's kin at the time of her marriage. Dowry has its root probably in the early vedic period. Though no dowry was demanded, the bride was given fine clothes, jewellery, and gifts at the time of marriage.

In the beginning, all these were given to the bride by her parents or elders for her own use, gradually the elders of the husband's family started receiving, controlling, and using this property. With the gradual fall of status of woman greater incidence of child marriage, anuloma marriage and the demand for dowry started increasing.

Max Radin has defined dowry as the property, which a man receives from his wife or her family at the time of his marriage. Dowry may be broadly defined as gifts and valuables received in marriage by the bride, the bridegroom, and his relatives.

The dowry is becoming an increasingly onerous burden for the bride's family. Antidowry laws exist but are largely ignored, and a bride's treatment in her marital home is often affected by the value of her dowry. Increasingly frequent are horrible incidents, particularly in urban areas, where a groom's family makes excessive demands from the bride's family even after marriage and when the demands are not met, the bride is harassed, sometimes leading to mortality.

Causes of Dowry

- Greed factor
- Urge to show off
- Social status
- Lack of education
- Weak implementation of anti dowry laws
- Religious constraints
- Illiteracy
- Propulsion towards adhering to customs.

Dowry Prohibition Act, 1961

Attempts have been made to eradicate the evil of dowry system. **Mahatma Gandhi** was much against, and he educated the youth to become self-dependent and take pledge not to have any dowry. Various efforts have also been made by teachers, voluntary workers, and young people themselves. Because of increasing public opinion against dowry system, Dowry Prohibition Act was passed by the central government in 1961. Presents given at the time of marriage are not included in Dowry Prohibition Act. This is a drawback of this Act.

Changes in Family

Family has been undergoing changes under the impact of following factors:
- Industrialisation
- Western education
- Urbanization
- Legislative measures
- Modern education
- Quarrels in family

Family has undergone some radical transformations in recent period. Its structure has been changed, its functions have been altered and its natures have been affected. Various factors like social, economic, education, legal, cultural, scientific, technological development, etc. are responsible for all these changes in the modern society.

- **Decreased control of the marriage contract**: Marriage is the basis of family. In traditional family the marriage was settled by the parents. The marriage ceremony was based on the principle of male dominance and female obedience. In modern families, it is very difficult to see this type of parental control regarding marital affairs. The marriage is now settled by the partners themselves. It is the choice of mate by mate usually preceded by courtship or falling in love. Today more stress is being laid on romantic love, marriage also has become a civil contract rather than a religious sacrament. It can be dissolved easily at any time as it is settled by mutual consent of the partner. The authority of religion over the conditions of marriage has markedly declined. Divorce, desertion, and separation are frequent occurrence in modern family whereas it was rare phenomenon in traditional family.

- **Changes in relationship of man and woman**: In a modern family, the woman is an equal partner in life with equal rights. When they are not interested in maintaining their marital relationship, they may file for divorce. The morality of the struggle for women's liberation has been aggressively questioned. More freedom and rights are being demanded for the family, society, and the entire nation. The availability of employment has allowed women to support their families financially and has given them the freedom to work in places like offices, factories, banks, and schools. Although her standing has improved due to her economic independence, her attitude towards her family and society has also been impacted.
- **Reduced size of family**: Due to industrialization and urbanization the family size has been reduced and parents no longer desire more children rather develop a tendency to have a smaller family with the help of modern contraceptives.
- **Decline of religious control**: The modern family is secular in attitude. Now-a-days, people prefer to watch mythological TV shows or series rather reading spiritual books like Ramayana, Bhagwat Gita etc.
- **Parent-youth conflict**: Interpersonal conflicts in the family are increasing. The conflicts are growing between the parents and their adolescent children. **Kingsley Davis** says, 'The stress and strain in our culture is symptomatic of the functionless instability of the modern small family.
- **Separation of nonessential functions**: The modern family has given up many functions which were performed by the traditional family. Educational, procreation and care of sick person functions have been shifted to certain external agencies like hospitals, maternity homes, nurseries kindergarten and schools, etc. Movies, clubs, are providing recreation to people. People leave home for commercialized recreation center, which

has affected the cohesion of family. Protective functions of family have also declined. Some families are not providing protection for the physically handicapped, mentally retarded, aged, diseased, infirm, and insane people. Other agencies have taken over this function.

However, in spite of structural and functional changes, the family still plays a significant role in ensuring socialisation of children and providing emotional support to its members. The task of procreation and upbringing of children is done almost satisfactorily by the family only. The psychological satisfaction and social respect earned through marriage and successful life is considered unparallel in terms of equality. Due to this, the family is still a universally indispensable institution.

MARRIAGE

Like family, marriage is another important social institution. Marriage is one of the most ancient, important, and universal social institution which has been in existence since the inception of human civilization. Marriage is a cultural phenomenon which sanctions a more or less permanent union between partners, conferring legitimacy on their offspring. As an institution, marriage is designed to satisfy the biological needs especially the sexual needs of the individual by legal and customary values.

The custom of marriage admits men and women to family life and fixes certain rights and duties in respect of children born of their union. As a stable social institution, it binds two opposite sexes and allows them to live as husband and wife.

But the term 'marriage' or 'Vivah' is a combination of two terms, i.e., 'Vi' and 'Vaha' which means the ceremony of carrying away the bride to the house of bridegroom. In some societies, it is considered as a religious sacrament whereas in other society it is a social contract.

Marriage is deemed essential for virtually everyone in India. For the individual, marriage is the great watershed in life, marking the transition to adulthood. Arranging a marriage is a critical responsibility for parents and other relatives of both bride and groom.

Marriage is an institution which admits men and women to family life. It is a stable relationship in which a man and woman are socially permitted to have children, the right to have children implying the right to sexual relations. The purpose of a marriage institution is:

- ❖ Establishing household
- ❖ Entering to sex relations
- ❖ Procreating
- ❖ Providing care for offspring

Definition

'Marriage is a contract for the production and maintenance of children.'
—**Malinowski**

'Marriage is a stable relationship in which a man and a woman are socially permitted without loss of standing in community to have children.' —**HM Johnson**

'Marriage is a relatively permanent bond between permissible mates.'
—**Lowie**

'Marriage is the approved social pattern whereby two or more persons establish a family.' —**Horton and Hunt**

'Marriage consists of the rules and regulations which define the rights, duties and privileges of husband and wife with respect to each other.'
—**Lundberg**

'Marriage is a socially approved way of establishing a family of procreation.' —**Gillin & Gillin**

Thus, from the above analysis it is concluded that marriage is both a biological, psychological, cultural and social affair. Marriage is a special type of relationship between permissible mates involving certain rights and obligations.

Characteristics of Marriage

- Marriage is a universal social institution. It is found in almost all societies and at all stages of development.
- Marriage is a permanent bond between husband and wife. It is designed to fulfill the social, psychological, biological and religious aims.
- Marriage is a specific relationship between two individuals of opposite sex and based on mutual rights and obligations.
- Marriage requires social approval. The relationship between men and women must have social approval.
- Marriage establishes family. Family helps in providing facilities for the procreation and upbringing of children.
- Marriage creates mutual obligations between husband and wife. The couple fulfill their mutual obligations on the basis of customs or rules of particular society.
- Marriage is always associated with some civil and religious ceremony. This social and religious ceremony provides validity to marriage. Though modern marriage performed in courts still it requires certain religious or customary practices.

- Marriage regulates sex relationship according to prescribed customs and laws.
- Marriage has certain symbols like ring, Mangalsutra, Sindur, special signs to a married woman.

Types of Marriage

Following are the main forms of marriage

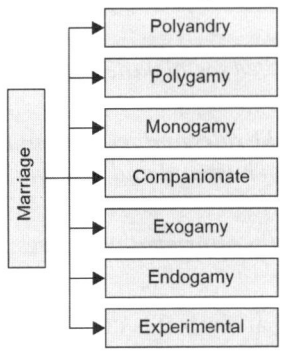

Polyandry

Marriage of women with more than one man is called polyandry. Polyandry in India is of two kinds:

- **Fraternal polyandry**: In this kind of polyandry, women become wife of all brothers if she is married to any one of them. It is more prevalent among class and some other tribes. The children are regarded as the offspring of eldest brother. It is also known as alelphic polyandry. It is prevalent among the Todas.
- **Non fraternal polyandry**: In this type of polyandry, it is not necessary that all the husbands of a women should be brothers. It is found in nayar tribe of India. The woman lives with her different husbands in turns and while she is with one of them, the children thus born is not known. The polyandrous unions of the nayar can hardly be called even from a non-legal point of view, considering that they were loosest and lost fugitive character.

Causes of polyandry

- **Population factor**: Lesser number of female than males in a tribe and the necessity of checking increase in population are some of its main causes of polyandry.
- **Economical factor**: In these tribes where custom of bride price is prevalent, poor condition of people becomes a cause of

polyandry. A single male finds it difficult to pay whole bride price, so more than one man jointly makes this payment.
- **Joint family**: Often for keeping solidarity and unity of a joint family polyandry is adopted. Special fraternal polyandry is due, chiefly to this cause.

Advantages	Disadvantages
• Population control is achieved through polyandry • It strengthens the economic conditions of family • There are less chances of dispute for property does not get divided	• This type of marriage has an impact on health of woman such as infertility, AIDS, pelvic inflammatory disease etc.

Polyandry is generally considered an obstacle in the way of social progress. It causes harm to married life and creates several other psychological problems. It is on this account that polyandry has come to an end in those societies also wherein it once prevailed.

Polygamy

When a man is married to more than one wife at a time, it is called polygamy/polygyny. In India, it is still prevalent among Muslims. It was present among Hindus at the time of rule of kings.

It is of two types namely:
- **Sororal Polygyny**: It is a type in which the wives are invariably the sisters. It is often called 'sororate'. The Latin word 'Soror' stands for the sister. When several sisters are simultaneously or potentially the spouses of the same man, the practice is called the sororate.
- **Non- Sororal Polygyny**: As the term suggests, it is a type of marriage in which the spouses are not related as sisters.

Causes of polygamy

- **Enforced Celibacy**: Men do not approach the women during the period of pregnancy and while the child is being breastfed. Due to this long period of celibacy, a second marriage was contracted.
- **Earlier aging of the female**: In the uncivilized tribesmen remarried a number of times because the women aged earlier.
- **Women as badges of distinction**: Among some tribal's, a man's social status is often measured in the terms of a number of wives. Greater the number, greater the prestige.
- **Taste of variety**: Men go after several women for they have a taste for variety.

- **The constancy of sex urge in men:** Unlike the woman, man is susceptible to sex stimulation throughout the year. Polygyny provides him an opportunity to enjoy sex life throughout the year.

On account of the greater harmful effects of polygyny on family life, polygyny has been declared illegal in civilized societies. The Indian government has declared polygyny an offense under Hindu Marriage Act, 1955.

Monogamy

When a male marries with a single female, the marriage is called monogamous type. Almost all civilized societies regarded this type of marriage as ideal one and is the leading form of marriage. It produces the highest type of affection and sincere devotion.

According to **Malinowski** *'Monogamy is, has been, and will remain the only true type of marriage.'*

Advantages of monogamy

Monogamy seems to be superior to other forms of marriage. It enjoys certain merits over other forms and these merits are now well recognized. Some of them are:

- **Universally Practicable**: Since there is a one-to-one ratio in almost all the societies, only monogamy can provide marital opportunity and satisfaction to all the individuals. No other forms can equally satisfy all.
- **Promotes better Understanding between Husband and Wife:** Monogamy produces the highest type of love and affection between husband and wife. It contributes to family peace, solidarity, and happiness. Vatsayana, remarked "At best a man can only please one woman physically, mentally, and spiritually. Therefore, the man who enters marriage relations with more than one woman, voluntarily courts unhappiness and misery".
- **Contributes to stable Family**: Monogamous family is more stable and long lasting. It is free from conflicts that are commonly found in polyandrous and polygynous families. **Herbert Spencer** has said that monogamy is more stable, and the consequent family bond is stronger.
- **Aged parents are not neglected:** It is only in monogamy that old parents are protected and looked after properly.
- **Provides better status for Women:** Women are given only a very low position in polygyny. Their rights are never recognized. They

can be divorced at will. But in monogamy, women enjoy better social status. In modern societies, they enjoy almost equal social status with men.

Thus, some cultures value monogamy as an ideal form of family organization. However, many cultures prefer other forms of family organization. Anthropological data suggests many societies prefer polygamous marriage as a cultural ideal. There are multiple forms of non-monogamy that are used to organize families, as well as multiple forms of monogamy such as marriage, cohabitation, and extended families.

Group Marriage

Group marriage is that type of marriage in which whole group of men is married to a whole group of women. Each man of male groups is considered to be the husband to every woman of female group. This type of marriage is found only in polyandrous societies. In brief, group marriage is not a marriage at all but a kind of sexual communism.

Companionate Marriage

It is a type of marriage in which marriage is done on the basis of understanding that marriage can be dissolved by mutual consent as long as there are no children. Its purpose is founded on companionship rather than a marriage's traditional functionalities of raising children, gaining financial support, or having security.

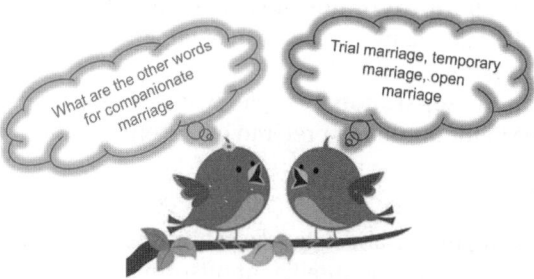

Endogamy

Endogamy is the rule that one must marry within one's own caste, or other group. However, it seldom permits marriage of class kin. Endogamous marriage is that which is controlled within the group. Actually, endogamy and exogamy are relative words. In subcaste exogamy of Hindus the marriage is contracted outside the subcaste but the same marriage would be endogamous from the viewpoint of the race or nations.

Forms of endogamy

In India following forms of endogamy are to be found:
- **Divisional or tribal endogamy:** In which no individual can marry outside his own or tribe or divisions.
- **Caste endogamy:** In which marriage is contracted within the caste.
- **Class endogamy:** In which marriage can take place between people only one class or of a particular status.
- **Subcaste endogamy:** In which choice for marriage is restricted to the subcaste.
- **Race endogamy:** In which one can marry in the race only. People of the veddah race never marry outside the race

Causes of endogamy

The following can be causes of endogamy:
- **Policy of separation:** An important cause of endogamy is the policy of separation meaning thereby the will to live in separation from others.
- **To keep wealth in the group:** When any women of group marries into another, her children also belong to the other group and in this way the numerical force of the first group suffers.
- **Religious differences:** Generally, marriage between people of dissimilar religion is not considered good.
- **Racial or cultural difference:** Racial exogamy does not take place due to racial and cultural difference.
- **Sense of superiority or inferiority:** At the root of caste endogamy and racial endogamy is the sense of superiority or inferiority of one group from another.
- **Geographic separation:** People who are separated by long distance naturally do not prefer to marry one another

Exogamy

Exogamy is progressive and is approved from the biological viewpoint. This leads to healthy and intelligent offspring. But this fact applies only to marriages outside the group. This benefit cannot be derived by forbidding sagotra, an sapravara marriages. In higher hindu castes, some relatives are neglected by disallowing marriage in 7 generations on the paternal side and 5 on the maternal side.

Forms of exogamy

In India the following forms of exogamy are to be found
- **Marriage outside the gotra:** Among the Brahmins the prevailing practice is to marry outside the gotra. People who marry within

the gotra has to repent and treat the woman like a sister or mother. This restriction has been imposed since people of same gotra are believed to have similar blood relation.

- **Marriage outside the pravara**: Besides forbidding marriage within the gotra the Brahmins also forbid marriage between persons belonging to the same pravara.
- **Marriage outside gotras among the kshatriya and vaishyas**: Among Kshatriyas and Vaishyas it is the gotra of the 'purohit' which is taken into consideration. In these the ancestry is carried on not through to saint but some follower. In the Rajput the gotras start from the victors or the first name of the ancestry. Sometimes gotras take the name of the village where the first person lived. In this way thousands of gotras have come into being.
- **Marriage outside the totem**: Totem is the name given to any specific vegetation or animal with which a tribe believed it has some specific relation. In most tribes of India it is customary to marry outside the totem. Among the same totem the marriage is forbidden.
  - **Pravaras**: The pravaras are also in the name of ancient saints. The gotras of Brahmins are pravaras.

According to **PV Kane**—'Gotras' are the names of those ancient saints who have been traditionally believed to be ancestors of an individual, but 'Pravaras' are those very old saint who were very learned and great and were the ancestors of even those who introduced gotras.

The word 'Pravara' comes from the root meaning 'selection'. Pravara is name of those selected saints which were uttered of his own volition by a religious sacrifice. Later on, the number of saints of pravaras was counted and determined. The number is believed to be 'forty-nine'. The saints so chosen of one's own free will were called 'pravars'. It is evident from the opinion that the words gotras or pravaras are not indicative of any blood relationships. Pravaras and gotras are confined only to Brahmins. The gotras and pravaras of Kshatriyas are accepted to be as that of their priests. The history of gotras and pravaras is so ancient that it seems meaningless to forbid marriage on the basis of gotra and pravara when there have been hundred of generations in the interval.

Inter-caste Marriage

Inter-caste marriage means the union of a man and women belonging to two different castes. According to sociologist, inter-caste marriage existed in ancient India. The strict laws of endogamy came into force only when the varna system transformed into the caste system. This led to difficulties in finding a bridegroom as a consequence of which such malpractices as dowry, unsuitable marriages, etc. came into existence. The sole means of putting an end to such malpractices is the encouragement of inter-caste marriage. Two forms of inter-caste marriage have been accepted 'anuloma and pratiloma marriage'.

Anuloma and Pratiloma Marriages

In the Anuloma marriage system, men of higher castes wed women of lower castes. Pratiloma marriages is also form of inter-caste marriage in which men of lower caste marry women of superior castes. The rejection and prevention of inter-caste marriages is based upon the notions of purity and cultural differences between various castes. But as a result of the influence of Western culture, the cultural differences between various castes in India are generally being eliminated.

Widow Remarriage

The second problem concerning Hindu marriage is widow remarriage. It is one of the main restrictions of Hindu marriage that a woman cannot remarry after her husband's death. The following are the main reasons which prohibited widow marriages:

- **Ideas of Kanyadan**: According to this concept, the girl is donated to a suitable candidate. One who acts kanyadan cultivate punya for his next birth.
- **Idea of sacredness**: According to Hindu religious texts 'A woman can retain faithfulness to her husband in all aspects namely by her mind, body and intellect.' Therefore, a Hindu widow cannot render her body to another man.
- **Emphasis on racial purity**: After the Mohammedan settlements in India, Hindus recognized the necessity of maintain the racial purity. This feeling strengthened the restrictions upon women.
- **Concept of eternal relationships**: A Hindu marriage is not only a social contract, but it also recognizes that marriage relations are eternal. Therefore, almost all Hindu widows never accept to remarry.
- **Economic dependency**: One of the most important factors is the hindrance of widow marriage lies in economic dependency of women. Their economic dependency is the main factor which discourages them for taking a step towards this direction.

Reformation Movements

In late, social reforms and various organizations have striven to remove the ban on remarriage of widows. Arya Samaj has a great contribution in this direction. This Organization among their other activities have started a widow remarriage society. Though there is strong opposition from the higher caste Hindus but the social attitudes are changed.

Hindu Widow Remarriage Act, 1856

- The introduction of widow remarriage act was a major change in the state of women that prevailed during that period. **Ishwar Chandra Vidyasagar** played a major role in the establishment of the act. Before this act, the sati custom was also abolished by **Lord William Bentick**.
- According to the prevalent customs in some parts of India, widows, especially upper caste Hindu widows were expected to a lead a life of austerity and extremities. They were boycotted from festivals and even shunned by family members and society.
- Ishwar chandra cited Hindu scriptures to show that widow remarriage was well within the folds of Hinduism. Through his efforts, Lord Cannings enacted the Widow Remarriage Act throughout British India.
- As per the law, 'No marriage contracted between Hindus shall be invalid, and the issue of no such marriage shall be illegitimate, by reason of woman have been previously married or betrothed to another person who was dead at the time of such marriage, any custom and any interpretation of Hindu Law to the contrary notwithstanding.'

LEGISLATIONS ON INDIAN MARRIAGE

Hindu Marriage

The institution of Hindu marriage occupies a prominent place in the social institutions of the civilized world. A Hindu marriage can be defined as a religious sacrament in which a man and woman are bound in a permanent relationship for physical, social and spiritual purposes of dharma, procreation and sexual pleasure. Thus, Hindu marriage is not merely a social contract but a religious sacrament.

It results in a more or less permanent relationship between a man and a woman. Its aim is not merely physical pleasure but spiritual advancement. It is not merely an individual function but has social importance. Its ideals are the fulfillment of Dharma, procreation, and enjoyment of sexual pleasure. It exhibits an integral approach to this social institution.

Aims of the Hindu Marriage

- **Fulfilment of Dharma or religious duties**: According to the Hindu scripture's marriage is the basis of all religious activities. In the words of **K.M. Kapadia** "marriage being thus primarily for the fulfilment of duties, the basic aim of marriage was Dharma." According to Mahabharata, "wife is very source of the Purusharthas , not only of Dharma, Artha and Kama but even of Moksha. Those that have wives can fulfil their due obligations in this world; those that have wives can be happy, and those that have wives can lead a full life."
- **Procreation**: In the Hindu family, the child is given a very important place. According to Rigveda, the husband accepts the palm of the wife in order to get a high breed progeny. According to Manu, the chief aim of marriage is procreation.
- **Sexual Pleasure**: According to Manu, marriage is an asocial institution for the regulation of proper relation between the sexes. The Hindu scriptures have compared the sexual pleasure with the realization of divine bliss. According to Vatsyayan sexual pleasure is the chief aim of the marriage. A maiden who has attained youth should herself get married without waiting for the assistance of elders.

Forms of Hindu Marriage

The Hindu scriptures admit the following eight forms of marriage:
- **Brahma marriage**: In this form of marriage the girl, decorated with clothes and ornaments, is given in marriage to a learned and gentle bridegroom. This is the prevalent form of marriage in Hindu society today.
- **Prajapatya marriage:** In this form of marriage the daughter is offered to the bridegroom by blessing them with the enjoyment of marital bliss and the fulfilment of dharma.
- **Aarsh marriage:** In this form of marriage a rishi used to accept a girl in marriage after giving a cow or bull and some clothes to the parents of the girl. These articles were not the price of the bride but indicated the resolve of the rishi to lead a house-hold life. According to **P.K. Acharya** the word aarsh has been derived from the word rishi.

- **Daiva Marriage:** In this form of marriage the girl, decorated with ornaments and clothes, was offered to the person who conducted the function of a Purohit in yajna.
- **Asura marriage:** In this form of marriage the bride-groom gets the bride in exchange of some money or articles given to the family members of the bride. Such form of marriage was conducted in the case of marriage of Pandu with Madri.
- **Gandharva marriage:** This form is marriage is the result of mutual affection and love of the bride and the bride-groom. An example of this type of marriage is the marriage of the King Dushyanata with Shakuntala. In this form of marriage the ceremonies can be performed after sexual relationship between the bride and the bride-groom. In Taittariya Samhita it has been pointed out that this type of marriage has been so named because of its prevalence among the Gandharvas.
- **Rakshas marriage:** This type of marriage was prevalent in the age when women were considered to be the prize of the war. In this type of marriage, the bride-groom takes away the bride from her house forcibly after killing and injuring her relatives.
- **Paisach marriage:** This type of marriage has been called to be most degenerate. In this type a man enters into sexual relationship with a sleeping, drunk or unconscious woman. Such acts were regularised after the performance of marriage ceremony which took place after physical relationship between the man and woman.

Hindu Marriage Act of 1955

The Hindu Marriage Act of 1955 has not regulated the marriage among Hindus. Section of the Act lays down: A marriage may be solemnized between any two Hindus if the following conditions are fulfilled, namely:
- Neither party has a spouse living at the time of marriage.
- Neither party is an idiot or a lunatic at the time of marriage.
- The bridegroom has completed the age of eighteen years and the bride the age of fifteen years at the time of the marriage. It has now been raised to 21 and 18 respectively.
- The parties are not within the degrees of prohibited relationship, unless the custom or usage governing each of the permits of a marriage between the two.
- The parties are not sapindas of each other unless the customer or usage governing each of them permits of a marriage between the two.

❖ Where the bride has not completed the age of 18 years, the consent of her guardian in marriage, if any, has been obtained for the marriage.

Hindu Marriage Based on Exogamy

Under the usage and custom of Hindu law no two persons tracing their common ascendancy through their father within seven degrees of ascendancy can at all marry among themselves, while on the mother's side the restrictions extend up to the fifth degree. Under the Hindu Marriage Act, the degrees have been reduced to five on the father's side and three on the mother's side. The Hindus are the only civilized people whose marriage laws are based on the principle of exogamy. From the highest Brahmins to the rudest tribes of the Nilgiri Hills and Assam, the system of exogamy is prevalent. Among the Brahmins and Viashyas the name of the exogamous unit is known as 'gotra'. Males and females having the same gotra shall not marry.

Marriage Rites: 'Saptapadi'

'Saptapadi which meant taking seven steps by the bride and bridegroom jointly round the consecrated fire. When the seventh step has been taken the marriage becomes under laws complete and binding. Before the seventh step is taken marriage is incomplete and may be revoked. Thus, the performance of 'saptapadi' is an essential condition of Hindu marriage.

Muslim Marriage

In the Muslim community marriage is universal for it discourages celibacy. Muslims call their marriage Nikah. Marriage is regarded not as a religious sacrament but as secular bond. The bridegroom makes a proposal to the bride just before the wedding ceremony in the presence of two witnesses and maulavi or kazi. The proposal is called ijab and its acceptance is called qubul. It is necessary that both the proposal and acceptance must take place at the same meeting to make it a Nikah. It is a matter of tradition among the muslims to have marriage among equals though there is no legal prohibition to contract marriage with a person of low status, such marriages are looked down upon. The run-away marriages are called kifa when the girls run away with boys and marry them on their own choice are not recognized. Marrying idolaters and slaves is also not approved. There is also provision of preferential system in mate selection. The parallel cousins and cross cousins are allowed to get married.

Marriage that is held contrary to the Islamic rules are called Batil or invalid marriage. Muta is a special type of marriage for pleasure which is for a specific period only. Iddat is the period of seclusion for three menstrual periods for a woman after the death/divorce by her husband to ascertain whether she is pregnant or not. Only after this period she can remarry.

Muslim marriage can be dissolved in the following ways: Divorce as per muslim law but without the intervention of the court. They are of two types: Kula where divorce is initiated at the instance of the wife and Mubarat where initiative may come either from the wife or from the husband. Talaq represents one of the ways according to which a muslim husband can give divorce to his wife as the Muslim law by repeating the dismissal formula thrice. Talaq may be affected either orally by making some pronouncements or in writing by presenting talaqnama. Divorce as recognized by Shariah Act 1937 provides for three forms of divorce: Ila, Zihar and Lian. There is also provision of divorce as per the dissolution of Muslim Marriage Act 1939.

Tribal Marriage

- Marriage by exchange.
- Marriage by capture is where a man forcibly marries to a woman.
- Marriage by probation allow a man to stay at woman place for weeks together after which if they decide to get married.
- Marriage by purchase or giving bride price. A man is required to give an agreed amount of cash/kind to the parents of the bride as price which usually varies according to physical beauty and utility of the bride.
- Marriage by service is where the man services at his father-inlaws before marriage.
- Marriage by trial.
- Marriage by elopement

Modern Changes in the Hindu Marriage

Due to the influence of Western culture and English education the Hindu marriage system has undergone considerable changes. Some of the important ones are:

- **Marriage is not held as compulsory**: In the Hindu society formerly, marriage was considered to be absolutely compulsory for both male and female. According to Hindu scriptures, a person who does not beget a son through marriage cannot attain heaven. No man could perform 'yajna' without a wife. Marriage therefore was necessary even for religious purposes. But, due to influence of Western culture many males and females do not consider marriage to be necessary these days. Due to economic difficulties also, some persons do not enter into matrimony. The modern educated Hindu girl is not ready to accept the slavery of male. The educated men and women do not believe in the ancient religious values and therefore do not consider marriage to be necessary. Breaking of the taboos of Sagotra and Sapravar marriage: Ancient Hindu tradition forbids the marriage of persons belonging to same Gotra and Pravar. This very much restricts the field of choice of mate. Therefore, at the present the educated persons are gradually violating the restriction. It has been also rejected by law.

- **Opposition of Child Marriages**: In medieval India the custom of child marriage was very much in vogue. After the passing of Sarada Act child marriages have become illegal. Another factor leading to the restriction of child marriage in Hindu society is the tremendous increase of women education. The boys do not marry early because of late settlement in career.
- **Permission of Inter-caste Marriage**: Formerly, inter-caste marriage was considered to be wrong in the Hindu society. It has now been legally permitted. With the increase of co-education, women education and the democratic ideal of equality and liberty, inter-caste marriages are now considered to be signs of forwardness.
- **Permission of Widow Remarriage**: Due to the untiring efforts of the social reformers and educated persons widow remarriage is no more considered to be wrong in Hindu society. Consequently, its incidence is now on the decrease.
- **Prohibition of Polygamy**: Formerly, a man was allowed to marry several women in order to get a son. With the increase of women education, the ladies are demanding equal rights in marriage. The Hindu Marriage Act of 1955 has declared polygamy to be illegal. No one can marry a second time, while the former spouse is alive.
- **Provision for Divorce**: The Hindu Marriage Act of 1955 has introduced a significant change in the institution of Hindu marriage by permitting divorce under certain specific circumstances.

INFLUENCE OF FAMILY AND MARRIAGE ON HEALTH

- Joint family pays more attention of taking care of geriatric group.
- The members take sick persons adequate care in the joint family.
- Children emotionally, so attached to their relatives in the joint family.
- In the modern family parents are well aware about contraceptives, so they can plan very well about their family.

- The standard of living is high in nuclear family. That's why the members of the nuclear family immediately seek the healthcare.
- Mental illness due to lack of emotional closeness is higher in modern family comparing to joint families.
- There is less chance of developing deficiency diseases in nuclear families because it is less in number, and everyone gives more importance for their food and clothing.
- Marriage among minors may cause physical problems like adolescent pregnancy and may lead them to develop emotional disturbances also.
- Superstitious beliefs and practices are common among joint family system because of the old members.
- Some of the traditional families, still practices child marriages, and taboos regarding death, rituals and fasting are in practice.
- Women develop many health problems in the joint families because of their hard work without taking rest.

Both nuclear and joint families have their own advantages and disadvantages. But the small family norm has more value than large family. It helps the nation controlling the population. Small family is considered as happy family and leads to a prosperous nation.

- Family word is derived from the Roman word famulus which means a servant. According to Elliot and Merrill, Family is a biological social unit composed of husband, wife, and children.
- Mating relationship, rearing, and caring of children, protection, affection and satisfaction of sexual needs are the functions of family
- Family is classified on the basis of marriage, nature of residence, descent, size, and structure.
- Marriage is one of the most ancient, important, and universal social institution which has been in existence since the inception of human civilization. According to HM Johnson, Marriage is a stable relationship in which a man and a woman are socially permitted without loss of standing in community to have children.
- There are many forms of marriage like polyandry, polygamy, monogamy, companionate, exogamy, endogamy etc.
- Family and marriage play an important role in health and disease- care during pregnancy, postnatal period, care of new-born, diseased, aged and socialisation.

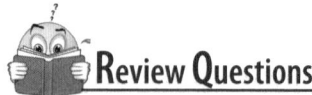

Review Questions

Short Answer Questions

1. Define family.
2. Define marriage.
3. Write down the functions of family.
4. Discuss the types of family.
5. What are the types of marriage?

Long Answer Questions

1. Define marriage. Write down the various types of marriage.
2. Define family. Write down the types of families.
3. Explain the characteristics of different types of family.

5 UNIT

Social Stratification

Chapter Outline

- Introduction – Characteristics & forms of stratification
- Function of stratification
- Indian caste system – origin and characteristics
- Positive and negative impact of caste in society.
- Class system and status
- Social mobility-meaning and types
- Race – concept, criteria of racial classification
- Influence of class, caste, and race system on health.

Learning Objectives

After reading this chapter, students will be able to:
- Define social stratification
- Explain the forms of stratification
- Enlist the functions of stratification
- What is the positive and negative impact of caste in society
- Discuss the concept of class system and status
- Elaborate the concept of race and the criteria of racial classification
- How class, caste, and race system influence health

Unit 5: Social Stratification

> **Key Terms**
> - **Social stratification:** Process of forming social classes
> - **Caste system:** A system in which people are born into a social standing that they will retain their entire lives
> - **Class:** A group who shares a common social status based on factors like wealth, income, education, and occupation
> - **Class system:** Social standing based on social factors and individual accomplishments

MEANING AND TYPES OF SOCIAL STRATIFICATION

Social stratification is in fact a social process in which the society is divided into various groups or classes. These groups have their own characteristics, status, roles, etc. Their relationship with one another is also determined on the basis of this stratification which confused to undergo change. As a result of this change the status and roles of various classes and strata also change. This change brings about certain changes in the social setup.

Indian caste system is typical example of social stratification. There is a hierarchical arrangement between different strata in which society is divided. Sometimes this stratification is known as caste system and sometimes as a class system. This stratification carriers with it contain privileges and also disabilities.

Every class or stratum has a place in the society which enjoys on its certain privileges and obligations. It may be called a division of society in groups, classes or categories that are linked with each other by relations of superiority than inferiority.

Different social thinkers and sociologist have defined it in different ways.

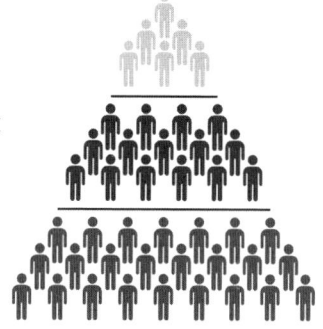

Definition of Social Stratification

Various social thinkers and sociologists have defined social stratification in different ways. 'Social stratification is the division of society in permanent group or categories linked with each other by relationships of superiority and subordination.'

'Stratification' is a horizontal division of society higher and lower social units.

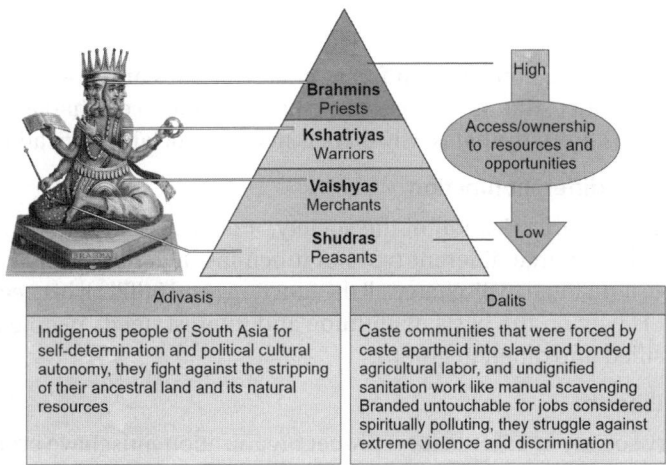

Hierarchical order or difference between high and low: In the process of social stratification there are difference on the basis of superiority and inferiority because members of a particular group belongs to higher class, they enjoy certain privileges and facilities. These facilities and privileges are not available to the members of the lower class.

Factors of Social Stratification

Certain factors are responsible for stratification. These factors are:
1. Difference in human being
2. Need for different functions
3. Equilibrium

Differences in Human Being

Man differs from one another not on account of biological characteristics but also on account of social, cultural, economic, psychological and other characteristics.

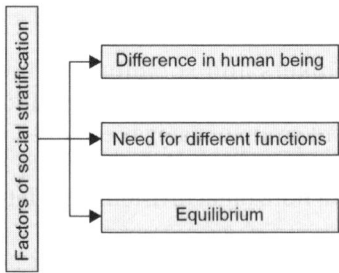

If all the persons have different characteristics and are pleased in one group, stratum or class, they shall not able to discharge their functions properly that is why there is need for social stratification.

Need for different function

For proper organization of the society, it is necessary that people should discharge different types of functions. It is not possible for single individual to discharge all the functions and fulfill all his needs. That is why on the basis of aptitude and interest needs people are classified into different groups.

Equilibrium

Every society in order to have proper organization must have proper social equilibrium. It means one proper group should not dominate over theirs. This cannot take place if the society is divided into various groups and people have different functions to discharge. Because of these functions they shall be mutually dependent and this mutual dependence shall be responsible for maintaining the social equilibrium.

Main Basis of Social Stratification

Biological Basis of Social Stratification

In an ordinary setup, the society is divided into different groups or states on the basis of biological characteristics.

It is an account of the biological basis that Whites consider themselves to be superior group than colored people and Aryans consider themselves to be superior from others particularly Dravidians.

Biological basis comprise of the following characteristics and social stratification may be based on them.

Stratification of the society on the basis of sex

This is an age old and quite simple classification. There are two types of social order, matriarchal or patriarchal.

In the matriarchal society, it is the women that is considered superior and has control over political and social institutions. But in patriarchal society, man is considered powerful. On the basis of superiority of man or woman the society is divided into various groups.

Stratification of the society on the basis of age

In Indian society elders are respected by younger people and people who have grown quite old are given all sorts of respect. Here the whole social system is under the control of elders and in Australia the role of elders is superior which is known as Gerontocracy. From the point of view of age, a society may be divided into four classes: Children, adolescent, youth, elderly. Classification on the basis of the age old practice.

Stratification of the society on the basis of birth

Here, by birth a person is considered superior or inferior. A person born in Brahmin family is considered superior or and a person born in family of Sudras is considered inferior. Caste system is nothing but a classification or stratification on the basis of birth or heredity.

Social stratification on the basis of race

Some people have tried to classify the society into different stratas on the basis of their racial characteristics.

People belonging to a particular race and possessing a particular characteristics are considered superior to others. In America whites are considered superior to colored. People that is why there are separate hostels, places of recreation, congregation, etc. for the colored people. Hitler considered the Aryan race to which he belongs superior to other races.

Sociocultural Basis of Social Stratification

Stratification of society is also based on social and cultural factors. This type of stratification is seen in various types of societies.

Important basis of this type of stratification as follows:

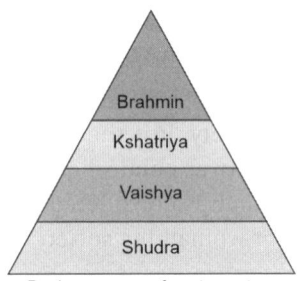

Basic structure of caste system

Economic basis of social stratification

Society is divided into various classes on the basis of their economic conditions or equipment. Those who possess a good deal of wealth are known as rich people. Those who do not have anything and earn their livelihood by selling their labor known as poor people and the class, which is in between the two and is known as middle class.

Concept of rich as well as poor class changes according to the change of value of the society. Those who possess land and cattle are considered rich. While ordinary farmers who live at the mercy of feudals or landlords are considered poor.

According to **Karl Marx** there is a class of capitalist or Bourgeoisie which controls the means of production. Then there is a class called petty bourgeoisie or middle class. The other class is the class of proletariat who sell their labor and earn their livelihood. They have no private property worth the name.

Religious basis of social stratification

In certain societies, social stratification is made on the basis of religion. In such stratification, certain persons are considered at the top of the society, because the religion has given them certain privileges for example amongst Roman catholic the pope is at the top and according to the religious order below may be the people belonging to different classes of groups.

In Hindu society also because of religious factor, Brahmins are considered to be superior most.

Political basis of social stratification

People are also classified into various groups or stratas on the basis of their political position or the political power that they enjoy.

For example, in a democratic setup elected representatives are considered superior to their people, bureaucratic setup it is the bureaucrats who occupy higher status.

In a political party, certain people are considered superior while others are considered inferior to them. In fact the basis of this type of sociocultural stratification is the political power or the political consideration.

Forms of Social Stratification

Stratification is generally two types or forms. First stratification is based on external factors or the factors over such people who do not have a control and the other is the stratification that is based on birth, race and religion, etc.

Normally this type of classification is based on birth or traditions this is known as caste and the second type of classification which known as class stratification which is based on occupation, in some and other personal or individual equipment or attainments.

Stratification of the former type or caste stratification are generally found in a traditional or primitive society.

Generally, the following forms of social stratification are three section in different types of societies:

Caste Stratification

In this type of stratification the hierarchical order of different classes is determined on the basis of birth. Apart from it, the membership of groups are also determined on the basis of birth.

Normally in Hindu society there are four classes *viz* Brahmin, Kshatriya, Vaishya, and Sudras. These castes have further been divided into subcastes.

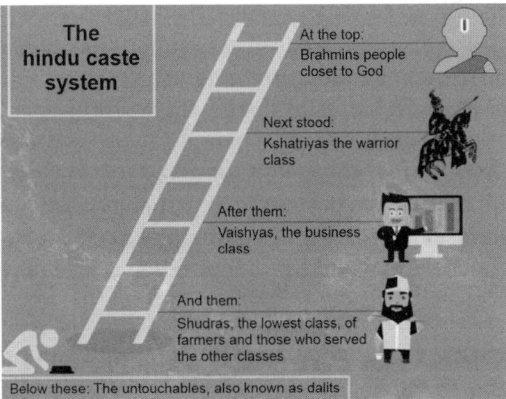

In South Asian Muslim society a distinction is made between the ashraf, who are supposedly descendants of Muslim Arab immigrants, and the non-ashraf, who are Hindu converts.

The ashraf group is further divided into four subgroups:
1. Sayyids, originally a designation of descendants of Muhammad through his daughter Fatimah and son-in-law Ali,
2. Shaykhs (Arabic: "Chiefs"), mainly descendants of Arab or Persian immigrants but also including some converted Rajputs
3. Pashtuns, members of Pashto-speaking tribes in Afghanistan and northwestern Pakistan
4. Mughals, persons of Turkish origin, who came into India with the Mughal armies.

The non-ashraf Muslim castes are of three levels of status: at the top, converts from high Hindu castes, mainly Rajputs, insofar as they have not been absorbed into the Shaykh castes; next, the artisan caste groups, such as the Julahas, originally weavers; and lowest, the converted untouchables, who have retained their previous occupations.

In such type of stratification, it has not been possible for a person to leave the membership of one group or join others. Here the membership is predetermined.

Racial Stratification

This is another form of social stratification for which hierarchical order or the superiority of one class is relevance to the other is determined on the basis of the membership of a particular race.

In such type of stratification, it is not possible for people to leave one race and join other.

Class Stratification

This type of stratification is based on economic consideration and other personal and individual attainments.

In such a society, it is possible for the members of a particular class to move into another class, as also people are considered superior or inferior to one another.

As a result of this type of stratification, people also have different roles and statuses. It mean the members of a particular class have status attached to them and they have to play a role in relevance to the society.

THE INDIAN CASTE SYSTEM: ORIGIN AND FEATURES

The Meaning of Caste: Origin of the Word

The word 'Caste' owes its origin to the Portuguese word casta which means breed, race, strain or a complex of hereditary qualities. The

Portuguese applied this term to the classes of people in India known by name of *jati*.

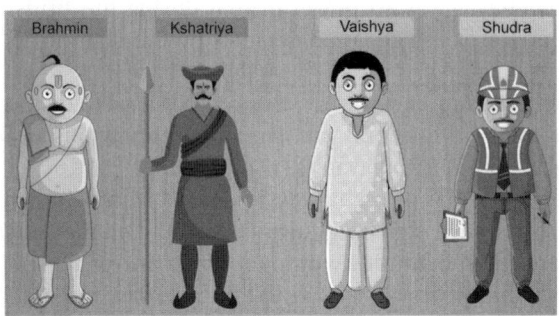

The English word 'Caste' is an adjustment of the original term. **CH Cooley** says 'when a class is somewhat strictly hereditary, we may call it a caste.'

According to **Green**, *'Caste is a system of stratification in which mobility, up and down the status ladder, at least ideally does not occur.'*

According to **Megasthenes**, two elements of caste system are (i) there is no intermarriage and (ii) there can be no change of possession.

Ketkar says *'Caste is a group having two characteristics, membership is considered to those who are born of members and forbidden by an inexorable social law to marry outside the group.'*

According to **Dharmashastra** *'Caste means social exclusiveness with reference to diet and marriage, birth and ritual are necessary.'*

The meaning of caste is better understood by analyzing its origin and special features, that by its definition.

Segmental division of society:
- The society is divided into various castes with a well-developed life of their own, the membership of which is determined by its consideration of birth.
- The status of a person does not depend on his wealth but on the traditional importance of the caste in which he had the fortune of being born.
- Caste is hereditary, no amount of wealth and no amount of penance or prayers can change his caste status.
- Status is determined not by vocation but by birth
- The governing body of a caste is called panchayat which literally means body of five members, but in fact there are many more who meet whenever decisions are taken. It takes cognizance of the offences against the caste labor which prevents members of the caste from eating and drinking or smoking with members of other castes.

- Against sex regulation which prohibits marriage outside the caste. It decides civil and criminal matters.
- The panchayat was so powerful that during the British regime it retired cases which once decided by the state in its judicial capacity.
- Its chief punishments were (i) the sin's (ii) feast to be given to the caste's men (ii) corporal punishment (iv) religious explanation like taking bath in holy waters (v) outcasting.

In short 'caste has its own rules.' It is small complete social world itself and quasi sovereign body, all inclusive and marked off from one another and yet substituting within the larger and wider society.' The citizen own their moral allegiance to this caste first, rather than to the community as whole.

Origin and Development of Caste System

Caste system is supposed to be sophisticated form or varna dharma. In **Rigveda**, there is reference to three main classes—Brahman, Kshatriya and Vaishya, Sudra is considered to be dasa, a class recognized in later period.

According to **GS Ghurye**, *'caste in India must be regarded as a brahminic child of the Indo-Aryan culture, cradled in the land of Ganges and then transferred to other parts of India by the Brahmin and prospects.'*

Rigveda mentions that *'Brahmin is created from the mouth of Purusha, Kshatriya from his arm and Vaishya from his thighs.'*

It stresses the difference between arya and dasa not only in color but also in speech, physical features and religious practice.

The Dasa are mixed born out of intercaste marriage of other three classes and considered as sudras or nishadas.

The classes mentioned in Rigveda are based on division of labor *viz*, occupations adopted by the groups, but they were not stratified or rigid. They were of an open system of changing from group to group.

During the **post vedic period** and **medieval periods**, caste system developed into a rigid and stratified institution based on birth, imposing several restrictions on the relations between them.

During the **modern period**, several changes have taken place in the structure and function of caste.

An exact origin of caste cannot be easily traced as it is a complex phenomenon prevailing since many ages. Several thinkers have attempted to explain its origin by formulating certain theories of caste system. The most important of these theories are traditional theory, occupational theory, religious theory, political theory, racial theory and evolutionary theory.

Features of caste in India Changing Trends in Caste System

Caste in India is supposed to be a rigid institution with many stratified groups in the form of sects and sub-castes.

The emergence of a large number of jaties or sub-sects is due to violations of caste regulations in the original four fold system.

Caste rigidity is more stringent among sects and sub-sects than among four groups. Many sub-sects have given up traditional occupations and also citied from caste obligations.

During the pre-independence period British administration had tremendous influence on the institution of caste. British rulers introduced several laws in order to bring about fundamental changes in traditional caste system.

They applied equity in matters of administration and introduced certain legal norms to abolish the caste hierarchy. The lower caste groups became conscious of their legal rights and fought against higher groups to avoid exploitation.

But the higher caste groups by their superior knowledge and economic resources thwarted their attempts.

Western types of education in schools and colleges was liberal and secular to alter the traditional religious education of caste groups.

Increasing opportunities of employment for both men and women and public offices and industries broke the barriers of caste.

Occupation became pursuits of individuals choice instead of being hereditary and traditional. Impact of new occupational patterns on caste created cultural diffusion and economic classes.

Industrialization during the 19th century provided new uniform work styles and division of labor and several unions were started during 20th century.

Migration of rural people from rural to industrial cities caused break of traditional caste ideas.

Ascribed status of caste occupations changed to achieve status by performance of work. Family and kinship groups which were once units of production affected by new industrial system.

Industrialization caused by urbanization in which people of all caste groups mingled with new ideas of commercialism, economic enterprise, leisure and entertainment.

Along with sanskritization, westernization has to a great extent affected the traditional caste system. There are various changes at different levels, the new technology, institute ideology, and values, rationalism, individualism, nationalism, humanitarianism and secularism are the new concept of westernization which lead to a series of changes in institutions and outlook of the people. It led to various reforms cutting across the barriers of traditional caste system.

Changes in Caste System During Postindependent Period

Indian constitution inaugurated on 26th January 1950 proclaimed India as sovereign democratic republic with main aim of creating a casteless and classless society.

Hindu caste system based on inequalities of birth and social status was condemned by the fundamental rights incorporated in Indian constitution. India as sovereign democratic republic establishes equality to all citizens irrespective of caste, creed or religion.

There has been a tendency towards formation of caste association particularly among lower caste groups.

Casteism has developed in much narrower sense by group loyalty converted into politics.

Institution of caste has secured new fields of activity in politics. Elections in many administrative bodies clearly reveal the caste element is a decisive factor.

At present caste is a political structure with a series of changes from its traditional imperatives.

SOCIAL CLASS SYSTEM AND STATUS

The social classes are the fact groups not legally or religiously defined and sanctioned. They are relatively open not closed. Their basis is indisputably economic but they are more than economic groups. They are characteristics groups of the industrial societies which have developed since 17th century. The relative importance and definition of membership in a particular class differs greatly over time and between societies, particularly in societies that have a legal differentiation of groups of people by birth or occupation.

In the well-known example of socioeconomic class, many scholars view societies as satisfying into a hierarchical system based on occupation, economic status, wealth or income.

According to **Ogburn** and **Nimkoff** a social class in the aggregate of persons having essentially the same social status in given soeity.

Marx defined class in terms of the extent to which an individual or social group has control over the means of production.

Class are seen to have their origin in the division of social product into a necessary product and surplus product.

Marxists so plan history in terms of a war of classes between those who control production and those who actively produce the goods or services in society and also developments in technology and the like.

In the Marxist view of capitalism, this is a conflict between capitalists (bourgeoisie) and wage workers (proletariat).

Class in Marxism are not static entities but are regenerated daily through the productive process.

MacIver and **Page** defines social class as any portion of the community marked off from the rest by social status.

Max Weber suggests that social classes are aggregates of individuals who have the same opportunities of acquiring goods the same exhibited standard of living.

He formulated three component theory of stratification with social status and party classes (or politics) as conceptually distinct elements.

Social class is based on economic relationship to the marked (owner, renter, employer, etc.).

Status has to do with non-economic qualities such as education honor and prestige.

Party class refers to factors having to do with affiliations in the political domain.

Difference between Class and Caste

Caste	Class
According to Max Weber, castes are perceived as hereditary groups with a fixed ritual status	A Class is based on social status, wealth and power acquired, level of education and other achievements.
A person belonging to certain caste has to follow certain traditions, rituals and customs	A person belonging to a certain class is not bound by customs, rituals, or traditions.
According to Louis Dumont & Edmund Leach, caste is unique to the Indian sub-continent	Classes are usually found in highly industrialized countries located in Europe, North America.

Contd...

Contd...

Caste	Class
The caste system does not promote democracy, since it severely limits equal opportunity to rise from an individual's station	Class system does not necessarily act as a barrier to democracy, since classification is based on education, social status, and the work one does.
Caste System is static	Class system is dynamic
Caste system works as a political force.	Class system does not act as a political force.

STATUS

Status is a term used to designate the comparative amount of prestige deference or respect accorded to persons who have been assigned different roles in group or community.

The status of a person is high, the role he is playing is considered important by the group. If the role is regarded less high, its performer may be accorded a lower status. Thus the status of a person is based on social evaluation.

Status is a position in the general institutional system, recognized and supported by the entire society spontaneously evolved rather than deliberately created in the folkways and mores.

Status means the location of the individuals within the group, his place in the social network.

Ascription and Achievement of Status

Ascribed Status

The status, which a child receives at the time he is ushered into the process of socialization is his ascribed status.

The status is ascribed to him at a time when society knows least about the potentialities of the child. Therefore, the society ascribes to him a status on the basis of its own rules, generally at this time. The society considers the following factors.

Sex

All societies prescribe different attitudes and roles to men and women. The genetic difference between men and women are not great enough to explain the social difference between them. The social difference themselves are not fixed but change from one society to another and from one time to another.

Though in our society the status assigned to women have changed greatly yet, it is doubtful if the ascription of status according to sex will ever disappear from society.

Age

Age is an important factors used by all the society for role assignments. Generally a society recognizes at least five age periods infancy, childhood, adolescence, adulthood and old age. Sometimes in addition they have two more peculiar period to which they attach importance, namely the unborn and the dead.

The society ascribes status to a child on the basis of his relations to his parent and siblings. His status is identified with that of his parents.

The ascriptions of citizenship, religious affiliation and community membership is in most cases a matter of identifications with parent social factor, sex, age and kinship do not exhaust all the bases for the ascription of status.

All societies classify their member into a number of group or categories and ascribe to such categories differ in degrees of status. These groups may originate in many different ways. They may arise out of difference in technical skill or other abilities. They may also originate through the formation of some social units such as ' teachers, fraternity or officers, club.

In India, both the family and caste has ascription characteristics play a crucial role in the placement of person.

Achieved Status

Achieved status previous for an orderly and legitimate change of status according to the individual's manifestation of talent and effort. If the society does not do so and allow its members to change.

In order to make use of their capacities for common social ends the society must institutionalize the achievement of status.

Social Needs of Status System

The social status is of great importance both for individual and the society. An individual wins respect in society by virtue of his status. Entitled him to more respect than before.

Role and status go together. The role of an individual determines his status and his role changes along with its status structure. Status entitles a person to enjoy prerogatives. Thus an individual's gets many direct and indirect advantages from social status.

SOCIAL MOBILITY: MEANING AND TYPES

Meaning of Social Mobility

Individiuals are recognized in society through the statuses they occupy and roles they enact. The society as well as individuals is dynamic. Men are normally engaged in endless endeavor to enhance their statuses in society, move from lower position to higher position, secure superior job from an inferior one. For various reasons people of the higher status and position may be forced to come down to a lower status and position. Thus people in society continue to move up and down in the status scale. This movement is called social mobility.

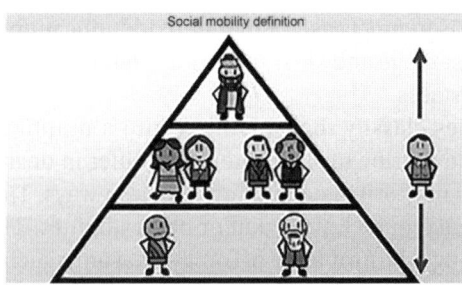

The study of social mobility is an important aspect of social stratification. In fact, it is an inseparable aspect of social stratification system because the nature, form, range and degree of social mobility depends on the very nature of stratifications system.

Stratification system refers to the process of placing individuals in different layers or strata.

According to Wallace and Wallace social mobility is the movement of a person or persons or group from one social class or social stratum to another.

Types of Social Mobility

Horizontal and Vertical Social Mobility

A distinction is made between horizontal and vertical socials mobility.

Horizontal social mobility refers to change of occupational position or role. If an individuals or group without involving any change in its position in the social hierarchy.

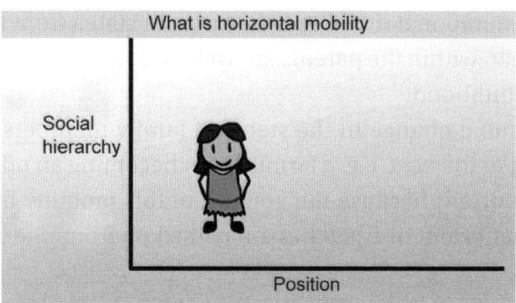

Vertical social mobility refers essentially to changes in the position of an individuals or a group along the social hierarchy.

When a rural laborer come to the city and becomes an industrial worker or manager takes a position in another company there are no significant changes in their position in the hierarchy. Those are the examples of horizon a mobility. It indicates a change in position within the range of the same status.

Vertical mobility is a movement from one status to its equivalent.

If an industrial worker become a business man or lawyer he has radically changed his position in the stratification system. This is an example of vertical mobility.

Vertical mobility involves change within the lifetime of an individual to a higher or lower status than the person had to begin with.

Forms of Vertical Social Mobility

The vertical mobility can take place in two ways—individuals and groups may improve their position in hierarchy by moving upwards or their position might worsen and they may fall down in the hierarchy.

When individuals get into seats of politicals position, acquire money and expert influence over others because achieved individuals mobility.

Like individuals, even groups also obtain high social mobility, e.g. when a dalit from a village becomes an important official it is a case of upward mobility.

On the other hand an aristocrat or a member of an upper class may be dispossessed of his wealth and he is forced to enter a manual occupation. This is an example of downward mobility.

Inter-Generational Social Mobility

Time factor is an important element in social mobility. On the basis of the time factor involved in social mobility there is another.

Inter-generational mobility is a change in status from that which a child began within the parents, household to that of the child upon reaching adulthood.

It refers to a change in the status of family members from one generation to the next, e.g. a farmer's son becoming an officer.

It is important because the amount of this mobility in a society tells us what extent of equalities are passed on from one generation to the next.

If there is very little inter-generational mobility, inequalities is clearly deeply built into the society for people life chance are being determined at the moment of birth.

When there is mobility people are clearly able to achieve new status through their own efforts regardless of the circumstances of their birth.

Intra-generational Mobility

Mobility taking place in personal terms within the life of the same person is called intra-generational mobility.

It refers to the advancement in one's social level during the course of one's lifetime. It may also be understand as a change in social status which occurs within a person's adult career.

For example, person working as a supervisor in a factory becoming its assistant manager after getting promotion.

Structural Mobility

Structural mobility is a kind of vertical mobility.

Structural mobility refers to mobility which is brought about by changes in stratification hierarchy itself.

It is a vertical movement of a specific group, class or occupation related to others in the stratifications system. It is a type of forced mobility for it takes place because of the structural changes and not because of individuals attempts.

For example, historical circumstance or labor market changes may lead to the rise of decline of an occupational group within the social hierarchy.

An influence of immigrants may also alter class alignments expecially if the new arrivals are disproportionately highly skilled or unskilled.

RACE

Race or group of people that have many characteristic, geographical position on certain other traits.

In fact, it is stratification of or particular social order or social making. In ordinary sense it is used for different things in different fields.

From the point of view of phychology, people having common and similar physical and bodily features are called a race.

From the point of view of linguistics those who use one language are said to belong to one race.

But for scientific study it is necessary to have the correct definition of the term race that would indicate its real concept.

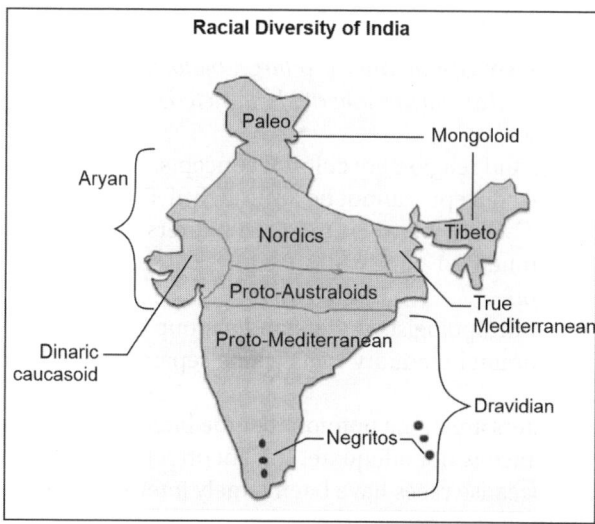

Definition

According to **AW Green**, *'A race is a large biological human group, with a number of descriptive inherited characteristics which vary within a certain range.'*

According to **Biesanz** and **Biesanz,** *'A race is a large group of people distinguished by inherited physical differences.'*

According to **Paul AF Walter**, *'A race is a large division of human beings distinguished from others by relatively obvious physical characteristics, presumed to be biologically inherited and remaining relatively constant through numerous generations.'*

Characteristics of Race

The common characteristics and elements may termed as the element of race. Their characteristics are:
- Race is a large group of common origin.
- Their groups of people possess certain common biological characteristics that they have inherited.
- These inherited characteristics although varying within a certain range, passion from one generation to another.
- These members of a large group have system of in breeding and related amongst themselves.
- They sometimes have common geographical origin.

Race as Biological Concept

According to **AW Green,** *'race is a large, biological human grouping with a number of distinctive inherited characteristics which vary within a certain range.'*

Language and religion are cultural concepts, on their basis race a physiological concepts cannot be accurately defined.

Ethnic difference between men are matters of blood. They are biologically inherited along with such physical characteristics as eye, skin and color.

By race anthropologists understand a group of individuals who possess common hereditary traits which separate them from other groups.

Some writers are of the opinion that the biological interpretation of the term race is not adequate. It is incorrect to attribute race to hereditary because races have been largely intermixed. So the term should be used in its genetic sense.

According to **Penniman**, race is a genetic class in which there are many indefinite and mutually related genetic characteristics by means of which it can be distinguished from other classes and on the basis of which the conditions of continuous separation among the offspring and future generation can be distinguished **Julian Huxley** also does not subscribe to the biological meaning of race. He wanted the term race to be substituated by the word ethnic group.

Race ethnicity is biological category the people of a given race have all certain inherited physical features that distinguished their race from other race.

There is variation within the race and there is overlap in regard to some of the specific features among races.

These unique inherited features have resulted from thousands of years of endogamy so that a racial group has a common and distinguishable ancestry.

Horton and **Hunt** are of the opinion that is wrong to define race only as a biologically distinct group. According to them it is a socially significant concept also.

Accordingly they define race 'as a group of people somewhat different from other groups in a combination of inherited physical characteristics but race is also substantially determined by popular social definition.

Traits for Racial Groups

It is the combination of traits that is used to distinguish racial groups.

A Negro, for instance, has curly hair, dark complexion, a big head with a small nose and thick lips. He differs from a Chinese who has straight hair, flat nose and yellowish complexion.

But as said above, sometimes it becomes difficult to tell whether the difference of traits are hereditary or environmental. Such attributes as stature, weight and color of the skin can be greatly modified by the environment and as such they are little value in distinguishing races, hair form and eye color are considered to be more stable genetic factors. However, there is no one trait which can be regarded as fundamental.

When anthropology was first developing, it was thought that head form was the best criterion of races, since the skull approaches its full growth early in life and was no subject to environmental changes.

But since base discovered that the cephalic index may be materially altered by the environment into which the individual is born, this trait is no longer considered as the principal criterion of race.

Thus, anthropologists have used different basis for their classification of races, now one character or combination of characters is regarded as fundamental and now another, some anthropologists regard color as the proper basis, others prefer hair form, head shape, or some other.

It may also be noted that within same race there may be some variations of physical traits or people of two races may possess a similar physical trait. This much can be concluded that:

- There are in mankind real physiological traits by which individuals differe from each other. Some of these traits are widely predominant in certain groups, especially among primitives.
- These traits are biologically transmitted, these groups of men are known by the name of race or races.

Classification of Races-criteria of Racial Classification

Anthropologists have suggested numerous schemes of classification which differ widely from each other.

Huxley in 1870 giving five principal types, i.e. Negroid, Australoid, Mongoloid, Xanthochroid and Melanochroid, while others use a four fold division into Caucasian, Mongolian, Negroid and Australoid.

The Caucasian is subdivided into Nordic, Alpine and Mediterranean.

Although there is no clear cut lines is separating them, there are being considerable overlapping, each stocks is marked by certain characteristics which are more or less common to all its members each of these three racial division may further be divided into sub- races.

A brief description of the importance of characteristics of the above races is as follows:

- **Caucasoid:** This is known as white race, but in fact it is of light color. It has hair ranging from brown to black, eyes light blue, hair upon chest, arm, legs, medium light structures, thin lip, etc.
  The important subraces of caucasians are:
  - *Nordic:* The important characteristics of this race are high forehead, leptorrhine nose, thin lips, blue eyes, yellow hair, white or red color of the skin with average heights 5.8. They are found in cardinavian Baltic and British Island.
  - *Alpine:* This race is found in Central Asia, its important racial characteristics are broad and small forehead, small eyebrows, medium nasal index, medium cephalic index, medium lips deep gray eyes and light white skin and height 5 feet and 5 inch.
  - *Mediterranean:* These are found in Spain, Portugal, Italy and France. Their racial characteristics are long head, head circumference is less than 75 inch, small eyebrows, medium lips, leptorrhine nose, light gray eyes, curly hair, gray skin and height 5 feet and 4 inch.
- **Mongoloid**: This race is mostly found in Asia particulary in central Asia. Its physical characteristics are gray eyes, yellow complexion, black hair on the body, flat nose, broad face and medium height. This group includes the following races.
  - *Asian Mongols:* These are found in China, Japan, and Northeast india.
  - *Micronesian:* Polynesian. These are found in the Eastern Island of Malansia:
- **Negroid**: These are found in Africa, their important characteristics are black skin, wooly hair, broad nose, thick lips, high head and

average height 5 feet and 6 inch. The important sub-division of this race are negro.
- *Far estern pygmy:* These are found in Andaman and Nicobar, and Philippines.
- **Malenesina**: These are found in Pacific Islands.
- **Bushman and Hottentots**: These are found in Kalahari Desert of Africa.
- **Australoid**: These are found in Australia. Their racial characteristics are high head, low forehead, big and broad nose, medium lips, gray eyes, wavy hair and average height.

Races in India

Indian population is polygenic and mixture of various races. Sir Herbert Risley a British ethnographer, in his book, a attempted to classify Indian races as:
- Pre-Dravidian type surviving among primitive tribes upto India Gangetic valley.
- The Dravidan type living in southern peninsula upto Indo-Gangetic Dravidian valley.
- The Indo-Aryan type found in the Punjab, Kashmir and Rajasthan.
- Arya–Dravidian type found in Indo-Gangetic valley.
- The Sethio-Dravidian type founds in Eastern India.
- The Mongoloid type found in Assam and foothills of eastern Himalaya.
- The Mongoloid Dravidian type found in West Bengal and Odisha.
- BS Guha has identified six major racial elements in the population of India namely the Negritos, Proto-Australoids, Mongoloids, Mediterranean, Western Brachycephals and Nordic.
- Out of these, first three are the oldest residents of the subcontinent. They are confined to the small pockets in the south, the Kadars, the Irulas and Paniyan and Honge and Jarwar in Andaman Islands have the definite Negritos characteristics.
- Some of the traiber of this group are found among the Angami Naga and the Bagadi of the Rajamahal hills.
- The Proto-Australoid groups numerically more significant. Most of the tribcs of central India belong to it.
- The Mangoloid groups are sub-divided into Paleo mongoloid and Tibeto Mongoloid.
- Tribal groups in the Himalayan region and North Eastern are the Mongolian stock.

- The latter are rivals were the Mediterranean, the Western Brachycephals and the Nordic (India-Aryans). The Mediterranean are associated with the Dravidian language and culture.
- The Nordian were major ethnic element to arrive in India and make profound impact on Indian.
- Psychologists and sociologist have conducted an intellectual ability.
- In words of Hooten is as follows, ' There is no objective scientific techniques for the measurement of intelligence, temperament, economic capacity, etc. that are capable of indiscrimination application to people.
- Possessing different cultures and living under diverse conditions of economic and social environment difference whether physical or mental which have been observed among various racial groups do not necessarily indicate inferiorities or superiorities.

RACISM

Racism is nothing but a type of social conscious that grows out of the feeling of belonging to a particular race. The feeling of racism found its place in the 19th century. Since then the term racism has become an important part of the dictionary of the social sciences.

People belonging to one particular race considered themselves superior to another race and this resulted into social conflicts. Some of these conflicts brought world wars.

Hitler prepared his countrymen for a war on the slogan of the superiority of the Aryan race which German people claim today. The result of this feeling of racial superiority was the Second World War.

Suppression has caused havoc in international field as well as the social field. It is necessary to study it in proper manner.

Definition

Racism has been defined by various social thinkers in different ways.

According to **Jacob** and **Stern**: Racism holds that our population is characterized by a cluster of inherited physical mental and temperamental features, peculiar to it are other environment influences that there are innately superior or inferior races and ethnic sub-divisions, and that hereditary factors determine every phase of people's cultural life.

According to **Benedict**: One group has the characteristic of superiority and the other has those of inferiority.

Theory of Racism

The theory of racism or theory of racial superiority and inferiority is psychological myth, pure and simple.

In the world today there is no pure race. Race have been so much intermingled and intermixed that to talk of racial purity is simply living in fool's paradise. Theory of racism is wrong is proved on the basis of the following factors:

- **Scientific tests:** On the basis of scientific tests, it has been proved that no race is superior or no race is inferior. Racial traits and characteristics have nothing to do with mental and intellectual development. This has been proved by scientific test on researchers.
- **History believes the theory of racial superiority:** On the basis of history it can be said that no race whether it be Aryan or Nordic is superior. All these races in their early days were barbaric and they have achieved civilization from barbarism. The principle of cultural superiority of certain races is completely false.
- **No purity of blood:** Theory of purity of blood has also been proved wrong on the basis of scientific researchers. Blood has no relation with heritage and no blood can claim cultural and intellectual superiority.
- **No pure race in the world:** In the process of history, now there is no pure race in the world. The theory of purity of race is completely wrong. Even in India it is wrong to say that there are pure Aryans. Aryans married dravidians and so on and so forth.
- **Mixture of races is not detrimental to breed:** It is believed that inbreeding maintains the purity of the blood and race. It is also believed that when there is inter mixing of the blood, it leads to down fall of the race. This is wrong theory. Now psychologists have proved that marrying outside the race, mixing the race, lead to improvement in the race.
- **Confusion of the race with culture and nationality:** Those who talk of the superiority of race confused with culture and nationality.

Culture, nationality and race are not identical. It is not necessary that all who belong to one particular nationality may also belong to one particular race or those having one culture may belong to one particular race. Many people who are not Aryan from the point of view of race speak the Aryan language.

INFLUENCE OF CASTE, CLASS AND RACE ON HEALTH AND HEALTH PRACTICES

Caste, class and race are the major components of social stratification. The differences in these three aspects resulted in inequalities among the social groups. These factors are closely associated with the determination of one's health and health practices. Even though health is a fundamental right of an individual, all groups do not achieve it in many occasions because of individual differences.

Important factors related to caste, class, race and health are discussed below:

- In some of the castes, they follow strict food restrictions. For example, Brahmins won't take non-vegetarian foods. If they are not substitute with other nutrients for restricted food items, they are in risk of developing certain deficiency diseases.
- Some castes in India, still practicing joint family system. This joint family system gives a good opportunity to take care of sick and elderly people comparing to modern family.
- In certain castes, the superstitious beliefs are more common. Even though much advancement is taken place in these scientific areas, certain castes strictly adhere with their own traditional superstitious beliefs regarding health practices.
- The high and middle class people give more importance for taking balanced diet and exercises. Most of them are very much concerned towards their bodily health.
- Middle and high class people are well aware about the challenge regarding health and health maintenance. They are getting more chance to know about health aspects, from their educational and occupational institutions.
- In high and upper middle classes the economy is not major concern. They are well affordable for all the health care facilities. Even for minor ailments they go to health care centers. But poor socioeconomic people they are not affordable for their minor health problems.
- Upper class people accept scientific advancement and current trends in medicine. Most of them are not stick to the traditional practices and superstitious beliefs. They pay more attention towards health and health practices.
- Certain races, the body physique itself, like athletes. Broad shoulders, long arms and legs are the certain features of them. They develop positive self-attitudes and morbidity rate also less comparing to other races.
- Racial differences make much impact in enjoying the health facilities. As a result of racism, the health care worker will deliver

the best care for patient who belongs to his own race. Some way, some person's patients will not accept the care which is delivered by another racial person.
* In India, the caste system is more prevalent. The health team while delivering health care show the difference to other caste people. The health team members give more attention to a patient who belongs to his/her own caste.

+ Social stratification is the hierarchical arrangement and establishment of social categories. It refers to patterned inequality in the division of society.
+ Caste is the hierarchical endogamous group having common name, common traditional occupation, common culture, relatively rigid in matters of mobility.
+ Caste system have the features like segmental division of society, hierarchy, restrictions on food, drink, and smoking.
+ Social mobility is the movement of a person or persons from one social status to another. Change in mobility occur due to urbanization and westernization.
+ Race draws attention not only of skin colour and physical attributes but also of language, nationality and religion.

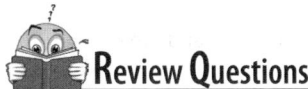

Short Answer Questions

1. What do you mean by social stratification?
2. Write down the types of social stratification?
3. What are the features of caste system?
4. Write down the functions of family.
5. Define social mobility.

Long Answer Questions

1. Discuss the origin of caste system in India.
2. Define caste. What are the features of caste system.
3. Define social mobility and its types.
4. Define race. Explain the classification of race.

UNIT 6
Social Organization and Disorganization

 CHAPTER OUTLINE

- Social organization—meaning, elements and types
- Voluntary associations
- Social system—definition, types, role, and status as structural element of social system.
- Interrelationship of institutions
- Social control—meaning, aims and process of social control
- Social norms, moral and values
- Social disorganization—definition, causes, Control, and planning
- Major social problems—poverty, housing, food supplies, illiteracy, prostitution, dowry, Child labour, child abuse, delinquency, crime, substance abuse, HIV/AIDS, COVID-19
- Vulnerable group—elderly, handicapped, minority and other marginal group.
- Fundamental rights of individual, women, and children
- Role of nurse in reducing social problem and enhance coping
- Social welfare programs in India

 Learning Objectives

After reading this chapter, students will be able to:
→ Define social organization.
→ Discuss its elements and types
→ Explain about the social system
→ Understand the interrelationship of institutions

Contd...

Contd...

- Define social control
- Describe the process of social control
- Understand the concept of social norms, morals, and values.
- Discuss social disorganization
- Identify the major social problems
- Recognise the vulnerable groups
- Enlist the fundamental rights of individual, women, and children
- Understand the role of nurse in reducing social problem and enhance coping
- Enumerate the social welfare programs in India

Key Terms

- **Role:** Duty which is expected to have
- **Norms:** A pattern or trait taken to be typical in the behavior of a social group
- **Social disorganization:** A state of disequilibrium among members of the groups
- **Social problem:** A set of conditions which are defined as wrong by society

SOCIAL ORGANIZATION

According to the perspective of social organization, the social history of India is the oldest of any country in the world. The world at that time was living in ignorance and cruelty, about 2000 years B.C. Indian culture was diverse and civilised. Indian society had gone organized on the principles of knowledge, purity, and truth. There was respect in the society for unity, prosperity, and human qualities.

A society is a group of individuals who have common bond of nearness and common goal. The individuals need the group for all needs to meet. Different groups perform different functions as they need are established with different purposes. These groups comprise social organizations.

Social organization indicates the state in which there is a peaceful interaction among the different elements of society. They word according to pre-fixed and recognized aims. In other words, the existence of definite role and status is necessary for social organization. Besides there should be uniformity in the aims, goals, and programs among the members of society. A process of harmony and adoptability continues with the changing conditions of society. There is also harmony between the individual aims of the person and the collective aims of society.

Social organization makes social habits which develop because of collective experiences as the medium of thinking and action and established harmonious relations between different institutions and committees. Social organization depends upon the degree of harmonious relationship among institutions and committees and this direct is dependent upon the structure of society. Consensus of all the members on a social subject, consensus of a collective subject and adaption of one method for the achievement of common points and one definition of all main social institution are only the viewpoints based on conjecture. These states may take comparatively more or less time. The given social hypothesis of social control, values and social structure appears to be impossible. All the social values cannot be viewed from one point view. The age today's individualistic whether the society lives in villages or industrial centres.

Social structure can never remain static in any condition. The Hindu society is completely different from Hindu society of past. Collective habits can also never remain static.

Meaning and Definition

Social organization is a state wherein various institutions in the society are functioning in accordance with their recognized or implied purposes.

According to **Ogburn** and **Nimkoff**, '*An organization is an articulation of different parts which performs various functions. It is an active group device for getting something done.*'

'*Social organization is a system by which the parts of society are related to each other and to the whole society in a meaningful way.*'
—**Earnest Jones**

'*Organization is a state of being a condition in which the various institutions in a society are functioning in accordance with their recognized or implied purposes.*'
—**Eliott and Marrill**

Characteristics of Social Organization

Social organization have the various characteristics-

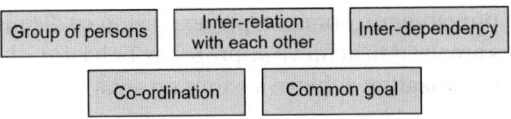

Elements of Social Organization

An organization has a social structure. Within the organization individuals hold various positions and abide by the set rules to achieve common goals or objectives. The elements of social organization are-

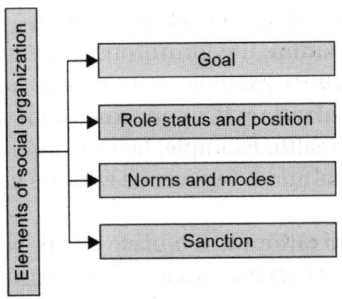

- ❖ **Goal**: Members in an organization are inter-related to each other and display unity of interest. All members try to achieve a common goal. For example- A family where all the members are inter-related and perform activities to achieve happiness
- ❖ **Role status and position**: Within an organization every member has an assigned role to perform and a position and status to occupy. Members are prepared to accept one's role and status. For example- In the College of Nursing, Principal is the designation, and role in which she has to do administration, management and teaching. She enjoys her status as principal because of the value of her role.
- ❖ **Norms and modes**: Every organization has their certain modes and norms which control its members through discipline, regularity, and punctuality. An organization functions smoothly if its members follow these modes and norms. For example- Few norms of College of Nursing are-
    - ♦ Students should be regular
    - ♦ Nursing students must maintain their dignity
    - ♦ Staff members need to be punctual
    - ♦ Discipline must be maintained by all.

- **Sanction**: Every organization follows a system of sanctions. If a member does not follow the norms, he is compelled to follow them through sanctions (conditions) which may range from warning to physical punishment. For example, expulsion or dismissal. These sanctions are used to achieve appropriate behavior which in turn help the organization achieve a common goal.

Types of Social Organization

In a social organization people work together with division of work, co-operation, and co-ordination. Members are related to each other on the basis of status and position in order to accomplish a common goal. Based on the goal to be achieved and the role to be performed social organizations can be classified as follows-

- **Political organization**: This form of organization is more concerned with political matters. Example, state, nation, rural, urban, etc.
- **Economic organization**: It is concerned with the production and distribution of wealth. Example, factory, industry, etc. As factory produces material and is concerned with the benefits on the basis of economy.
- **Religious organization**: It is a place where people offer prayers and carry out religious rituals. The main goal of religious organizations is to meet spiritual needs of the people, to achieve mental satisfaction and happiness. Example- church, temple, mosque, gurudwara.
- **Financial organization**: It deals with money matters such as depositing or withdrawal of money. Example, bank, post offices, provident fund organizations.
- **Educational organization**: It is concerned with providing education and dissemination of knowledge. The main goal is to make society literate. These organizations provide knowledge, skills as well as change the behavior of individuals. Example- Schools and colleges.

All these organizations are considered as social organizations. Social organization refers to co-ordinated social relationships among inter-dependent parts or groups.

VOLUNTARY ASSOCIATIONS

The term 'voluntarism' is derived from the Latin word 'voluntas' which means will, freedom. Therefore, voluntary association means freedom of association. It means people have legal right to combine for the promotion of the purposes in which they are interested.

Unit 6: Social Organization and Disorganization

Article 19 (1) (c) of constitution of India, confers on the Indian citizens, the right to form association.

The voluntary associations are called as non-governmental organization in the UN (united nations) terminology. The other names of voluntary associations are VOLAGE (Voluntary Agencies) and AGS (Action Groups).

Definition

According to **Michael Banton,** *'Voluntary organization is a group organized for the pursuit of one interest or of several interests in common.'*

According to **David**, *'Voluntary organization is a group of persons organized on the basis of voluntary membership without state control for the furtherance of some common interests of its members.'*

Characteristics of Voluntary Associations

Voluntary associations perform number of functions for the welfare of its members, the development of the nation, integration of the society and solidarity of the country. Voluntary associations registered under the Societies Registration Act, 1980, the Indian Trust Act, 1882, the Cooperative Societies Act, 1904 or the Joint Stock Companies Act, 1959 depends upon the scope of its activities to give it a legal status.

The main characteristics of voluntary organization are as follows:
- It has definite objectives and purposes and programs for their fulfilment and achievement.
- It is governed by its own members on democratic principles, without any external control.
- Voluntary association has its own administrative structure and a duly constituted management.
- It collects and save fund for its activities in the form of contributions of subscription from the member of local community and abroad.

According to **Norman Johnson**, voluntary organization has 4 characteristics:
1. Method of formation
2. Method of government
3. Method of financing
4. Motive

Functions of Voluntary Association

- Voluntary association formed for the promotion of cultural, social activities, recreational and encourage the professional interests.

- Voluntary association act as a buffer between the individual and state. They involve the citizen in noble affairs and avoid concentration of powers in the hands of Government and serve as power brokers.
- Voluntary organization enables the individuals to learn the fundamental of groups and political action through the participation in the governing of private or non-governmental organization.
- Well-organized voluntary action helps the individuals with diverse interests, contributes to strengthening of national solidarity and promotes participative character of democracy.
- Voluntary associations can raise the additional resources locally and meet the uncovered needs to enrich local life.
- Voluntary association helps to the state in the areas of limited sources and performs such functions in much better ways comparing to the state organization.
- Voluntary associations work for progress, development and consequently in course of time and help the state to expand its activities over wider areas.
- Voluntary associations help the individuals to utilize their talents, experience, and spirit of service to bring about changes in the society.
- Voluntary associations act as stabilizing force by connecting the people who are not politically motivated and not interested in other areas but interested only in national integration and concentration on non-political issues.
- Voluntary associations perform the functions of educating the public about policies of government about their welfare, their rights, and their obligations.
- Voluntary association helps to meet the requirements of special groups such as aged, handicapped, women, children, etc. which cannot be adequately met by the state for the reasons of financial security.

Voluntary Health Associations

- Indian Red Cross Society
- Hind Kusht Nivaran Sangh
- Indian Council for Child Welfare
- Tuberculosis Association of India
- Bharat Sevak Samaj
- Central Social Welfare Board

- Kasturba Memorial Fund
- Family Planning Association of India
- All India Women Conference
- All India Blind Relief Society
- Professional Bodies
- International Agencies live case, FORD foundation, Rockefeller Foundation.

SOCIAL SYSTEM

A system is an orderly arrangement of various parts which are inter-related with each other and interact upon one another on functional relationship. Interactions occurring in various groups in systematic way is social system.

Social system is a network of relationships and an orderly and systematic arrangement of social interactions. Social system is made up of a plurality of individuals. They interact with others according to shared norms within the social system

A social system is based not on the action of a single individual or group but rather on the interaction between various individuals or groups. These interactions are directed towards attaining certain goals or value and are guided by expected patterns of behavior or norms.

For example, in a larger social system or in a subsystem like in family where materialistic desires are given prime importance and are regarded with highly valuable individual's actions will be motivated and directed towards fulfilling such desires. In such attempts there must always be an agreement on means and ends.

Institutional norms always keep a guard on the activities of individuals and regulate their behavior. Consensus on shared means and on ends channel social action and help to promote integrated system of action, and development in the social system, e.g., consensus between production units of economic system and policy making units of political system.

The social system involves three major basic concepts. They are values, norms, and interaction pattern. These three major concepts bear a close relationship with those which are used for the personality system. That is for a better understanding of a social system, it is necessary to deal with values, norms and interaction pattern besides referring to its individual member's goal's, expectation, and pattern of action. The reverse is not true since only some of the individual goals which shared by others in the social system

Types of Social System

Social system has been classified by different authors in different ways. Following are the important classifications of a social system:
- **Morgan and other evolutionists** divided the social system into three basic stages based on the evolution of human culture:
  - *Savagery social system:* This type of social system is represented by uncivilized people. It is further classified into-
    - Lower savagery: Fruits and nuts subsistence, invention of language ate uncooked food, living in prosniscuity with no real family.
    - Middle savagery: Fish subsistence and fire
    - Upper savagery: Bow & arrow
  - *Barbarian social system:* This type of social system is represented by uncivilized people. It is further divided into-
    - Lower barbarism: Pottery
    - Middle barbarism: Domestication of animals, cultivation of maize,
    - Upper barbarism: From tools
  - *Civilized social system:* This type of social system is represented by the modern society. Phonetic alphabets, writing, intensive agriculture production and monogamy.
- **Gerhard and Jean Lenski** classified the social system into four types based on means of livelihood in the society:
  - *Hunting and gathering social system:* The social system tends to be organized around a nomadic culture.
  - *Horticulture and Pastoral social system:* This type of social system is found in horticultural societies which use hand tools to cultivate crops. In regions where horticulture was impractical, there pastoralism emerged. These societies were based on domestication of animals. Both societies have more complex social organization and increased specialization.
  - *Agrarian social system:* This type of social system is based on agriculture, domestication of animals and other related activities such as weaving, pottery and small occupations like blacksmiths, carpenters, etc.
  - *Industrial social system:* This type of social system is characterized by sophisticated machinery with advanced source of energy developed during this period.
- **Durkheim's** classified the social system into two types based on type of population:
  - *Mechanical social system:* ancient societies thrived on mechanical form of social system which was characterized by

small homogeneous population with no specialization. The social links were based on customs, obligations, and emotions. The status is determined by kinship and there is little individual freedom.
- *Organic social system:* Modern societies are found based on organic social system. These are characterized by a large population with complex division of labor. The social links are based on individual status and occupation. Individual status is determined by occupation rather than kinship ties.

❖ **Sorokin** classified the social system into three types based on cultural systems:
- *Sensate:* In this form of cultural system material happiness is given primary importance.
- *Ideational:* In this form of cultural system spiritual happiness is given primary importance.
- *Idealistic:* In this form of cultural system both material happiness and spiritual happiness are given importance

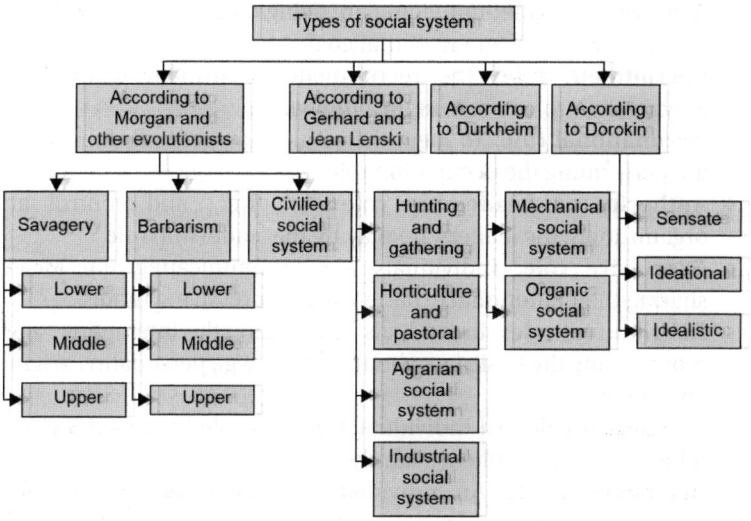

ROLE

Each and every individual has a role to perform. They are expected to perform their roles properly. Roles are very much helpful for an individual to achieve a status in the society. The individuals may play many roles in a society. Some may play a task oriented; some may play a relation oriented and other may play self-oriented roles. An individual is expected to play many roles at the same time in a group, e.g., a boy is a son to his parents, student to his teacher, husband to his wife and father to his children.

Definition

According to **Lundberg**: Social role is a pattern of behavior expected of an individual in certain group or situation.

According to **Kimbell Young**: What the individual does or performs we call as 'Role'. In the process of social organization both roles and status are the vital factors. When an individual is not performing his role properly may lead to change in his status, these alterations are automatically affecting the equilibrium of the social organization. Roles are not static and limited. They are continuously changing and multiplying in nature.

Different Types of Roles

- **Achievement Role**: Individual are fixing their goals and working towards the achievement of that goal.
- **Recruitment role**: The recruitment department people are playing their role to recruit the employees.
- **Occupational role**: To meet the economic needs all individuals are performing the occupation role.
- **Authority or Leadership role**: To direct and control an organization, the leaders are playing the leadership role.
- **Expressive role**: Individuals are communicating the ideas, sharing their emotional experience by expressive symbols.
- **Distributive role**: Individuals are indirectly interacting and representing the basic fact about all roles, e.g., personality, origin, and belief.
- **Dependent role**: An individual performs role by depending on others, e.g., wife's role in a family.
- **Independent role**: An individual alone performs certain roles without anybody's help, e.g., researcher conducting a research project.

Significance of Role

It is the role that influences the functioning and the working of the society. Once of person has been separated from status or a position, he loses the position and status that he enjoyed while he was occupying the position. In fact, with the status, there goes a power and prestige. This power and prestige can be maintained with the help of the role that a person plays.

Role is a system of distribution of responsibilities based on ability and capacity. Every society, no matter how simple, or complex, meets different persons in terms of both prestige and esteem. Roles leads to distribution of work and division of responsibilities. Due to roles, it is possible to maintain the organizationally set up and the integrity of the society. In short, social roles are quite important for society

STATUS

Social status is a place of individual or person in society. It is placing an individual is the intricate system of social relations.

Definitions

According to **Ogburn and Nimkoff**, *'Status represents the position of the individual in the group.'*

According to **Lapiers**, *'Social status is commonly thought of as the position which an individual has in the society.'*

Characteristics of Social Status

- It is nothing but a place of an individual within society or group.
- There is an element of prestige attached with every status, the higher the element of prestige, the higher the status.
- Work and sometimes birth determines the status.
- Influence that a person exercise on other members of the group and determines his or her status.
- Culture also determines the social status

Types of Status

- **Ascribed status**: It is not based on one's own effort, his capabilities, and his abilities. It is based on one's caste, family background, etc.
- **Achieved status**: An individual is achieving his status by his own efforts and capabilities, e.g., an individual position in an institution.
- **Assumed status**: By this status we mean the status that is acquired by an individual by his own self. The duties and responsibilities that are attached to this status are also chosen by the individual himself.

Factors Determining Ascribed Status

- **Age**: Age in an important factor in determining the status. In traditional societies, the elders are respected, and the younger generation is under the control of the elder generation.
- **Sex**: In most communities' males always acquire a high status in the family.
- **Physical characteristics**: Physical characteristics like well build physique in males and beauty in females are the important determinants.
- **Kinship and Family**: In a society there are poor respected family, ordinary families, and high respected families. Individuals ascribe status according to the family to which they are born. The status of the person's judged based on the name of the family.
- **Caste**: Caste determines the status of an individual in our Indian society. In India Brahmins will be given high status followed by kshatriyas, Vaishyas and sudras.
- **Race**: Race is one of the status determining factors in the western society. In western society countries, white race is considered superior compared to blacks and mongoloids.

Determinants of Achieved Status

- **Education**: The level of education is an important factor to determine the social status. A highly educated, qualified and trained person has greater respect and honor in the family.
- **Occupation**: Individual's occupation determines the social status. In our Indian society doctors and engineers are more respected in the society compared with others.
- **Wealth**: In modern world, the wealth plays a vital role. It gives power to an individual who is having more wealth can exert more control on other individuals.
- **Political authority**: A political authoritative man has a very high status in the society. The governmental ministers, MP, MLAs, and other political dignitaries have high status in a society.
- **Marriage**: Through marriage an individual achieves the status of a husband or wife, daughter in law, son in law, brother-in-law, and other status. In marriage not only two individuals are getting united, but also two families are united.
- **Achievement of an individual**: In the modern society, individual achievements are significant in determining the social status. Now people are getting lot of chances to show their potentialities. An individual can achieve in the field of education, occupation, art, literacy, sports, science, and others.

Importance of Social Status and Social Behavior

Social status has an important role to play in society and social behavior. If a person of higher status, guides other correctly, he may lead the society to proper place. There are certain symbols of respect that bring recognition to social status. This gives an opportunity to others acquire those symbols. Role of an individual's also changes with the status. Those who have higher social status have to work more and discharge greater responsibilities towards society. It also leads to division of labor. Through social status people are able to divide their work and responsibility.

Social Significance of Status

Individuals get respect by virtue of social status in society. The role is basic element of status because the status of individual is determined status because the status of individual is determined by the role of an individual. The role change of an individual determines the changes in the social status also. An individual enjoys many advantages from the social status.

Social systems are universal phenomenon. The status promotes a sense of responsibility and dependability for cooperative living. The social system should be flexible. A rigid social status system may produce strain upon the individual and exercise a deleterious effect upon the life of an individual.

Comparison between Role and Status

Role	Status
Role is expected specific performance in a group, based on one's position. Roles help the individual to achieve the status in the society	Status is mainly determined by the socioeconomic and cultural activities and related to all members of the group. Almost all societies have the similar status.
Roles are properly established on the needs of the society	Status is established based on the social aspirations and ambitions
Roles are different from one individual to another. Roles are not dividing the society into various categories and ranking them	Status represents only a part of social setup
Role discharges in relation to the prestige and values attached with the status	Status adds prestige and respect

Role and status are closely related. Both role and status are very much needed in an individual life. Role and status help an individual to lead a successful life. Both are considered as two sides of same coins.

INSTITUTIONS

Institutions means for fulfilment of certain social and psychological desires. In fact, those universal desires, customs, and ways and means that are essential for maintenance of the society are called institutions. They are responsible for organizing people fulfilment of certain social desire. Social institutions are essential to maintain the ordered arrangement of social structure.

Definition

The term institutions have been defined by **MacIver** as the established forms or conditions of procedure characteristic of group activity.

According to **Summer**, *'All institution consists of a concept (idea, notion, doctrine, or interest) and a structure.'*

According to **Ginsberg**, *'Institutions are definite and sanctioned forms or modes of relationship between social beings in respect to one another or to soe external object.'*

The institutions are collective modes of behavior. They prescribe a way of doing things. They bind the members of the group together; some thinkers have distinguished between 'institution' and institutional agencies.'

According to them the term 'institution' refers to the normative patterns of behavior, whereas institutional agencies are the social system through which these express themselves. But since there is a close integration of these normative complexes and the systems through which their mode is effective, therefore most of the writers do not distinguish between them. The common practice is to refer to family, school, church, state, and many others as the institutions of society.

Characteristics of Institutions

The main characteristics or elements of the institution are given below:
- **Symbol**: Every institution has a symbol which can be material as well as non-material.
- **Definite objectives or purpose**: Every institution is organized with some specific object or aim. Without this object or aim the institution cannot exist.

- **Rules and discipline**: Every institution has certain rules which symbolized the discipline of that institution, and these rules have to be followed compulsion by individuals.
- **Collective functions**: Every institution depends on the collective functions of the individuals. Without this collective function, institution has no meaning and existence.
- **Definite procedures**: It has been evident from the definitions given above; every institution has certain procedures. These procedures are formulated on the basis of custom's dogmas and traditions.
- **Social control**: Every institution apart from fulfilling certain objectives is based on certain principles of social control. In other words, it exercises social control also.
- **Fulfilment of primary needs**: Institutions are formed for the fulfilment of the primary needs.
- **Stability**: Institutions are more stable means of social control. They exist in one form of non-generation to generations.
- **Sanction**: Every institution enjoys the social sanction; this sanction is the result of the right and powers given to the institution by the group or the society.

Types of Institutions

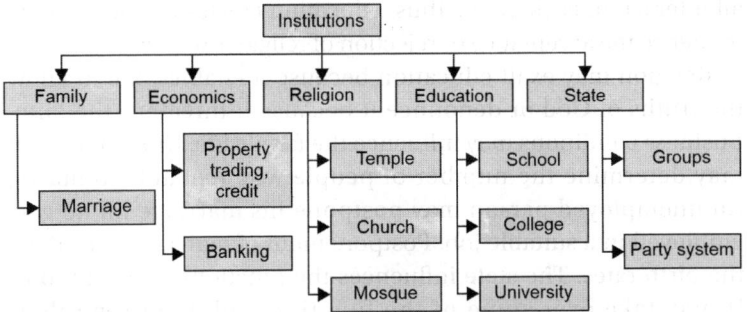

An important feature in the growth of institutions is the extension of the power of the state over the other four primary institutions (e.g., family, economics, religions, education). The state now exercises more authority by laws and regulations. Sometimes, folkways and mores are incorporated into laws, e.g., monogamy, sometimes, new laws may be enacted, e.g., Hindu Code Bill.

Today the family is being regulated and controlled by the state in scores of ways. A number of traditional functions of family have been taken over by the state. An institution never dies. The state has enacted laws regulating divorce, marriage, adoption, and inheritance. New institutional norms may replace the old norms, but the institution goes on, e.g., the modern family has replaced the norms of patriarchal family, yet family is an institution continues. When feudalism died, government did not end. The government and economic functions continued to be fulfilled, although according to changed norms. All the primary institutions are thousand years old, only the institutional norms are new.

Importance of Institution

- Unites the people to achieve the goal, causing cooperation among workers
- Controls the activities of people within social structure
- Transfers culture from one generation to another
- Provide status and role to people
- Maintains unity and harmony in society.

Inter-relationship of Institutions

A social structure owes its stability to a proper adjustment of relationships among the different institutions. No institutions work in a vacuum. Religion, education, family, government, and business all interact on each other. Thus, education creates attitudes which influence the acceptance or rejection of religious dogmas.

Religion may exalt education because it enables one to know the truths of God or denounce it because it threatens the faith. Business conditions may influence the family life. Unemployment may determine the number of people who feel able to marry. An unemployed person may postpone his marriage till he gets employed in a suitable job. Postponement of marriage may affect the birth rates. The state influences the functions of institutions. It may take over some of the function and determine their institutional norms. The businessmen, educators, clergy men and the functionaries of all other institutions also seek to influence the acts of state, since only state action may obstruct or help the realization of their institutional objectives. Thus, social institutions are closely related to each other.

The inter-relationships of the various institutions can be likened to a wheel. The family is the hub while education, religion, government and economic are spokes of the wheel. The rim would be the community within which the various institutions operate.

SOCIAL CONTROL

The term social control is generally referred to the regulation in which appeal to values and norms reduce and mitigate tensions and conflicts among individuals and between groups. Our behavior in day-to-day life is quite disciplined. We respect elders, we pay taxes to the government. Thus, we follow the norms and values of society to which we belong. But there are some people in society who do not follow these rules/ norms. There are measures of social control in society.

Society exercises its control through state, educational institutions, civic bodies, and other such institutions. The regulation of behavior of individual or group in a society is referred as social control. It happens either using force or by institutions through norms and values. In other words, concept of social control is for maintaining order in society.

French sociologist **Emile Durkheim** maintained that the essence of social control lay in the individual's sense of moral obligation to obey a rule --- the voluntary acceptance of duty rather than a simple exterior conformity to outside pressure.

Definition

According to **Mannheim**, *'The sum of those methods by which a society tries to influence human behaviour to maintain a given order'.*

EA Ross stated that, *'System of devices whereby society brings its member into conformity with the accepted standards of behaviour.'*

According to **Parsons**, *'Social control is a process by which, through the imposition of sanctions, deviant behaviour is counteracted, and social stability maintained.'*

Horton and Hunt stated that *'Sociologists use the term social control to describe all the means and processes whereby a group or a society secures its members' conformity to its expectations.'*

Kimball Young defines social control as the *'use of coercion, force, restraint, suggestion, or persuasion of one group of over its members or of persons over others to force the prescribed rules of the game.'*

According to **Lapiere**, *'Social control is a corrective measure for inadequate socialisation.'*

According to **Landis**, *'Social control is a social process by which social organization is built and maintained.'*

From the above definitions, it can be concluded that social control is an influence which is exercised by society for the promotion of welfare of group as a whole.

Need for Social Control

The reason is probable that social structure cannot continue to exist without a long period of order and stability in human behavior. Two elements of the normative dimension—norms (which are crucial for social control and stability) and the enforcement of these norms—make it possible for humans to repeat and behave in predictable ways. Both in childhood and as an adult, these norms are fostered through the socialization process, which involves the transmission of culture, and through sanctions, or actions intended to ensure norm compliance.

Aim of Social Control

The aim of social control according to **Kimball Young** is to bring about conformity, solidarity and continuity of a particular group or society.

Purpose of Social Control

Social control is to control individual behavior. No two individuals are alike in this attitudes, ideas, interests, and habits. People believe in different religions have different cultural backgrounds. There is every possibility of clash between them. But socially control them to unite and live together. Social control would establish social unity by regulating behavior of the individuals in accordance with established norms. It provides social sanction to the social wages of behavior. It checks the cultural adjustment. If any individual violates the cultural practices immediately the social control corrects the individuals

Importance of Social Control

Social control is required for the existence of society as conflicts, frustration, violence can be at rise in society without social control. There is difference in the nature, ideas, attitudes, personality, culture, eating habits etc. among the individuals in a heterogenous society. If each one behaves and acts according to their own opinion due to unregistered freedom, it will cause social disorder. So, to have an organised orderly social life and to have conformity, solidarity of a particular group in a society, we need social control.

Nature and Process of Social Control

Social control is the control of society over the individual. The control is over the undesirable and harmful tendencies of man. The society controls the individual and his parts on the right plan. The system of social control by the society changes in accordance with the changes in society. Social control is a collective term for those processes, planned or unplanned, by which individuals are taught, persuaded, or compelled to conform to the usages and life-values of groups.

Social control occurs when one group determines the behavior of another group, when the group controls the conduct of its own members, or when individuals influence the resources of others, social control consequently, operates on three levels from over group, the group over its members, and individual over their fellows. In other words, social control take place when a person is induced or fixed to act according to wishes of others, whether or met in accordance with his own individual interests.

It occurs in every aspect of the society such as in the family, peer groups, administrative organizations, non-governmental organizations, and in the government. It operates at three levels:

Group to Group	Group over its members	Individuals over fellow members
There are certain variations from the predetermined standards in every group. Any deviation that goes beyond what may be tolerated poses a risk to the group's well-being. The group then uses rewards or punishments to control the behavior of the individual and bring the non-conformists to line. The group's actions are collectively referred to as social control.	Every social group makes mistakes when attempting to socialize a new member. The individual's own preferences could not quite line up with the social norms of his group. Social control operates on the basis of individual's desire for social status, induces him to conform to group standards of conduct whatever his personal temptations.	In the process of socialization the growing child learns the values of his own groups as well that of the larger society. The individual learns ways of doing and thinking that are thought to be right and proper. He internalizes the social norms which become a part of his personality. People have strong, ingrained emotions that make it easier for them to work together with other members of the community to promote social welfare. Sometimes these sentiments by themselves are not enough to suppress the impulses of the individuals. Society has to make use of its mechanism to accomplish the necessary order and discipline. This mechanism is termed as social control.

Types of Social Control

- ❖ **Karl Mannheim** categorized social control as direct and indirect social control

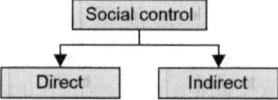

- ♦ *Direct social control:* This type of social control directly regulates the behavior of individual. Direct control is exercised upon the individual by people living in proximity. For example, primary groups such as family, neighbors, peer groups, play mates, etc., directly control the behavior of an individual. The impact of direct social control is more and durable.
- ♦ *Indirect social control:* This type of social control is directed by secondary groups. For example, traditions, institutions, customs, and social mechanisms control the behavior of an individual. These means are invisible and subtle. The impact of this social control is less and short lived.

- ❖ **Gurvitch** categorized social control into four types:

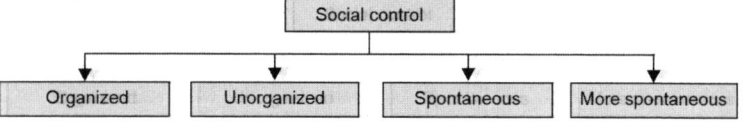

- ♦ *Organized social control:* This type of social control is directed by law, social organizations, etc.
- ♦ *Unorganized social control:* This type of social control is exercised by values, traditions, fashion, symbols, etc.
- ♦ *Spontaneous social control:* This type of social control is exercised by ideas, rules and regulations, norms, etc.
- ♦ *More spontaneous social control:* This type of social control is exercised by aspirations, decisions, desires, etc.

- ❖ **Kimball Young** categorized social control into two types:

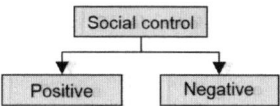

- ♦ *Positive social control:* In this type, positive steps such as rewards, praise, appreciations are used to control individual behavior. Here society encourages individuals by giving social recognition, fame, and respect.

- *Negative social control:* In this type, negative steps such as punishment, criticism, fine, and restraining are used to control individual behavior. Here the society discourages individuals by inculcating a fear of punishment either in a physical or verbal form.

❖ **Hayes** categorized social control into two types:

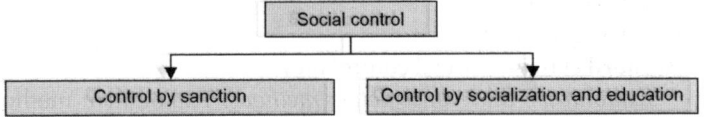

- *Control by sanction:* In this type of social control, those who follow societal norms are rewarded while those who act against are punished.
- *Control by socialization and education:* This type of social control is exercised through education and socialization.

❖ **Lumbey** categorized social control into two types:

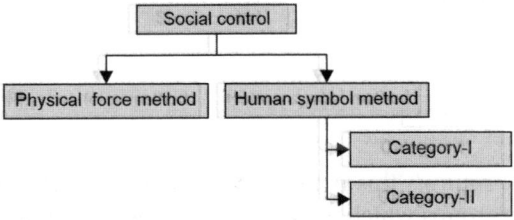

- *Physical force method:* In this type of social control, physical force such as police or law or legal system is used to control the individual behavior.
- *Human symbol method:* In this type of social control, values of society such as traditions, customs, religion, rituals are used to control individual behavior. It is further divided into-
    - Category I: It includes rewards, praise, education etc.
    - Category II: It includes gossips, satire, criticism, threat, punishments etc

❖ **Cooley** categorized social control into two types:

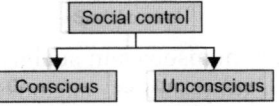

- *Conscious social control:* In this type, society forces an individual to act according to its accepted objectives such as law, education, etc.

- *Unconscious social control:* In this type, society uses unconscious methods such as religion, customs, traditions, etc. to control individual behavior.
- ❖ **EA Ross** categories into:
  - Laws
  - Custom and Religion
  - Suggestions
  - Folkways and mores
- ❖ **Bernard** classifies social control into:
  - *Exploitative and constructive methods*: Exploitative methods are punishment, repression, and intimidation whereas constructive methods include laws, education, custom and nonviolent coercion
  - *Positive and negative type of control:* Positive control includes appreciation, praise, reward etc are better ways to achieve social control than negative which includes punishment, restraining etc.
- ❖ **General classification**:

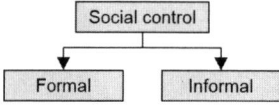

- *Formal social control:* This type of social control is exercised by secondary groups which an individual is forced to accept. These are recognized and deliberate agencies of social control such as law, education, army, constitution, etc.
- *Informal social control:* This type of social control is exercised by primary groups. These include beliefs, customs, social norms, mores, and folk ways.

Means or Ways of Social Control

Some important means of social control are divided into formal and informal means.

Informal Means of Social Control

Informal means of social control grow themselves in society. It exercised through customs, traditions, folkways, mores, religion, etc. They are very powerful particularly in primary groups like family, neighborhood, etc. Thus, informal means like praise, ridicule, boycott effectively control behavior.

Belief

Belief influence man's behavior in society. The belief is unseen power leads a man to right action because he believes that his action is being watched by an unseen power. Thus, the belief in re-incarnation, the belief in nemesis, the goddess of vengeance, the belief in the existence of hell and heaven and belief in the immortality of soul leads a man to right actions. These beliefs are categorized under the following five heads:
- Beliefs regarding accepted behavior
- Beliefs regarding penances
- Beliefs regarding immortality and re-birth
- Beliefs regarding heaven and hell
- Beliefs regarding the souls of the forefathers and ancestors.

These beliefs exercise a good deal of control on the behavior of the individual and make them act according to social values and norms.

Ideologies

Ideology is a theory of social life which interprets social realities. It influences social life which interprets social realities. Ideologies are powerful dynamic forces of contemporary social life. They are motivators of social action and makes life meaningful. For example: Leninism, Gandhism, and fascism are ideologies which are analysed and laid down to ideals before people.

Social suggestions

Social suggestions are also powerful means of social control. Suggestion is the indirect communication of ideas, feelings and other mental status communication may be made through various methods.
- Permitting life examples of great man, e.g., anniversaries movement of great people like Mahatma Gandhi, Jawaharlal Nehru, Vivekananda, etc.
- Through literature, e.g., journals, books, autobiographies, newspaper, etc.
- Education: Educational curriculum, etc.
- Advertisement, e.g., magazines, influence, attitudes, and actions.

These all-communication methods influence the human mind indirectly and changes behavior and make them as disciplined citizens.

Folkways

Folkways are patterns of behavior of everyday life which arise spontaneously and unconsciously in a group. It exercises powerful influence over man behavior in society. They are socially approved and, they have some degree of traditional sanction. Folkways are foundation of group culture, so they cannot be easily violated. If an individual does not follow them, he may be socially boycotted by his group, e.g., greeting others when met in morning. The way by which we clean our rooms and cooking food, etc.

Mores

When folkways grow to the stature of having moral obligation on these members of the society, they become mores. Mores are important for the welfare of the society. They are always molding human behavior and they are the instruments of control, e.g., prohibition, endogamy, antislavery, etc.

Customs

Customs are well-established habits of people which have been passed down from generation to generation. They arise and grow spontaneously and gradually. They are accepted by society and have been followed in the past. They are so powerful and regular social life to a great extent.

Customs bind people together and control selfish impulses, e.g., form of family, marriage, worship, religious festivals, rituals, are part of customs, dowry and bribe are also customs. Therefore, it is difficult to change them.

Religion

Religion is very important method of social control. It is a bundle of our beliefs and practices in certain powers, beings, and things. Religion exerts a powerful control over human behavior. It is found in all human societies like tribal, rural, and urban. It exerts a powerful control over human behavior.

Religion encourages the development and good virtues and ideals like love, sacrifice, modesty, honesty, mercy, forgiveness, and social services. Further unnecessary conflicts between various religions may result in violence and social disorganization. Today religion is losing its important fact. This is so because of growth of science and technology and predominance reason over faith.

Art and literature

Fairchild states that 'Art is one of the primary social institutions attempting to answer symbolically the riddle of life.' Both art and literature influence the imagination and exert control on human behavior.

Art: Art in its narrow sense includes painting, sculpture, music, dance, etc. Art is a method of sublimation and re-direction of the baser instinct of an individual. It is a combination of religion, morality, ideal and so many things. In short, art is an indirect and inadvertent manner trains the child or an individual for either way of life. Thus, it is an important method of social control.

Gillin and **Gillin** have rightly said that its uses are common to all men. It is used in war, in religious and the establishment of a new order or things. For example: A classical dance creates appreciation of your culture. The status of Mahatma Gandhi teaches us the virtue of simple living and high thinking. An excellent painting may arouse a feeling of sympathy and affection, etc. An artist has been called an agent of civilization.

Literature: Literature also influence the human behavior in society. Literature includes poetry, drama, and fiction, e.g., Ramayana, Bhagavad Gita, Mahabharat are classical works of great social values. For example: Detective literature effect, on crime, romantic literature gives passionate feelings and religious literature is superstitious, etc

Humor and satire

Humor is also a means of social control. Sometimes it often services to relieve a tension, anxiety, jealousy, it is also used to gain a favorable response. Humor controls by supporting the sanctioned values of the society. Satire employs wit and scorn as indirect criticism of actions felt to be vicious and tries to use it as the most effective means of social control.

Public opinion

The importance of public opinion as a means of control is great in simple societies. But when in modern complex societies, public opinion is very powerful. The desire for recognition to a natural desire, human praise is the sweetest music. Every individual wants to win public praise and avoid public ridicule or criticism. Thus, public opinion is one of the strongest forces influencing the behavior of people and fear of public ridicule and criticism we do not indulge in immoral or antisocial activities.

Fashion

In modern set up, fashion plays an important part in social control. It controls the ideas, the dress, beliefs and so many things. It is through fashion that man is able to mold his way of life. Fashion is nothing but exhibition of the ways of the society. It balances the society and the desire for distinction individuality and differentiation.

Recreation and play groups

After family, it is recreational or play groups that play an important role in socialization. It is not only bringing about exhibition and development of the instinct of the children and in note tendencies, but also trains them in accordance with the society. Through play groups or recreational groups, a man is able to control his animal instinct and also exhibit them in proper form. This play group brings about the development of the personality of the individual and on the other hand they exercise control.

Hayers has rightly remarked 'by supervised play children learn by experience that civilized life is happier for all concerned than savagery

Family

Family is a very important instrument of social control. On the one hand it socializes an individual and on the other it trains him about social behavior family prescribes rules and regulations that the members have to follow. These rules and regulation form a part of social control. In fact, family is also an important instrument and agency of social control.

Non-violence

The non-violence is just the opposite of physical force. It is a moral force that compels an individual to submit to a court. Mahatma Gandhi, father of Indian nation has given this important instrument of social control to the world. In non-violence, moral force plays its part and compels an individual to behave in a manner which is conceive for social betterment and better social organization.

Manners and ceremonies

In every society there are number of ceremonies, these ceremonies make the individual realized the importance of the social welfare and his social obligations. It also teaches them the way of social behavior and behavior with other individuals. Similarly, there are certain manners in society. These manners and ceremonies are the repeat exercise, a good deal of control over society and social behavior of man.

Leader or leadership

Leaders of the society have not only directed the easy of the members of the society, but they have also exercised a great control over him. Their ideas, their actions and their views influence the individuals so much that they try to keep them.

Formal Means of Social Control

Law

Law is a body of rules enacted by legally authorized bodies and enforced by authorized agencies. It clearly defines rights, duties as well as the punishments for their violation. The modern societies are large in size. Their structure is complex consisting of a number of groups, organizations, institutions and vested interests.

Informal means of social, controls are no longer sufficient to maintain social order and harmony. In modern society, relationships are of secondary nature. Security of life and property as well as the systematic ordering of relationships make formalization of rules necessary.

Law prescribes uniform norms and penalties throughout social system. Whatever were in mores and customs earlier has now been formalized into a body of law. Law prohibits certain actions, for example, anti-touchability act prohibit untouchability in any form and a person practicing, untouchability is liable to punishment, prohibition act forbids drinking at public places. In this way, law exercises a powerful influence upon the behavior of people in modern societies. It is most important formal means of social control. Early society depends upon the informal means of social control. But nowadays in modern society, people have defined rules and regulations to be followed to set required behavior and if violated leads to punishment.

Law is the body of rules formed by legally authorized people. Law defines rights, duties and punishments if violated clearly. Law describes uniform norms and penalties throughout a social system. Nowadays the body of law in every state is being increased in every state. The body of law is nothing but mores customs in earlier days. Some acts which formed for social control are:

- ❖ Hindu Marriage Act
- ❖ Anti-untouchability Act
- ❖ Prohibition Act.

In this way, law exercises a powerful influence upon the behavior of the people in modern societies and takes even larger part in total control.

Education

Education is a process of socialization. Education aims at moulding or changing the behavior of the growing individuals. Education prepares the child for social living. Education teaches disciplines, value, belief, social cooperation, tolerance, sacrifice, good behavior conduct, knowledge, honesty, fair play, and tense of right and wrong. The importance of education as a means of social control is being increasingly realized. Education is process of socialization. It prepares the child for social living. It reforms the attitudes wrongly formed by children. The importance of education for creativity, right social attitudes among youth cannot be overlooked

Coercion or force

Coercion means the use of force to achieve a desired end. Coercion may have immediate effect upon the offender, but it does not have enduring effects. It may be physical and non-violent. It is the ultimate means of social control when all other means are failed. Physical coercion may take the form of bodily injury, imprisonment, and death penalty. Physical coercion is without doubt the lowest form of social control. Non-violent coercion consists of strike, boycott and non-cooperation, e.g., like student may go on strike to ensure better hostel facilities. Boycott is the withholding of social or economic interaction with others to express disapproval and to force acceptance of demands. Non-cooperation is refusal to cooperate, e.g., teacher may refuse to cooperate the management over the payment of salaries, non-violent coercion can be successful way of effecting social control. Mahatma Gandhi also used non-violent force to grant independence to India.

SOCIAL NORMS

Norms

The concept of behavior has been turned into social norms. The concept of norms is centralized in sociology.

Meaning of Norms

Norms are standards of group behavior, when a number of individuals interacts, a set of standards develop that regulate their relationships and modes of behavior. These standards of group behavior are called social norms.

Norms incorporate value judgment: They represent 'standardized generalizations. They are concepts which have been evaluated by the group and incorporate value judgement. Thus, it may be said that norms are based in social values which are justified by normal standards or aesthetic judgement. A norm is a platform setting limits on individual's behavior.

Norms are related to factual world: Sociologists are interested mainly in operative norms, that is norms that are sanctioned in such a way that violations suffer penalties in the group. For example, most of the norms, are not sanctioned are not promised socially for refusing to turn the other cheek. Norms in order to be effective must represent correctly the relations between real events.

Definition

According to **Secord and Buckman**, *'A norm is a standard of behavioural expectation shared by group members against which the validity of perception is judged and the appropriateness of feeling and behaviour is evaluated.'*

Importance of Norms

Norms are of great importance to society, without norms behavior would be unpredictable. The standards of behavior contained in the norms give order to social relation interactions go smoothly if the individuals follow the group norms. Man is incapable of existing alone. His dependence on society is not derived from fixed innate responses to mechanical stimuli but rather from learned responses to meaningful stimuli. Hence his dependence on society is ultimately dependence upon a normative order.

Norms give cohesion to society, group without norms would be solitary, poor, nasty, brutish and short Norms influence individual's attitude and motives. They are specific demands to act, made by his group. They lead to the phenomenon of conscience, of guilt feelings, of elation and depression. They are deeper than consciousness. Becoming a member of a group consists of internalizing the norms of the group. Through internalization they become a part of himself automatically expressed in his behavior. The normative system gives to society a cohesion without which social life is not possible.

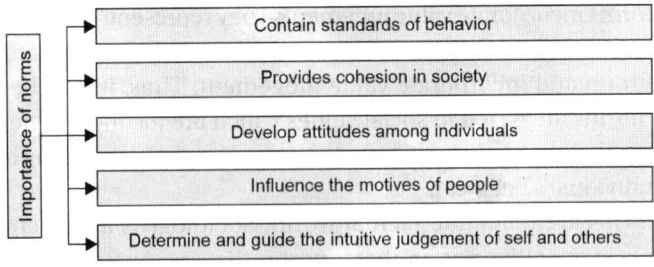

VALUES

The cultural standards of a society are called social values. Social values provide a meaning for our social behaviors. These values consist of all the sentiments and ideas of the group. The primary focus of the values is encouraging the right social behaviors. A group shares social values. This is different from individual values. The man himself enjoys individual value. It is forcing only the individual welfare. But social values are organized within the personality of an individual and it always seeks the others welfare. Values influence and regulate the thinking and the way of behavior of an individual. Examples for social values are non-violence and charity. They are general and shared by a large group. The norms are based on these social values. So, in day-to-day life, all individuals are conscious about the values. The basement of the value is culture. Culture is reflected by the social values. For example, the American values are based on American culture and that is belief in material progress, where an Indian value based on Indian culture marked by the spiritualism.

FOLKWAYS

Meaning

Folkways as the term indicates, is a sum total of the ways and pattern of behavior of a particular folk or a group of people. As a social being every individual has to undertake different types of behavior from morning till evening. Some of these behavior's are general and normal while the others are specific and particular. These specific and particular behaviors have their origin in the way of the folk or the group in the society.

Definition

According to **Horton and Hunt**, *'Folkways are simply customary normal, habitual ways of doing things.'*

According to **Gillin and Gillin**, *'Folkways are behavior patterns of everyday life which generally arise unconsciously in a group.'*

Important Feature of Folkways

- **Spontaneity in Origin**: Folkways are not planned. They are the recognized ways of behaviors arises automatically and spontaneously. They are developed out of experience.
- **Folkways Arise Spontaneously**: They are not deliberately planned or designed. They are developed out of experience. They are unplanned and uncharted.
- **Accepted by Group**: Folkways are a group behavior or response. Folkways are the recognized ways of behavior. The group accords recognition to certain ways while rejects others. Only such ways of behavior are folkways as have been approved by the group to which they relate.
- **Vary from Society to Society:** There are wide variety of folkways. But each group has different folkways. There are numerous folkways in different societies. The folkways become related to a particular group. There is considerable variation in the folkways between groups.
- **Folkways are Transformed Through Hereditary**: Folkways are passed from one generation to another through ancestors. Folkways are the important informal agencies of social control.

Customs and traditions are the origin of the folkways. These folkways differ from place to place, and they differ from group to group. The members of this group may catch an individual, who fails to follow the folkways. That is why most of the individuals are very conscious about the folkways of their own group.

MORES

Mores are standardized and regulators of human behavior. They develop from the folkways and customs. They are more powerful than folkways. They are more stable and obligatory. The term 'mores' is derived from the Latin word 'Mos', which means customs. More are the important aspects of social control and social life

Definition

According to **MacIver**, *'When the folkways have added to them conceptions of group welfare, standards of right and wrong, they are converted into mores.'*

According to **Gillin and Gillin**, *'Mores are the customs and groups routines, which are taught by the members of the society to be necessary to the groups continued existence.'*

Characteristic of Mores

- **Concepts of group welfare**: All mores are the element of group or social welfare attached to it. This element of social welfare converts a folkway into mores.
- **Determines modes of our day-to-day behavior**: Mores determine modes of our day-to-day behavior as social beings. For example, our behavior towards our parents and elderly is very much determined by our mores.
- **Helpful in social adjustment**: Mores are guided by the elements of welfare of the society or the group. They are, therefore based on the values and the attitudes of the society. They therefore play a vital role in the social adjustment.
- **Uniform in social life**: Mores are the standards of the behavior, their violation brings punishment. They, therefore, are very helpful in bringing out uniformity of social behavior. Because of the fear of punishment most of the members of the society, behave the manner as prescribed by mores.
- **Helpful in social change**: Mores can be instrumental in social change also. They are basically conservative and once they have persisted for a very long time, individuals grow restive and try to bring out a social change.

Other Important Features of Mores

- Mores always aim the group welfare.
- Mores judge the human behavior as right or wrong.
- Mores are natural, develops gradually and slowly.
- An individual who breaks the mores are punished.
- Mores are included in the laws of the nation.
- Mores most deals with the needs of the society.

Functions of Mores

According to **MacIver** following are the functions of Mores:
- They both compel behavior and forbid it. They are forever moulding and restraining the tendency of every individual. In other words, they are the instruments of control.

- In society there are innumerable mores like monogamy, antislavery, democracy and prohibition, conformity to which is regarded necessary.
- By conforming to the mores, the individual gains identification with this fellow and maintains those social bands which are essential for satisfactory living.
- The mores hold the members of the groups together. The members of the group though characterized by the consciousness of the kind and competing with one another by the good things of life and status. They are held in line by the constraint of mores.

There is a sense of unreflecting solidarity among people who share the same mores because their sentiments are alike. It also implies that there is a sense of resistance and antagonism towards anyone with different mores. There are mores for each sex for all classes and for all groups whose function is to maintain the solidarity of the group.

LAW

Meaning

Law is the expressed will of the higher political authority in the society for proper maintenance of peace and order in society. It is necessary for maintaining of the integrity and organization of the state.

Definition

Different social and political thinkers have defined it in different ways.

According to **Holland**, *'Law is a principle or rule of conduct so established as to justify a prediction with reasonable certainty that it will be enforced by the courts if its authority is challenged.'*

Characteristic of Law

- It is the rule or law of the external behavior of man.
- It is enforced by the state.
- It is followed and observed by the majority of the people.
- Its violation leads to some punishment or the other by the state.

Importance of Law in Social Behavior

Laws are framed for our society. The political authority of the state is enforced through these laws. These are intended at maintenance of the integrity of the society. They influence the society in the following aspects:

- **Regulate the behavior of the individuals:** Through laws the behavior of the individuals is regulated to such a manner that it conforms to social norms and political ideas.
- **Help in maintaining the organization of the society:** Laws keep the individuals within their limits. Those who do not observe them are punished. Thus, the integrity of the society is maintained.
- **Keep the criminals away from the society:** Evolution of laws leads to punishment. This fear keeps the individual criminals away from the society.

The importance of the law as an agency of controlling the social behavior has very well been summed up by the **Ross** in the following words: Law is the most specialized and highly furnished engine of social control employed by society.

CUSTOMS

Meaning

Customs are nothing but accepted and common ways of acting. They are very much responsible for maintenance from one generation to other get strengthened by new generation. These strengthened traditions are called customs.

Definition

The term 'Custom' has been defined by different sociologist in different ways. **Ross** has defined the custom in the following words: 'By customs is meant the tradition of a way of doing; by tradition is meant the transmission of a way of thinking or believing.

Characteristics of Customs

- **Social base:** Customs are formed spontaneously because of society. They are part of social inheritance and are not formed by individuals.
- **Customs are transmitted from one generation to another:** They are followed by individuals because many individuals or groups of individuals have followed them.
- **Customs are traditions:** That have been prevalent for several generations and have been strengthened because of the experience of the generation.
- **Conservative:** Customs are conservative, and it is not easy to change them.

- **No organized machinery to punish the evolution of customs:** Society does not possess organized and effective machinery to punish the evolution of customs.
- **More effective to regulate the behavior of individuals as compared to traditions:** Customs influence the behavior of the individuals from birth to the death. They have great capacity to influence the behavior of the individuals more effectively and in a more comprehensive manner as compared to traditions.

Origin of Custom

A custom does not grow suddenly. It is a result of a gradual development and takes good deal of time. In fact, it is a means to strengthen the existence and the values of the society. 'Folkways grow into traditions and traditions grow into customs.

Role and Importance of Custom in a Society

- **Simplifying the process of learning:** Customs provide readymade pattern of behavior and so the process of the learning of the individual becomes simplified.
- **Make social adjustments easier:** Through the readymade pattern of behavior it is easy of individual members to establish adjustment with the social situations or meet the new social situations in an easier manner.
- **Social utility or usefulness:** Customs have a social utility. Although they are not based on logic and reason, but they are helpful in the integration and maintenance of the society and its values.
- **Bring about uniformity in social life and behavior:** Through customs element of uniformity introduced in the social behavior of the individuals as members of the society.
- **Important agencies of social control:** Customs control the behavior of the individuals. They force them to act according to the prescribed patterns. They do not allow the individuals to go astray. Thus, these customs act as important agencies of controlling the behavior of the individual members of the society and also collective behavior of the society.

FASHION

All fields of life are fashion. It is an important means of social control. In civilized societies, the dress, literature, recreation, jewellery, decoration of house, way of talk, music art, are items of fashion. These spread to a greater range with the development of transport and communication. Fashion influences the imagination and exert control of human behavior. The martial music of the military band arouses feelings of determination and strength. Literature, the Autography, teaches the simple thing.

Difference between Folkways and Mores

Folkways	Mores
Folkways are narrower have a limited range of application	Mores are relatively wider and more genera
Folkways are less compulsive and more flexible	Mores are more compulsive regulative and rigid
Conformity the folkways through expected into strictly insisted on	Mores are effective and influential in molding character
Folkways only suggest which type of behavior is more relevant or appropriate in particular situation	Mores tell what is right and what is wrong. They prescribe the behavior
Violation of folkways is often ignored or tolerated	Violations of the mores brings the person strong disapproval and often severe punishment
Disobedience to ordinary folkways may not incurs every punishment most of the time	It is not tolerated or ignored, but seriously dealt with
Most of the folkways are ordinary rules of behavior and not backed by social support.	Mores are more sublime and serious for they have the support and the justification of values system
Folkways are subjects to frequent changes as we find it in fashions fads and crazes	Mores changeless frequently for they are more deeply in the society

Difference between Customs and Laws

Customs	Laws
Customs are the laws of society, and they enjoy the political sanction	They are prescribed by the state and enjoy political sanction
Evolution of customs leads to beings censored by the society and losing the status of a member of the society	Evolution of law leads to punishment by the political authority
Customs are the products of the society, and they grow in a spontaneous and natural manner.	Laws are manmade and prescribed by the state

Contd...

Contd...

Customs	Laws
Customs deal with the internal behavior of the members and also affect the conscience	Laws determine the external behavior and they are followed because of the fear of punishment.
Customs are informed means of regulating the behavior of individuals and the society. Generally, they affect the primary social such as family	Laws are formal agencies of enforcing good behavior and they regulate secondary social groups
Customs are not based on logic, and they are for all the members of the society	Laws are based on logic, and they are meant only for those who violated them
Customs are unwritten and soon voice is raised for their change.	Laws are written and clear out and generally voice is raised for their change.

Difference between Customs and Habit

Customs	Habit
Custom is a social phenomenon	Habit is an individual
Custom is socially recognized	Habit is not socially recognized
Custom is normative	Habit is not normative
Custom has got great social significance	Habit is more of personal importance
Customs has an external sanction	Habit has no external sanction

Difference between Fashion and Custom

Fashion	Custom
It is imitation of contemporary persons and so it is shortlisted and temporary	It is the imitation of ancestors and so more stable and permanent
Fashion reappears even after becoming out mode. In other words, fashion moves in a cyclic order	Customs does not appear after it has once become extinct
It is against dogmas and is inspiring by the feeling of novelty and originate	Customs is dogmatic and has a tendency towards ancient

Contd...

Contd...

Fashion	Custom
Fashion is based on self-ostentation and imitation	Custom is no doubt based on elders but is traditional in outlook. It is a habit
It is related to insignificant and temporary needs of the society and not all traditional	It is related to important and more stable needs of the society.
It changes rapidly and is facile.	Custom does not change rapidly. It is not facile
Fashion is based on self-expression and desire to be distinguished from others. It may not necessarily be related to culture.	It is certainly related to culture and is established with the in tension of bringing about conformity to cultural values.

Role of Nurse in Social Control Measures

Nurses are working in hospitals, community and other settings. They are dealing with different kinds of human beings. All individuals are not same. They also are having different background, different culture and their own way of life. But they are all controlled by certain factors in the society. These controlling factors are formed informal in nature. Social control guides and controls the individual's behavior, which will enable them to lead a successful social life.

Nurses should consider the individual customs, folkways, rituals, values, beliefs and practices. These are closely associated with one's culture. While she is planning out the nursing care, she should consider all the culture norms.

Nurses should respect their religious beliefs. They should consider their educational status. But they should not show inequality or partiality based on the socioeconomic status while they are implementing care. The nurses should be well-aware about the law and entire legal system. All patients are having the right to get fair treatment, privacy, maintain confidentiality and also accept or reflect the treatment pattern. While dealing with a traditionalized individual, nurses should always anticipate the culture log. This is very common among the geriatric group. Currently most of the Indian nurses are getting the opportunity to work in the foreign countries. They should be able to adopt the new atmosphere, because the control agencies are changing from one society to another.

The basic ideology itself it is different from our community to western community. Our ideology is based on religious beliefs, western ideology based on material culture.

As conclusion the nurses should have thorough knowledge about all agencies of social control, which belongs to a particular society.

SOCIAL DISORGANIZATION

Organization and disorganization are essential accompaniments of a society. No dynamic society either fully organized or disorganized does not lack elements of disorganization. In fact, social organization and social disorganization are anonymous each other and they influence the society and its progress. Different societies have different types of social structures, which have their own status and roles to play. When these individuals and social groups or social institutions do not get there deserved status and fail to play their role, there is disorganization.

In short, disorganization is that process as a result of which various social institutions and the individuals are not able to play their roles according to the objective and their status.

Social disorganization

It has been defined by various social thinkers in various ways. Given below are a few definitions of social disorganization:

According to **Elliot and Merrill**, *'Social disorganization is the process by which the relationship between members of a group is broken or dissolved.'*

According to **Ogburn and Nimkoff**, *'Social disorganization refers to the disruption of the functions of some social unit such as group or institution or community.'*

From the above definitions, it can be concluded that social disorganization is serious maladjustments rather than unadjustments in the society and due to this they are unable to satisfy the needs of individual.

Nature of Social Disorganization

The philosophically organic approach postulates the interdependence of culture and human nature. It must be included in the formulation of the nature of the social and personal disorganization. human nature reflects culture in the responses of the individual mechanism. Culture includes those response which are common to the group, and which are passed from generation to generation.

Characteristics of Social Disorganization

Social disorganization is a process which is governed by contain factors and situations. These result into certain qualities and characteristics of social disorganization that are given below:

- **Social disorganization is unconscious and unexpected**: Social disorganization is not a conscious process. It goes on unconsciously. People are not able to know that is going on.
- **Never absolute**: While social disorganization is unconscious in advertent, it is never absolute. Even during war and revolution, there is some elements or organization left in the society. In other words, it means that social disorganization is a process which is never complete and absolute.
- **Social disorganization takes place at the time of transition**: Social disorganization does not take place at a time when the society is properly organized. It takes place at a time when the society is posing from one stage to the other.
- **Social change in the basis of social disorganization**: In facts, social disorganization is indicative of social change. Social disorganization takes place only when there is some social change.
- **It is a transfer of function**: As a result of social disorganization, the functions of a particular group of the society are transferred to another, for example, as a result of industrialization the joint family system breaks. In order days the family was responsible for every function of the individual. Now it is not so.
- **Values and attitudes change and get dissolved**: As a result of social disorganization, the social values and attitudes get changed. They cease to have held him in high esteem and result into dissolution. In their place, new values are established for example, in India as a result of social disorganization the marriage system has indicated a lot of change.
- **Lack of influence of social laws**: Social disorganization, starts when the social law or the society starts losing its influence. It means that the customs and traditions cease to have any blinding

effect and the individuals find themselves free to do things that they deem proper.

- **Abnormal state**: Social disorganization is something from the normal state of the society. It is an abnormal state, which has been described by **Elliott and Merrill**. The study of social organization and disorganization has been associated traditionally with the concepts of normally and abnormally with the values and judgment which accompany these concepts. An organized society has been presumed to be normal and disorganization society as abnormal.
- **Physical or geographical factors:** The maladjustment of man and his culture to certain extraordinary physical or geographic conditions or situations may cause disorganization in society. This is especially true on the case of natural calamities such as storms, cyclones, hurricanes, famines, floods, epidemics, etc. which upset the social balance and bring in social disorganization.
- **Biological factor**: Population explosion or extreme scarcity of population, the instances of racial inter mixture, defective hereditary traits and such other biological factors may also cause disorganizing effects upon society.
- **Ecological factor**: Social disorganization is related to environment internal of regions and neighbourhoods.
- **Social problems leading to social disorganization**: Social problems and forces such as a revolution, social upheaval, a class struggle, a financial or economic crisis, a war between nations, mental illness and political corruption threaten the welfare of the society.
- **Degeneration of values**: Social values are often regarded as the sustaining forces of society. They contribute to the strength and stability of social order, but due to rapid social change new values come up and some of the old values decline. At the same time people are not able to reject the old completely and accept the new altogether. Hence conflict between the old and the new is the inevitable result of which leads to the social disorganization.
- **Disintegration and confusion of roles**: Members of society are expected to perform certain definite roles in accordance with their placements in society. Due to profound social change these expectations also undergo change, consequently people are confused with regard to their new roles.
- **Political subservience**: Political subordination of a country will result in social disorganization. The subordinate country is not permitted to develop its economy and institutions independently

and is made as a means to serve the interest of the dominant country.
- **Conflict of goals and means**: Conflicts of goals and means for achieving them may also cause disorganization. Most of the individuals share the dominant goals of the society and act accordingly. But lacking the means for achieving the goals by legitimate means some may resort to illegitimate and illegal means resulting in vice, crime and other expression of social disorganization.
- **Decline of social control**: The decline control of religion, morals, customs, traditions and other institutions on the behavior of men has also enhanced the process of disorganization. There is an increase in interpersonal conflicts, crimes, tensions, divorce, delinquency, mental derangement, etc.
- **Extreme divisions of labor**: According to **Durkheim** social disorganization is often brought about by extreme division of labor. In normal course, according to him, division of labor leads to social solidarity may become disturbed.
- **Disruptive social change**: Society undergoes change mainly due to the operations of physical, biological, technological and cultural factors. Sudden and radical social changes may disrupt the stability and the organization of the society. The result is social disorganization.

Types of Social Disorganization

Social disorganization takes several forms. It starts from the individuals and goes up to the entire nation, world that is why it is divided under the following heads:

Personal Disorganization

It means disorganization in personal life, such as child delinquency, youth delinquency, addiction to intoxicants, physical disabilities, suicide, etc.

Family Disorganization

It means that the social disorganization has affected the family life. It results into discontented relations between husband and wife and other members of the family. It exhibits in the form of indiscipline, family, tension, divorce, separations and other marital and family problems.

Community Disorganization

When the social disorganization affects the entire community or society, it is termed as community disorganization. Unemployment, poverty, political corruption, crimes, casteism, religious bigotry, anarchy, etc. are examples of community disorganization.

International Disorganization

The social disorganization is not limited to community. It affects the whole international structure. As a result of disorganization in the field of international world, wars, revolutions, dictatorship, imperialism, etc. come into existence.

Causes of social disorganization
1. Extreme division of labor
2. Violation of social rules
3. Degeneration of social values
4. Industrialization
5. Cultural lag
6. Ecological disturbances
7. War
8. Disruptive social change
9. Biological factors
10. Conflict of goals and means
11. Change in the role and status of the individuals

Measures to Control Social Disorganization

It is necessary to keep the society organized. Unless the society is kept organized, it may not be possible to keep the value of life. The best way to do away with social disorganization is find out the causes for it. After that, it is possible to bring out social disorganization, which is the best way for the removal of social disorganization. Following have been suggested as remedies of social disorganization:

- ❖ **Clear cut definition of social status and roles**: In order to avoid social disorganization, the best thing is to define clearly the status and the roles of various individuals and social groups. This would stop overlapping and check social disorganization.
- ❖ **Development of new social values and attitudes**: When the society acquires new values and attitudes, they should be allowed to have proper atmosphere for development.
- ❖ **Collective efforts to end social evils**: The entire society or group must be tried to check and do away with social evils. It will include crushing of all sorts of curve and social deformities.

- **Check on population**: When there is unchecked growth of population, it usually leads to social disorganization. Planning should be resorted to this regard.
- **Reforms of educational system**: In order to check social disorganization, it is necessary to have proper educational system. It would require its reform at every stage.
- **Minimize the religious, linguistic and group conflicts**: In order to check the social disorganization, it is necessary to minimize and lessen the differences that exist between different groups on the basis of religion, language, etc.
- **Regulated and planned industrialization**: In order to save the society from disintegrating and getting it organized, it is necessary to have regulated development of industry. These should be close co-ordination between villages and the cities. Small scale or collage or village industries should be developed in close co-operation and harmony. This would have a controlled urbanization and industrialization and check social disorganization.
- **Development of agriculture**: In order to feed people, it is necessary to have proper agricultural products. It can be possible by developing agriculture.
- **Elimination of casteism and untouchability**: In India particularly, if social disorganization is to be checked, casteism and untouchability must be eliminated completely.
- **End of unemployment and poverty**: Unemployment poverty led to several types of crimes that are responsible for social disorganization. Attempts should be made to do away with these economic evils.
- **Ending of economic disparities**: In our society, a good deal of economic disparities exists. They are very much responsible for all sorts of social and other types of disorganization. If social disorganization is to be eliminated completely, a socialist society has to be ushered in.
- **Elimination of the danger of war**: In fact, economic disparities and elimination of war go together. Once the lasting peace has been established, there is not possibility of social disorganization.

Social disorganization is an important aspect as sociology. If we want to have a properly organized society, we have to keep away the factors that are responsible for the social disorganization then only a balanced, properly organized and usual society and exist.

FUNDAMENTAL RIGHTS OF INDIVIDUAL, WOMEN, AND CHILDREN

Fundamental Rights of an Individual

Article in our constitution of India prohibits the discrimination of caste, sex, religions, race and place between citizens. It abolishes the untouchability. All individuals should be treated equally.

- **Right to Freedom** (Article 19) Article 19 (1) grants freedom to every citizen.
- **Right Towards Culture and Education** (Articles 29 and 30) Article 29 explains about provisions for minorities to preserve and promote their language, script and culture.
- **Rights Against Exploitation** (Article 23 and 24) Article 23 of constitution prohibits forced labor and declares use of women for immoral and other purpose is a punishable offence.
- **Right of Property** (Article 31) Article 31, 31 A and B grants the right of individual and trust town and administer their property.
- **Right Towards Religion** (Article 25 to 28) Article 25 explains about the freedom of religion. Every individual can practice and propagate their religion freely. Article 28 gives warning against imparting religious instruction in any educational institutes established and maintained by the state fund. But it is not applicable for the institutions established under any endowment or trust. Article 26 explains about the establishment of institutions for religious and charitable purposes and to acquire and own the property. Article 27 strongly prohibits raising fund through taxes to promote a particular religion.
- **Right to Constitutional Remedies** (Article 32) Article 32 of constitution provides for the enforcement of fundamental right by the court.
- **Right to Leisure** An individual has the right to spend leisure time freely based on his interest in a constructive manner.
- **Right to Work** Individuals have a right to opt all types of work based on his educational qualification, talents, capacities and interests.
- **Right to Freedom**: Article (19-22) Article 19 (1) grants freedom to every citizen. The important rights of freedom are as follows:
  - Freedom of speech and expression
  - Form association and unions
  - Assemble peacefully and without arms
  - To own or dispose property

- To reside and settle down in any part of India
- Free to have friendly relations with other countries, public order any decency and good conduct
- To practice any profession, trade, business
- The state is authorized to restrict freedom of the press in order to check standardized article and promotion of dissatisfaction towards contempt of court.

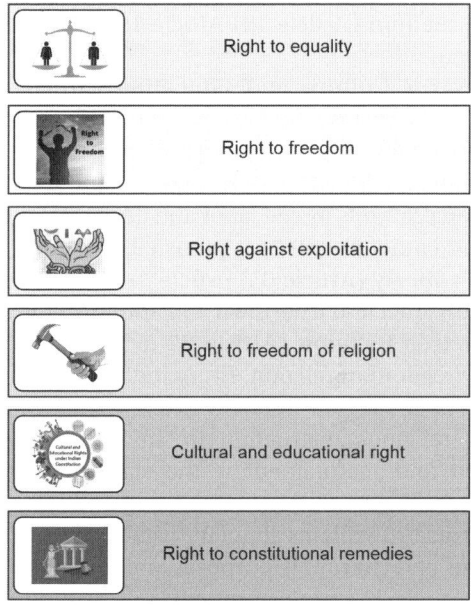

Fundamental Rights of Women

The privileges granted to women by the Constitution of India are as follows:

- **Equality before law:** Prohibition of discrimination on grounds of religion, race, caste and gender.
- **Equality of opportunity**: Equality of opportunity in matters of public employment and prohibition of discrimination on grounds of sex.
- **Humane conditions at work**: Directs the state to make provision for securing justice and humane conditions of work and for maternity relief.
- **Fundamental duty**: Enjoins upon every citizen to renounce practices derogatory to the dignity of women.
- **Reservation of seats for women in panchayats and municipalities**: Provides for reservation of not less than one-

third the total number of seats in panchayats and municipalities for women to be allotted by rotation to different constituencies.
- **Voting rights/electoral law**: Reservation of seats for women in municipalities is provided. The office of the chairperson in the panchayat at the village or any other level shall be reserved for SCs, STs and women.

Fundamental Rights of Children

- **Right to free and compulsory elementary education** for all children in the 6 to 14 years age group (Article 21A).
- **Right to be protected** from being abused and forced by economic necessity to enter occupations unsuited to their age or strength (Article 39).
- **Right to equal opportunities** and facilities to develop in a healthy manner and in conditions of freedom and dignity and guaranteed protection of childhood and youth against exploitation and against moral and material abandonment (Article 39).
- The **right to an identity** (Article 7 &8): Children are entitled to a name, legally registered with the government and a nationality. This ensures national support as well as access to social services.
- The **right to health** (Article 23 & 24): It includes medical care, nutrition, protection from harmful habits and safe working environments.
- The **right to education** (Article 28): Right to free primary education in safe and healthy environment to nurture child's physiological development.

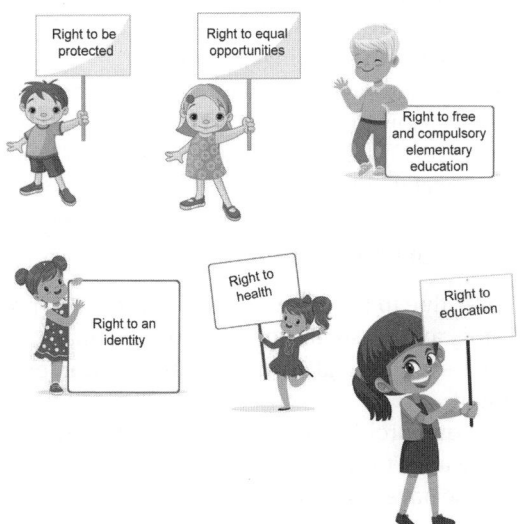

SOCIAL PROBLEMS

Social problems are the conditions threatening the well-being of society. Social problems are the result of the failure of a society to adopt its social institutions and culture to its growing needs.

Social problems are behavior pattern or conditions that are considered objectionable or undesirable by many members of a society.

With the increase in number of social problems the society cannot work smoothly or social progress is hampered/hindered and social disorganization exists.

When an individual or a group of individuals is disorganized and is not functioning according to the norms laid down by the society, the social problems exists.

Definition

According to **Green**: *'A social problem is a set of conditions which are defined as morally wrong by the majority or substantial majority within a society.'*

Nature of Social Problems

- Social problems are situations or conditions which are regarded by society as threats to its established ways or its well-being and therefore, need to be eliminated.
- Social situations are deplored by many people.
- Social problems are symptoms of social maladjustment. These cause dissatisfaction suffering and misery.
- Societies are not always harmonious. They face one another with hostility and suspicion.
- Therefore several cases of maladjustment and unadjustment present themselves in society.

Causes of Social Problems

No problems is due to a single or simple cause. Each problem has a complex history and is usually not due to one but many causes, which are sometimes even difficult to determine, e.g. war, poverty, crime, unemployment.

Sometimes one problem is interwoven with other problems that it cannot solve a part from them, e.g. to control crime, first control poverty, likewise poverty cannot be there without solving the problem of illiteracy.

A problem may be due to combination of biological, physical, mental, and cultural factors or any of them. No hard and fast rule can be laid down about the causes of social problems. However, social problems may affect different people in different way.

Classification of Social Problems

1. *Economic causes:* Poverty, unemployment, dependency, etc.
2. *Biological causes:* Physical diseases, physical defects.
   - *Bio-psychological causes:* Neurosis, psychoses, epilepsy, feeble-mindedness, suicide, alcoholism.
   - *Culture causes:* Aged, homeless, wounded, divorce, illegitimacy, juvenile delinquency.
- The causes of each social problems lie not in one source but in many sources and, therefore, to find an adequate solution to a problem it is necessary to investigate all the causes.
- Individual problems become social problems when they affect a large number of people amounting to a threat to the welfare or safety of the whole group. But all the individual problems are not social problems.
- Poverty, crime and disease are the common social problems.
- Many public health problems are social problems and vice versa.
- Narcotic addiction, alcoholism, venereal diseases and mental illness are both public health and social problems.

POVERTY

Poverty is the condition in which a person, either because of inadequate income or unwise expenditure, does not maintain a scale of living high enough to provide for his physical and mental efficiency and to enable him and his physical and mental natural dependents to function usefully according to the standards of the society in which he is a member.

Absolute poverty: It is one in which a person in not able to maintain a minimum decent standard of living or individuality poverty.

In a particular region or nation, if the resources available are not sufficient to meet the barest need of the people, then we call the entire people living in the region or nation as poor. Sometimes due to the failure of crops, industrial unrest, economic depression or for any other reason, the overall economic activities are at lowest ebb and the standard of living is shortly come down. This type of poor levels for living for a group is called *cyclic poverty*.

Poverty of an individual, not causes, either by the resources or levels of economic activity may be called individual poverty.

Poverty is a foremost problem, especially in the rural areas of India and other developing and underdeveloped countries. It basically depends on the economic status of the people. Poverty is a major problem leading to the sickness of people, personal, family and community disorganization.

Definition

According to **Gillin** and **Gillin:** Poverty is 'a condition in which a person either because of inadequate income or unwise expenditures does not maintain a scale of living high enough to provide for his mental and physical efficiency and to enable him and his natural dependents to function usually according to the standards of a society of which he is a member.'

Causes of Poverty

The major cause of poverty can be discussed under the following headways:

Physical Factors

Physical weakness or sickness like malaria, tuberculosis and other disease or physical handicapped can lead to decrease in income. Therefore physical illness, hereditary or accidents may cause or lead to poverty:

- Smoking, alcoholism, which is highly injurious to health, can lead to poverty by means of over-expenditure.
- Death of bread winner, the loss of life of the bread winner of the family lead the family to become poor.

Psychological Factors

Mental diseases and disability like autism and schizophrenia makes the person incapable of doing work. This affects the economic status of the person by decreasing his income.

Geographical Factors

- **Natural calamities:** Poverty may be caused due to floods, drought, famines, earthquake, tsunamis, etc. where there is a massive destruction of properties.

- **Destruction and lack of natural resources:** Destruction and lack of natural resources due to the improper usage of water and other natural products makes the country poor.
- **Adverse climate and weather:** The production of agriculture and industries depends on the weather and climatic conditions. Unfavorable weather and climate results in the decreased production which in term leads to low per capita income of the country.

Economic Factors

- **Agriculture:** Lack of high yield variety seeds, fertilizers, pesticides and insecticides, lack of tools and machines, absence of irrigation, landlessness, etc. lead to poor agricultural production, ultimately it result in poverty.
- **Unequal distribution:** Even though there is adequate production, unequal distribution of wealth and property leaves in poverty.
- **Unemployment and under development:** Rapid increase in population results in unemployment and underemployment. This affects this means of wages and income lands up in poverty.
- **Extravagancy:** Unnecessary expenditure for the occasion of festival, marriages, birthday and other social and religious functions may to poverty.

Social Factors

- **Types of family:** People living in joint families are at risk of developing 'home sickness'. So they will be unwillingly for job and studies. Thus unemployment occurs and farther ends in poverty. Also, in large families, the parents are not able to fulfill the needs of their all child due to poverty.
- **Traditions and customs:** Certain customs and traditions practiced in some of the societies also contribute to the poverty in the country, e.g. dowry system.
- **Caste system:** Vertical mobilization is not possible in caste system. The people belonging to a particular caste are supposed to do their traditional occupation. Since they cannot take up other jobs, they cannot improve their economic status, further leading to poverty.
- **Illiteracy and ignorance:** Poverty, illiteracy and ignorance are always interrelated. Due to poverty, the person becomes illiterate and ignorant. Simultaneously illiterate person is not able to earn more and finally lands up in poverty.

- **Overpopulation:** Overpopulation increases the demand of the society. Society has limited resources, whenever the demand is more, there will be a shortage of resources.
- **Religious concepts:** Some people believe that certain past of their wealth should be donated to their religion. Some feel satisfied when they are able to spend their earnings for their religions. At the same time, some believe that it is their fate to become poor. All these factors can contribute to poverty.
- **Lack of proper guidance:** Lack of proper guidance to the youth in choosing their profession causes unemployment and leads to poverty.
- **Improper health care delivery:** The health care services are mostly concentrated in urban areas. Whereas, in rural areas where more than 70% people live, are not able to reach these health services. Therefore, the diseases are not treated which may cause many disabilities and ultimately leading to poverty.

Political Factors

- **Improper organization of the government:** The economic planning of the government should be based on all types of citizens in a country. All the citizens in a country should be affordable for at least their fundamental needs. Financial planning and budgeting should not be done by the external forces. Problems like corruption and exploitation also lead the country to become poor.
- **War:** Due to war, the fertile land were destroyed. It also caused the total destruction of wealth and natural resources, which made the countries to land up in the poverty.

Measurement of Poverty

Poverty is measured to find the availability of goods that is to be consumed for the particular year.

The tools used for the measurement of poverty are the following:
- **Natural income:** It is the sum total of all income of the people in a country.
- **Net national product (NNP):** It is the total economic activity along with the net income from abroad in a particular time period.
- **Gross national product (GNP):** It is the value of output of goods produced by a nation during a particular period of time.
- **Per capita income:** It is the maintenance for a person in a country in a year. When the population of a country increases, the per

capita income of the country decreases. Therefore, the population is inversely proportional to the per capita income of the country.

Elimination of Poverty

Measures to be taken to control and eliminate poverty as follows:

- **Improvement in agricultural fields:** Provision of high yield variety (HYV) of seeds, adequate irrigation facilities, improvement in farming animal husbandry and poultry, redistribution of land, development of small scale and cottage industries are required to eliminate poverty.
- **Rehabilitation:** Rehabilitative services should be given to the people who are physically handicapped so that they can find a way to earn for their livelihood. Training facilities can be given to the family members of the diseased person.
- **Educational facilities:** Facilities for education should be provided for all children in rural areas. Compulsory education should be provided up to secondary level. This enables the youth to have vast outlook toward his or her life.
- **Health education:** Health education can be given to the people who love the unhealthy habits like smoking, drinking, and chewing tobacco. People should be taught about the harmful effects of smoking and alcoholism. Sex education and education regarding health should be given at the high school level to mould a healthy generation.
- **Family welfare programs:** It helps in preventing all unwanted births and reduces the overpopulation. Therefore, these programs should be implemented in rural areas for the betterment of country.
- **Equal distribution of health services:** Since a large percent of population in our country is in rural areas, more number of health centers, clinics and hospitals should be started in the rural and remote areas. The health care facilities should be increased in rural areas to improve health status of people.
- **Fixing minimal wages:** Minimal wages, should be fixed for all laborers, which can try to improve the living standards of the people.
- **Protection of natural resources:** Natural resources like water, minerals, land, and trees should not be wasted. The shortage of natural resources occurs if they are not properly used. Nationwide education should be given about conservation of natural resources.

- **Implementation of social security schemes:** Social security schemes like old age pensions, unemployment allowance, and allowance for handicapped, sickness assistance insurance should be provided to all people. Even in rural areas.
- **Improve the marketing facilities:** The marketing facilities should be improved and reasonable price should be given for the laborers for the production.
- **Provision of relief fund in disasters:** During the disasters or natural calamities, relief fund should be provided for the destitute, immediate measures should be taken to rebuild or renew the area affected.
- **Electrification:** Electricity and safe water should be supplied adequately to the rural areas. This improve the irrigation facilities for the farms.

HOUSING

Food, shelter and clothing are the fundamental needs of all individuals. Human beings organize their shelter in the form of houses. The ward households so much importance in an individual's life.

Definition

According to **WHO**: Housing can be defined as *'The physical structure that man uses and the environs of the structure including all necessary services, facilities, equipment and devices needed or desired for the physical and mental health and the social well-being of the family and the individuals.'*

Importance of House in Social Life

House is playing an important role in the social life. Housing has some goals in the society and at the same time it has to meet the needs of the individual.

Shelter: Housing provides a shelter to the individuals, which is the basic need of him.

Family life: House provides adequate space for family life and related activities like preparation of food, storage of food, sleeping for individual and to meet other basic needs.

Protection: Good housing provides protection from accidents, like fire hazards, electricity, poor flooring, etc.

Participation of family in community life: Family is the basic unit of community or society. Community is important to family in many ways like offers help in time of need.

Stability of economic status: Housing plays a form of investment of personal savings. It provides an economic stability and wellbeing to the family.

Health of the individual: Good housing, adequate water supply and adequate sewage disposal, etc. are the basic things to maintain the health status of the individual. A good housing prevents the spread of communicable diseases.

Accessibility to the community facilities: Some of the aim of housing is the accessibility to the community facilities like schools, shopping areas, worship places, health and other services.

Causes of Poor Housing

Poor housing is the result of a great number of causes. Most of the poor housing is present in the urban area. In cities the many people are living in a single room only.

- **Population explosion and industrialization:** Population explosion and industrialization made the people to migrate into the cities from villages. Because of the glittering nature of cities the migration is more nowadays, which results in over- population in the cities and hence the housing become a serious problem in the urban areas.
- **Proportion of population and house:** Number of houses per population is very less in the societies, especially in the cities, because of migration, the population is exceeded but the number of houses remains the same. New comer have to adjust in one room or two rooms. Thus the housing become a great problem.

Construction of houses in the cities become rapid, and in this case no attention is paid to health, privacy and other basic needs. The recommended standards of housing has become reduced and ultimately the houses become small in size and multi-storey. The people have to live in these unhealthy houses, because of the shortage of houses.

Standards of Housing

The standards of housing in India are the following:
- The site of the house should be elevated, free from nuisance and breeding places of mosquitoes and flies. It should have an access to the street.

- The house should be built in an open space.
- The floors should be pucca, smooth, impermeable and should not have any cracks or crevices.
- The walls should be smooth, resistible to weather and strong.
- Roof should be low heat transmittable.
- The number of rooms should be two or more than that in one room should be closed.
- The floor area per person, should be at least 50 sq ft and up to 100 sq ft.
- The room should provide adequate air space of at least 500 cu.ft per capita.
- One room should be provided with at least two windows. In that one should open towards the open space. Doors and windows should be at least two fifth of floor area.
- The house should have adequate lighting.
- Each house should have adequate kitchen and it should have adequate lighting.
- The house should have proper facilities for bathing and washing.
- The house should have safe and adequate water supply.
- Every house should have a sanitary privacy and the refuse should be removed at least daily from the dwelling and it should be disposed in a sanitary manner.
- Sanitary well should be there within half kilometer of area.
- Cattle shed should be at least 25 feet away from the house.
- House should provide safety from fire and other accidents.

Housing Problem in India

Housing became a major problem in both rural and urban areas in India. The attention should be given both to the quantity and quality of housing. India is still gapping with unmet basic housing needs of hundreds of thousands of citizens.

There were 0.9 million homeless people in urban India [Census 2011], in addition to a slum population of roughly 65 million (or 17% of urban India). People from India's rural areas, home to 833 million people, are migrating in large numbers to urban centres. As such, housing has gained paramount importance in government policies and private investments. Housing remains the biggest driver of economic growth with strong forward and backward linkages. Increasing the supply and quality of housing has a multiplier effect on the economy by boosting the primary sector (raw materials), manufacturing sector (construction materials) and the service sector (architects and engineers, skilled labours, banking and finance).

Governmental Approach to Overcome Housing Problems

House for All Project

Under this project the government targets to build, 20 lakh houses per year. According to the urban and rural shortage ratio (65:35) the project also changes its aim. That is out of this 20 lakhs houses they planned to build 13 lakh houses in rural and 7 lakhs in urban areas.

Indira Awas Yojana

The Indira Awas Yojana (IAY) was started in the year 1985-86 as part of Rural Landless, Employment Guarantee program. Under this program houses are allotted to the schedule castes and schedule tribe families. The houses will have one room, kitchen, attached with latrine, bathroom and smokeless chulha.

Subsidized Industrial Housing Scheme

The main objective of this scheme is to provide houses to the laborers. Under this scheme, the laborers will get housing loan at an extent of 65% co-operative societies, state government and urban housing boards are helping for the construction of the houses.

Low Income Group Housing Scheme

It was started in the year 1954, the person who has the annual income of at least 6000/- will get loan up to 80% for the construction of houses. The local bodies and co-operative bodies provides this loan.

Middle Income Group Housing Scheme

Based on this scheme, the people obtain loans from the LIC and various housing boards and societies for the construction of houses. It mainly focuses on the middle income group.

Slum Clearance Scheme

This scheme was adopted in the year 1956 by the Government of India, in order to provide financial assistance to state government and local bodies for improving the slum areas. Under this scheme both long term and short term schemes were started. But the implementation of this scheme is very low.

The Rental Housing Scheme

This scheme was launched in the year 1959, the main objective of this scheme, is the provision of houses or rent to the government employees. Under this, LIC and other financial loans are available and it can be payable in the next 10 to 20 years.

Land Acquisition and Development Schemes

Nowadays land values are high. It is very high in the urban and development area. The lower class and middle class people are not affordable for the lands to construct the houses. Land acquisition and developmental schemes was established in order to help the lower and middle class people. In this scheme, the state government could acquire land a suitable places and sell to the required people at reasonable price.

National Housing Policy

It has been launched in the year 1994, under this policy, houses are constructed for all income groups in the society by the housing society boards of states.

National Housing Bank, HUDCO, HDFC, SBI, ICICI and other Banks are giving housing loans. Also the government has given concession in income tax for encouraging the construction of houses. Due to lack of resources now the government invites the co-operative of private sectors, cooperative and NGO's for solving the magnitude of this housing problem

It is estimated that around 109.35 lakhs houses were likely to be built by the end of 9th five year plan. Also it is estimated that there will be possible shortage of 78.71 lakhs houses at the end of the five year plan.

Pradhan Mantri Awas Yojana (PMAY)

The government of India has a theme 'Housing for All by 2022. To achieve it, it has introduced the Pradhan Mantri Awas Yojana (PMAY) scheme. PMAY is a Central government affordable housing scheme for Lower Income Groups (LIG) and Economically Weaker Sections (EWS) and Middle Income Group (MIG) consumers. Take a look at the PMAY scheme both urban and rural.

ILLITERACY

Definition

Illiteracy can be defined as 'the inability to meet a certain minimum criterion of reading and writing skill.'

UN defines the illiteracy as *'the inability to read and write a simple message in any language.'*

Illiterate: It is a person over 10 years of age who is unable to read and write in any language.

Causes of Illiteracy

Illiteracy is not caused by a lack of intelligence. It is often a result of outside factor. The common causes include the following:

Poverty

Illiteracy is closely related to poverty that means the people under poverty line are commonly illiterates. The poor parents will not allow the children to go for education. Instead of that they will encourage them to go for work in order to meet their basic need such as food.

Because of this reason the people coming under poverty line will become illiterate.

Social Backwardness

Illiteracy is also related to social backwardness.

A large section of people belonging to schedule caste and schedule tribes are illiterate. These backward classes will be economically poor or will come under poverty.

Poverty and lack of knowledge regarding importance of education will make the parents to keep their children in the home itself.

Lack of Literacy within the Family

It is one of the major factors in the formation of illiterate in the society. If the parents are illiterate, they may not be knowing the importance of education. Here the parents will train the child in the traditional occupation, because they are having the feeling that some body should be there to follow the tradition after death.

Learning Disabilities

Some of the people will have some learning disabilities like short-term memory, difficulties, low IQ, physical disabilities, etc.

Even though the parents are willing to send their children for education or the children are not having interest in studies, they may not be able to achieve their goal because of their disability.

It is a known fact that number of children even if willing cannot go to school for various reasons and compulsion. These reasons may be non-availability of schools near residence, children, engaged in work (domestic chores like fetching water) attending to siblings, children dropped out from schools at one stage, and girls unable to attend school due to social conditions.

Importance of Education

- Education is the crucial element in social and economic development.
- World is moving very fast in science and technology developments. So our India is facing both external and internal challenges of development. And it is clear that education is the most effective instrument to meet challenges.
- Education is one of the most important prerequisites not only for successful working of a democratic system but also to achieve the goals of personal, social, political and cultural developments.
- Literacy is not merely mastering the art of reading and writing. It gives people self-confidence and strength.
- Literacy empowers the people with skills for productive work and above all a capacity to make decision, which is an important requirements for meaningful participating democracy.

Effects of Illiteracy

- Illiteracy keeps the people economically backward and also socially and politically unaware.
- The illiterates remain available for exploitation by caste, community and such traditional sentiments in elections and other social political activities.
- Illiteracy leads to the excessive population growth.
- Illiteracy results in the unemployment a major social problem in the society.
- Illiteracy can cause highest mortality rate because of unawareness of the spread of communicable diseases.
- An illiterate can be easily cheatable by others.
- Illiteracy makes the people to involve in various antisocial activities.

Interventions to Overcome Illiteracy

- National Policy on Education (NPE-1986) and the program of Action (POA-1992), envisages the provision of free and compulsory education to all children up to the age of 14 years before commencement of 21st century.

- The NPE emphasized two aspects of elementary education:
  - Universal enrolment and retention of children up to 14 years of age.
  - A substantial improvement in the quality of education.
- The government has allotted more funds in the field of education, in order to fulfill the commitment made by the government.
- Plan outlay of education increases from ₹153 crore in the first five year plan to ₹ 2038.64 crore in the 9th five year plan.
- Expenditure on education as percentage of GDP also rise from 0.7% in 1951-52 to 64.5% in 1999-2000. March 2002 budget allotted 3.8% GDP to education.
- Eighth five year plan has involved in various educational activities. As a result of that, more than 95% country's rural population has primary schools within one kilometer and 85% have upper primary schools within 3 kilometer.

  As a Result:
  - Enrolment of children 6-14 years of age in primary and upper primary school has gone up steadily to 87 and 50 percent respectively.
  - Significant improvements have taken place in enrolment of girls and SC and STs.
  - Number of upper primary and primary schools has gone from 2.23 lakh in 1950-51 to 7.75 lakh in 1996-97.
- Government has started various schemes to eradicate the illiteracy. They are:
  - District Primary Education Program (DPEP) initiative.
  - National program of nutritional support to primary education (Mid-day Meal Program 1995).
  - Operation blackboard.
  - National literacy mission.
- District Primary Education Program (DPEP) launched in the year 1994 as a major initiative to achieve the objectives.
- The Mid-Day Meal Program was started on 15th August 1995. It is aimed at improving enrollment, attendance and retention while simultaneously impacting on the nutritional status of students in primary classes. This program envisages provision of cooked meals for children studying in classes' I-V in all government, local body and government aided primary schools.
- Operation blackboard scheme launched in 1987-88 with a view to bringing about substantial improvement in primary school. This scheme has three components:

a. Provision of at least two all-weather rooms
b. Provisions of at least two teacher, one of them preferable woman.
c. Provisions of essential teaching and learning material including blackboards, maps, charts and small library toys, etc.

- Department of education has started 1979–1980, the program of non-formal education to provide elementary education into like children, those who are unable to attend the schools.
- National literacy mission was setup on May 1998, to impact a new scene of urgency and seriousness of adult education. Literacy campaign is taken as the dominant strategy for education of illiteracy.
- A special program for women was launched in 1989. It is called Mahila Samakhya (education for women quality). This program aims of creating an environment for women to seek knowledge and information with a view to bringing about a change in their perception about themselves and that of the society.
- Literacy in India was started to create awareness and strategies in the importance of education for the under privileged children and youth.
- Sarva Shiksha Abhiyaan (SSA-2003) is an effort to universalize elementary education by community ownership of the school system
- New India Literacy Programme, the objectives of the scheme is to impart not only foundational literacy and numeracy but also to cover other components which are necessary for a citizen of 21st century such as critical life skills, vocational skills development, basic education and continuing education

PROSTITUTION

Prostitution is an ancient social evil and is more common in urban areas. Prostitution is considered as one of the oldest professions.

Definition

Prostitution is the sale of sexual service. A person selling sexual services is a prostitute. Some of the definition for prostitution are as follows:

According to **Elliott** and **Merrill,** *'Prostitution involve illicit sex union on a promiscuous and necessary basis with accompanying emotional difference.'*

A prostitute may be defined as: An individual male or female who for some kind of reward (monetary or otherwise) or for some other form of personal satisfaction and a part or full time profession, engages in normal or abnormal sexual intercourse with various persons who may be of the same sex as or the opposite sex to be prostitute.

The **prostitution act** or immoral traffic act passed in India also lays on stress on the above aspects of prostitution.

Thus, four important constituents of prostitution are:
1. Lack of affection or personal interest
2. Mercenary basis, whether cash or in kind
3. Promiscuous sexual relationship and
4. Prostitution is tragedy of women who are illiterate, unfortunate and poor.

Causes of Prostitution

Most of the researchers indicate that majority of sex workers in India work as prostitutes due to lacking resources to support themselves or their children. Some of the major causes of prostitution are as follows:

Poverty

The number of prostitutes increase in poverty. Many people are coming to this profession to earn their livelihood.

Mental Illness

Women, whose intellectual capacity is low, are not able to foresee the dangers that occur in their life. These women can easily be fooled and exploited by others.

The number of rape cases among mentally retarded women is increasing day by day.

Uneducated Women

Many agencies give false promises of good jobs to the uneducated women. Unfortunately these poor women believes those words and finally exploited.

Prestigious Life

Some women who want to lead a prestigious life in the society may enter into this profession. They earn more in society and lead a highly luxurious life.

Over Sexual Desires

Some women who are over sexual in nature enter into this profession to satisfy their sexual drives.

False Hope of Marriage

Girls who are being cheated by the lovers, with false hope of marriage, may also land up in the prostitution.

Religious Factors

Religious practices like devadasi system forces a girl to become prostitute

Devadasi literally meaning female servant of god. In devadasi system a girl reached puberty is dedicated to a deity or a temple.

Types of Prostitution

The various types of prostitution are as follows:

Street Prostitutes

In street prostitutes the prostitute solicits customer while waiting at the street corners or 'walking on the street.' Some girls show their bodies off in poses in adult magazines that portray them as or mimicking prostitutes.

Escort or Out Call Prostitution

In 'escort' prostitution, the act takes place at the customer place of residence or more commonly at his or her hotel room (currently referred as to 'out call' or at the escort place of residence or in the hotel room rented for the occasion by the escort called in call.

This form of prostitution often shelters under the umbrella of the escort agencies, the amount of money that is made by an escort is different depending on race, appearance, age, experience, gender, services rendered and locations.

Sex Tourism

Sex tourism, partially or fully for the purpose of having sex, usually with prostitutes.

Some of the tourists, organize themselves around a number of websites where they boast about their conquests, share photos of their sex partners, discuss tips on finding prostitutes at the best possible rates in foreign countries and how to avoid detection both at home and aboard.

Ritualized Prostitution (The Devadasi System)

Devadasi system is a religious practice in parts of southern India, including Andhra Pradesh, whereby parents marry a daughter to a deity or a temple.

The marriage usually occurs when she reaches puberty. She then acts as a caretaker to the temple and deity she has been devoted to. In recent times, this practice has been used to push girls into prostitution.

Other Classification of Prostitution

Prostitutes can be classified into two major groups.
1. **The overt group:** It includes those who live in brothels.
2. **The clandestine group:** Includes a wide variety of women who enter into sex relationships for mercenary considerations.

Legal Aspect of Prostitution

Many Acts came into action for the prevention of prostitution. It has been started from the year 1923. The Acts are as follows:
1. Preventing of Prostitution Act (1923)
2. Uttar Pradesh Naik Girls Protection Act (1929)
3. The Bombay Devadasi Protection Act (1934)
4. Prevention of Dedication Act (1934)
5. Madras Devadasi Act 1947
6. Suppression of Immoral Traffic in Women and Girls Act (SITA)

The Sex Differences Coming Under Various Legislation in India

- Living on the earnings of prostitute
- Soliciting in the public places for prostitution
- Procuring girls for the sake of prostitution
- Importing girls for prostitution
- Knowingly permitting prostitutes to be in public places for the trade
- Unlawful detention for the sake of prostitution
- Managing or assisting use of premises for the brothel.

The current laws in India that legislate sex workers are fairly ambiguous. It is a system where prostitution is legally allowed to thrive but which attempts to side from the public. The primary law dealing with the status of sex workers is the 1956, law referred to as 'The Immoral Traffic Suppression Act (SITA).' This law came into action throughout India in May 1958.

Prevention and Control of Prostitution

As prostitution is a victim less crime and a labor profession we should take a great effort to prevent and control prostitution.

The measures to be taken to prevent or control the prostitution are given below:

Sex Education

There should be sex education lessons at schools and college levels. Especially the girls should be taught about the danger of sex exploitation.

Educate the individuals and society about the danger of venereal disease consequences of the prostitution. Also educate the youngsters about the self-control at homes and at schools. Encourage people to have a decent family life.

Change of Rigid Social Customs

There are some customs in our society, which always encourage the prostitution like prohibition of widow remarriage, devadasi system and higher demand of dowry.

If we are encouraging the widow remarriage, avoidance of devadasi system and avoidance of dowry system, we can prevent the prostitution at a certain level.

Job Opportunities

Most of the woman who are coming for prostitution are from the low social economic group. Sometimes they will be forced by family members or others to go for this profession, in order to improve their economic status.

Hence we should offer some employment opportunities for these women. It will improve their economic status, and prohibit them to join this profession.

Social Education and Propaganda

These are the improvement measures to fight against this evil.

Awareness should be done among the public regarding the legal aspects of prostitution and encourage the public to report any nuisance in their surrounding areas. Educate the public regarding the hazards of prostitution and the laws.

Others

- Educate the public especially the males to respect women and avoid exploitation of them sexually.
- Adequate implementation of existing legislation against prostitution.

Provision of

- Vocational and moral training facilities for women of lower economic stratum.
- Rescue homes, shelter homes and other facilities should be provided for the poor and destitute women.
- Males should be taught to respect women folk and not exploit them sexually.
- Unhealthy social customs such as devadasi system to be abolished immediately.
- Sex education at school and college levels. Girls should be taught the danger of sex exploitation by males.
- Social education and propaganda also are important measure to fight with this evil.
- A healthy public opinion should be created against illicit sex relations.
- Obscene films and pornographic literature should be immediately banned.
- Legislation against prostitution should be implemented.

Prohibitory measures for Prostitution

- Medical examination of all prostitutes should be conducted frequently.
- Any woman who is infected should be segregated immediately and should not be allowed to receive customers till she is cured.
- Licensing system of prostitutes will be helpful if it is permitted by law. This will facilitate to have constant check over them.
- The medical people who deal with them should be specially trained.
- Sympathetic, efficient, and free care should be provided to the prostitutes because many of them are very poor and helpless.
- Many of the brothels are situated near the market places and industrialization areas. Brothels should be declared illegal.

- Employment of women in hotels and similar institutions should be under close supervision.

Rehabilitation of prostitution

- A very important aspect of prostitution is the rehabilitation of those prostitutes who want to leave their profession.
- Unless unit society welcomes them back, gives shelter, assurance and security, we cannot expect these unfortunate women to leave their ways.
- There should be adequate provisions to train them in some other work, educate them and settle them especially young women.
- The older women should be assisted through social security schemes and free medical assistance.
- If prostitutes have children, they should be cared by the state, especially female children should be protected at least they should not follow the foot steps of their mothers.

FOOD SUPPLIES

The Food and Agriculture Organization (FAO) was formed in 1945 with headquarters in Rome. It was the first United Nation's organization specialized agency created to look after several areas of world cooperation.

The chief aims of FAO are:

- To help nations raise living standards
- To improve nutrition of the people of all countries.
- To increase the efficiency of farming, forestry and fisheries.
- To better the condition of rural people and through all these means, to widen opportunity of all people for productive work.

The FAO's prime concern is the increased production of food to keep pace with the ever growing world population.

The most important aspects of FAO's work is towards assuring that the food is consumed by the people who need it in sufficient quantities and in right proportions to develop and maintain a better state of nutrition throughout the world.

In this context, the FAO has organized a world freedom from hunger campaign (FFHC) in 1960. The main object of the campaign is to control 'malnutrition' and to disseminate information and education.

The FAO is also collaborating with other internal agencies in the Applied Nutrition Program.

The Joint WHO/FAO expert committees have provided the basis for many cooperative activities nutritional surveys, training courses, seminars and the coordination of research programs on brucellosis and other zoo noses.

The Government of India have launched several nutritional programs to tackle major problems of malnutrition prevailing in India. They are:
- Applied Nutrition Program
- School Mid-day Meal Program
- National Goiter Control Program
- Supplementary Feeding Program
- Prophylaxis against anemia
- Vitamin A prophylaxis for the prevention of blindness

Applied Nutrition Program

This project was launched by the Government of India in 1963 with aid from UNICEF, WHO/FAO for improving the nutrition of the nursing mothers means breastfeeding mothers and expectant mothers and children.

Applied Nutrition Program has now become an integral part of the community development program in different state of India.

This program broadly consists of following aspects:
- Production of protective foods such as eggs, fish, milk, vegetables, fruits by the community. Youth and Mahila Mandal are actively associated with the production aspects of the program.
- Consumption of the food especially by the vulnerable section of the population program. Through practical demonstration such as poultry keeping, inland fisheries, kitchen gardens and feeding programs are conducted by the Mahila Mandals.
- Nutrition education: The Applied Nutrition Programs is fundamentally an education program. Through practical demonstration such as poultry keeping, inland fisheries, kitchen gardens and feeding programs the community is educated on the importance of protective foods for good health.
- Mid-day Meal Program (MDMP): The MDMP is also known as school lunch program. This program has been in operation since 1961 throughout the country.

The major objective of the program is to attract more children for admission to schools and retain them so that literacy improvement of children could be brought about.

In formulating mid-day meals for school children the following broad principles should be kept in mind:
- The meal should be supplement and not a substitute to the home diet.

- The meal should supply at least one third of the total energy requirement and half of the protein need.
- The cost of meal should be reasonably low.
- The meal should be such that it can be prepared easily in schools.
- As far as possible, locally available foods should be used, this will reduce the cost of the meal.
- The menu should be frequently changed to avoid monotony.

Community Nutrition Programs

Nutrition Programs in India

Programs	Ministry
Vitamin A prophylaxis program	Ministry of Health and Family Welfare
Prophylaxis against nutritional anemia	Ministry of Health and Family Welfare
Iodine deficiency disorders control program	Ministry of Health and Family Welfare
Special nutrition program	Ministry of Social Welfare
Balanced nutrition program	Ministry of Social Welfare
ICDS program	Ministry of Social Welfare
Midday meal program	Ministry of Human Resource Development

Vitamin 'A' Prophylaxis

One of the component of the national program for the control of blindness is to administrate a single massive dose of vitamin 'A' daily.

Preparation orally to all preschool children in the community every six months through peripheral health workers.

An evaluation of the program has revealed a significant reduction of vitamin 'A' deficiency in children.

Prophylaxis Against Nutritional Anemia

The program consists of distribution of iron and folic acid tablets to pregnant women and young children (1–12 years).

Mother and child health centers in rural areas and ICDS projects are engaged in the implementation of this program.

The technology for the control of anemia has also been developed at the national institute of nutrition at Hyderabad.

Control of Iodine Deficiency Disorders

Nearly 145 million people estimated to be living in known goiter endemic areas in the country.

The National Goiter Control Program was launched by the Government of India in 1962 in the conventional goiter belt in the Himalayan region with the objective of identification of the goiter endemic areas to supply. Iodized salt in place of common salt and to assess the impact of goiter control measures over a period of time.

The iodine deficiency disorder (IDD) control program was mounted in 1986 with objective to replace the entire edible salt by iodine salt, in a phased manner by 1992.

Special Nutrition Program

This program was started in 1970 for the nutritional benefit of children below six years of age, pregnant and nursing mothers and is in operation in urban slums, tribal areas and backward rural areas.

The supplementary food supplies about 300 kcal and 10-12 gram of protein per child per day. The beneficiary mothers receive daily 500 kcal and 25 grams of protein. This supplement food is provided to them for about 300 days in a year.

This program was originally launched as a central program and was transferred to the state, sector in the fifth five year plan as part of the minimum needs program.

The main aim of the Special Nutrition Program is to improve the nutritional status of the target groups. This program is gradually being merged into ICDS program.

Balwadi Nutritional Program

This program was started in 1970 for the benefit of children in the age group 3-6 years in rural areas. It is under the overall change of the Department of Social Welfare.

Four national level organizations including the Indian Council of Child Welfare (ICCW) are given grant to implement the program.

This program is implemented through Balwadis which will provide preparatory education to these children. The food supplement provides 300 kcal and 10 gram of protein per child.

ICDS Program

Integrated Child Development Services (ICDS) was started in 1975 in pursuance of the national policy for children.

There is strong nutrition component in this program in the form of supplementary nutrition vitamin A prophylaxis and iron and folic acid distribution.

The beneficiaries are preschool children below 6 years, pregnant and lactating mothers.

The ICDS now covers more than 1000 community development blocks and an additional 1000 blocks will be covered during the seventh five year plan.

The state and union territories are encouraged to undertake ICDS projects on the central pattern to cover more beneficiaries.

The workers all the village level who deliver the services are called Anganwadi workers. Each Angawadi workers covers a population of about 1000.

A network of Mahila Mandals has been built up in ICDS project areas to help Anganwadi workers in providing health and nutrition services.

The work for Anganwadi workers is supervised by Mukhya Sevikas.

The field supervision is done by the child development project officer (CDPO).

Kitchen Gardens

Families should be encouraged to plant kitchen gardens. Such gardens should be located (*i*) near to the houses for easy care, (*ii*) near to the source of water, (*iii*) in rich soil, and (*iv*) on a land with gentle slope.

Kitchen gardens not only provide fresh vegetables and fruits but also help in the disposal of kitchen waste water (sullage water) in a hygienic manner. Kitchen garden can help to improve the diet in the family.

VULNERABLE GROUP: ELDERLY, HANDICAPPED, SOCIAL STATUS OF OLD PEOPLE IN INDIA

Elderly

Elderly is a major type of vulnerable groups in the society. Older adulthood begins usually between 60 and 75 years of age. The older adults have to face some special challenges because of great variation in the physiological, cognitive and psychological health status, old people will have reduced ability to stress.

Categorising the Elderly People

These are four categories of elderly people. They are:
Young old: From 65 to 75 years of age
Old: From 75 to 85 years of age
Old old: From 85 to 100 years of age
Elite old: Over 100 years of age.

Problems Faced by the Elderly

As one ages, physical appearance also will change, skin develops wrinkles, hair turns grey, teeth falls, etc. Therefore depression and complain of adjustment problems are developed within self and family.

The major problems faced by the elders are given below:

Retirement

Most of the people after the age of 60 are unemployed. However, some of them who are healthy continue to work on a full or part time basis. Few elders spend more time by resting or sleeping.

Post-retirement days can foster a sense of integrity and despair because of the loneliness and inability to carry out the household needs and their wishes.

Economic problems and economic dependency

The financial needs of elders vary in considerable rate. Problem with the economy are related to the low retirement benefits, lack of pension, plans for many workers are increased length of retirement years. Older women usually have low income than men and will be the poorest one.

Old people, who are having physical and mental disability, usually depend on caregivers or family members. It is important risk factors, which lead to elderly abuse. In general cases, the income becomes limited or fixed, as they are retired from the occupation. It is also a reason for depending on caregivers or family.

Relation

During old age, most of the people experience relocation.

Elders with decreased mobility want living arrangements like all the facilities in one floor and they need more accessible bath room facilities. Sometimes the house may be too large, which makes the elders to move a lot, often this movement is stressful. Some elders would like to go near their children for support and supervision. Some of them may relax to long-term care facilities or nursing homes.

Maintenance of independence and self-esteem

Most of the elders want to have independent. It is important to them, that they wanted to look after themselves even if they have to struggle to do so.

The nurses has to acknowledge the elderly clients ability to think, reason and make decision.

Most elders are willing to listen to suggestion and advice but no one wants to be wandered around.

Perception

Perception is the ability to interpret the environmental stimuli and in commonly depends on the awareness of senses.

In the aging process, senses become impaired. The ability to perceive the environmental stimuli and reaction towards the particular stimuli get diminished. Also the change in the nervous system will affect the perceptual capacity.

Coping ability

Coping ability of the elders changes based on their nature and previous lifestyle. Most of them are not ready to cope up with the situation during the old age. Many won't adapt to the retirement and adjust to the minor ailments.

Health and medical problems

Old age naturally developed with countless health problems physically and mentally. Some common diseases are depression, dementias, Alzheimer's disease, diabetes, hypertension stroke and cancer. Geriatric care is concerned about attending old people illness and giving timely medical treatment.

Social and psychological problems

Old people often feel neglected, marginalized and helpless. Mental disorders in old age are commonly due to loss associated with aging, comprised quality life, socio-economic problem, feeling of loneliness, unworthiness and feeling as burden. These feelings are very harmful for healthy social existence and mental peace of the elderly, leading to increased incidence of psychological disorders in the elderly.

Fear of death and grieving

Well adjusted couple usually thrives for companionship during old age. A great of affection and closeness may develop during this period of aging, together and nurturing each other. When a partner dies, the remaining partner experiences the feeling of loneliness, emptiness, and loss. Most of them are capable of leading their life alone but the reliance in younger family members increases on advancing age and occurrence of ill health.

Tasks to be Fulfilled by the Elders

- Adjust towards the decreased physical strength and health.
- Adjust to the retirement lower and fixed income.
- Adjust to the death of spouse and friends.
- Adjust to the new relationship with children.
- Adjust towards the leisure time.
- Adopt the lonely living.
- Take care of one's own health.
- Keep active and involve in various social activities.
- Safeguard the physical and mental health.
- Remain in touch with family members.
- Find meaning in life.

Intervention to Overcome Problems of Elderly

- Family relationship has to be tightened as a care provider in the society.
- Encourage social services and social support to reduce the stress in family with the dependent elders.
- Involve the status in all social programs to prevent social isolation.
- Establish and encourage the self-help group activites.
- Promote the long-term care facilities in the social institutions.
- Promote the activities of voluntary health organizations to meet the needs of the elderly to get emotional satisfaction, social security and self efficiency.
- Make sure that elders have sufficient income or asset to manage their life.
- Emphasize on empowerment and independence of elderly women.
- Identify the elderly abuse in the society in its early stage.
- Encourage mass media programs to protect the elderly from abuse.
- Provide facilities for the research on elderly.

- Ensure better quality life to the elders.
- Encourage the family members to provide warmth and support to the elders.
- Provide economic security by means of pension, old age allowance, free medical like counselor, guide, etc.
- Encourage counseling and treatment to elders to cope with familial and personal problems.
- Mobilize governmental and non-governmental organizations to strength the welfare services to the elders.

Handicapped

In every society, there are some persons who are handicapped:
- Blind
- Deaf
- Lame

And also who are physically weak owing to chronic ailments such as tuberculosis, leprosy and malaria. There are millions of people in the world and in India living in such handicapped conditions.

It is estimated that there are at least 2 million blind persons in India, and equal number of people may be suffering from other handicaps like deafness and lame.

The handicapped child is one, who deviates from normally, that is physically, mentally and psychologically.

Physically Handicapped

- Blind, deaf, dumb or cleft palate
- Crippled by cerebral palsy and poliomyelitis
- Burns affected
- Children with heart diseases.

Mentally Handicapped

- Feeble minded
- Mentally retarded.

Psychologically Handicapped

- Neglected orphans—deprived and abandoned
- Children deprived of parent's affection
- Maladjustment, delinquent with behavior problems.

Definitions

Handicapped can be defined as 'A person who deviates from normal health status either physically, mentally or sociallly and who require special care treatment and education.'

Because of various reasons a person can become handicapped, it is given below:

Disease/disorder → impairment → disability → handicap.

In case of disease it may be any neurological disorder, accident, etc. when it is explained under accident.

- Disease/disorder is the accident.
- Accident may lead to loss of extremities (impairment)
- Inability to walk or perform daily activities (disability)
- Unemployment or handicap.

Major Types of Handicaps

There are various types of handicaps in our society. The main five types of handicaps are given below:
1. Blindness
2. Deafness/muteness
3. Crippled persons
4. Mentally handicapped
5. Leprosy

Blindness

Blindness is a major form of handicap and largest proportion in India are suffering in this handicapped.

It is estimated that the blind population is increasing day by day. Lack of vitamin A in the food is responsible for half of the blindness in India.

Other major causes include the inflammatory disease of conjunctiva and corneal cataract. Glaucoma, malnutrition, syphilis, small pox and improper management of eye problems.

The blindness can be prevented if treated early. Other preventive measures include proper diet, vitamins, treatment of minor problems, hygienic habits and maintenance of proper working facilities.

Rehabilitation can be given to the blind people by employing them in cottage industries like basket making, weaving, spinning or other handicrafts. Other jobs like telephone operation, typing and physiotherapy can also them to have and independent income.

Causes

- Vitamin A deficiency in food.
- Inflammatory disease of conjunctiva and cornea.
- Cataract, glaucoma, malnutrition, syphilis, gonorrhea, smallpox, poor management of eye diseases.

Medical Measures

- Proper diet—vitamin A rich foods like fruits, papaya, carrot, yellow pumpkin, etc.
- Vitamin supplementation through syrup and other medicines.
- Treatment of minor problems from time to time.
- Hygienic habits.
- Maintenance of proper working facilities.

Rehabilitative Measures

- The blind people are given proper training in jobs like telephone operation.
- Typing, physiotherapy, cottage industries basket making, canning of chair, weaving, knitting, spinning and other handicrafts.
- India there are few centers where such training is given to blind people and also education can be provided through brail language.

Deafness/Muteness

Deafness is completely related to the hearing when a person is deaf he will not be able to develop the communication skills. The various reasons responsible for the deafness are otitis media, congenital defects, acute ear infection, congenital syphilis, malaria, mumps and cerebrospinal meningitis.

Early detection and treatment of ear infection can prevent the deafness with an effective training and guidance, the deaf can develop the communication skills. This handicappedness is related to sense of hearing.

When the child cannot hear because of deafness, he does not speak too.

Preventive Measures

- Proper care of ear aliments.
- For deaf proper training can be helped to develop the capacity to speak.

Crippled Persons

There are number of crippled people in our India. Various reasons are responsible for the crippling.

Some of the causes are congenital abnormalities, rickets, poliomyelitis, paralysis, accidents, arthritis, cerebral palsy, and tuberculosis of bones and joints.

Poliomyelitis is the major cause of crippling in India, it can be prevented by the administration of vaccine.

In India most of the crippled persons are engaged in the begging profession. By the provision of proper guidance, training and assistance crippled person can lead their independent life in the society. At a certain level he can fulfill his responsibilities towards the family. Even for crippled, no statistics were available but a large number of crippled adults and children are present in rural and urban areas.

Causes

The reason for crippling may be varied:
- Congenital anomaly, rickets, poliomyelitis, cerebral palsy, other form of paralysis, arthritis, accidents, TB bones and joints, etc.

Poliomyelitis is the most common cause of crippling in India. The dreadful and serious disability disease handicap can be easily prevented by family administration of vaccine, i.e. Polio vaccine orally.

Preventive Measures

- Most of the crippled persons are engaged in begging profession in India.
- With proper training, guidance, and assistance they can be helped as an independent person and also respected by others.
- To fulfill his/her responsibilities towards his family and community, those must be given a combination of medical, educational, social and vocational services work together as a team.

Mental Problems

Mental problems may be broadly classified into
1. Mental disorders
2. Mental deficiency

Mentally Handicapped

Mentally handicapped are more common in our country.

The mental problem can result from either mental disorder or mental deficiency. The causes of mental problems include hereditary congenital defects, organics neurometabolic disorders, perinatal complications, premature births and accidents.

Treatment of congenital mental deficiencies is very difficult. Most of the treatment facilities are absent in the mental hospitals in our country. Only the violent and aggressive patients are admitted to the hospitals.

Moreover that the uneducated and rural population believes that mental disorders are the result of demonical possession of God's curse, so they take the patients to the religious places or quacks to get rid from the demons.

In developed countries like Europe and America proper facilities are provided to take care of the mentally handicapped people.

Causes

These may be caused by birth injuries, congenital defects, or accidents, growth retardation, environmental causes, psychological disorders.

These patients are so ill looked and even death is common because of severe illness. These clients have social stigma and no need of admission unless they are violent and unmanageable. Exploitation is common in these cases.

The children with idiots, imbeciles and feeble mindedness and placed in foster homes or any other institutions. Arrangement of proper education and suitable employment like farm work, domestic services, etc. are useful.

Preventive Measures

Proper care and management, happy and healthy living conditions, control of population, family counseling and education, education of preventive diseases, sex and family life education, education about hazards of consanguineous marriages.

Leprosy

Leprosy is a disease as old as human society. India has approximately one million leprosy patients. Leprosy spread fastly. Most of the lappers are engaged in begging occupation.

The main causes of these diseases are poor living conditions, overcrowding, malnutrition and ignorance regarding mode of transmission.

In order to prevent the spread of leprosy it is important that infectious cases should be identified early and isolated them.

Today the treatment facilities are available in most of the hospital and it can be treated effectively and deformities are corrected.

Commonly the lepers are reflected by the family and thrown into the society. So education must be given to public regarding cause and spread of the disease, and include the family in the rehabilitation of lepers after the cure from leprosy.

Causes

Poor living conditions, malnourishment, overcrowding, prolonged drought conditions, ignorance of contamination and spread of disease.

Preventive Measures

- Infectious cases should be identified and isolated
- Proper education of public about the cause and spread of disease
- Lepers who are cured can be rehabilitated with the cooperation of the family
- Occupational therapy
- Physical therapy and special exercises.

MINORITY GROUPS AND OTHER MARGINALIZED GROUPS

Minority groups are other marginalized groups.

Definition

A minority group is a group of people who, because of their physical or cultural characteristics are singled out from the others in the society in which they live for differential and unequal treatment, and who therefore regard themselves as objects of collective discrimination.

—**Louis Wirth (Sociologist)**

Types of Minority Groups

There are various groups of minorities in the world. They include the following:

Racial or Ethnic Minorities

Every large society contains minorities. They may be migrant, indigenous or landless nomadic communities, but in some places subordinate ethnic groups may constitute a numerical majority, e.g. Blacks in South Africa under apartheid. International law can protect the rights of racial or ethnic minorities in a number of ways.

Gender and Sexual Minorities

The number of men and women are roughly equal in most societies, the status of women as a subordinate group has led some to equate them with minorities. In addition, various gender variant people can be seen as constituting a minority group or groups such as inter-sexual, transsexual and gender non-conformities.

Age Minorities

The elderly have in the modern age usually been reduced to the minority role of economically non-active group. Children can also be understood as a minority group and the discrimination faced by both young and the elderly is known as ageism.

Disabled Minorities

The disability rights movement has contributed to an understanding of disabled people as minority or a coalition of minorities who are disadvantaged by society. The deaf community is often regarded as a linguistic and cultural minority rather than a disabled and some deaf people do not see themselves as disabled at all.

Religious Minorities

It is one of the largest minorities present all over the world. Various religious minorities are present in our India. Much discrimination is faced by these religious minorities.

Religious Minorities in India

Following are the religious minorities in India:

Muslim

The Muslim population in India numbering million constituting 14% of the total population forms the largest minority in India. Muslims are the biggest minority group in India, accounting for 142 persons in every 1,000.

The feeling of insecurity, an aftermaths of partition, lingers on, strengthened each time when there is a communal orgy everywhere.

Muslims are inadequately represented in the various government services. In government offices Muslims representation is less than 5 percent. In the recruitment for jobs in foreign countries muslim doctors and engineers representation is below 2 percent.

Literacy rate among the Muslims is very low. Muslim literacy is less than half of other communities.

Governments have allowed minority communities to run their own institutions without hindrance.

Christians

The Christians form the second largest minority community in India with 28 million (2.3%) of the total population. They made a remarkable contribution in the field of education, health and social services.

Christians have chain of schools, colleges and hospitals.

All hospitals in India depend largely on Christian girls from Kerala for their nursing staff.

Whenever some part of India is hit by flood or some kind of natural disaster Christian association's aid to the victim and organize relief work. Christian educational activities are more prominent.

Christian enterprise in Kerala was largely responsible for producing the highest literacy rate in India twice as high as that of neighboring states. Among Christians a majority of whom are roman catholic constitute 22 percent of Kerala population.

The Christian missionaries established printing press and spread knowledge. Many of them mastered Indian languages, spoke and wrote in them.

Even the English language was regarded by them as a Christian tongue. The problems of the Indian Christians are many and varied. Major problems of the community are the right to propagate religion and the missionary activities.

It is generally alleged by the Hindu communal group that the missionaries indulge in conversions, through their education, medical and social service activities.

Sikhs

The Sikhs form the third largest religious minority in India with 20.8 million people (1.7 percent of the total population).

The undivided Punjab, the proportion of the Sikh population was 33.33 percent only after the re-organization of the state, it rose to 60.22 percent almost the double.

The Akali Dal a major political party of the Sikh community, February 1948 demanded a separate Punjabi sabha under the leadership of late master Tara Singh.

Since recognition of Punjab as a separate state, the character of the Sikh community as minority has been drastically changed. It is no longer a minority community in the state.

In spite of the fact that the Sikh community is in minority in all other states and union territories, no case of discrimination has come to light from any quarter, rather are reports and assertions that the community is treated very fairly.

Anglo-Indians

They form a microscopic minority in India with only just 125,000-150,000, living mostly in Kolkatta and Chennai. They have obtained some special safeguards in the constitution of India. The community enjoys political, social, economic safeguards under the constitution of India. It is a racial, religious and linguistically combine minority.

According to Article 330, the Anglo-Indian community have been provided with two seats in the parliament and they are nominated by the president of India.

The community enjoyed special transitory safeguards was in the matters of appointing in the railway, customs, postal and telegraphic services in the union. Thus the community has been given fair treatment.

The community is 100 percent literate and is essential urban.

Frank Anthony the undisputed leading of the Anglo-Indian community, had all praises for the Government of Indian in safeguarding the interest of the Anglo-Indians.

Parsis

In the 7th century AD, groups of Aryans high skinned, curly hair fled their homeland ran to escape religious persecution by muslim invaders and settled down in coastal Gujarat.

Today they constitute an eminent and affluent minority. According to the census of 2011, they constitute 0.006% of country's population nearly 70 percent of the Parsis concentrated in Mumbai alone.

Today this tiny community called the Parsis is being hounded by another one more devastating bio-extinction. There are one and half times more deaths in the community than there are births.

Another major difficulty besetting in the community is the excessively high incidence of intercommunity marriages, conversion to Zoroastrian is disallowed.

Parsis and Jews are the smallest minorities in India. Parsis even though formed the smallest minorities, have not only represented the core of the political struggle in India but have led the economic revolution in India.

The Dadabhai Naoroji is justly and greatful accredited with the first and the earliest inspiration of the cause of swaraj.

Every Indian will point to Jamsetji Tata is the pioneer of India's industrious in various field. He was the first to introduce foreign technology talent in the promotion of industry in India.

The members of the Parsis community are economically well-off and they are predominately urban.

CHILD ABUSE

Child abuse is harm to or neglect of a child by another person. Whether child or adult.

Child abuse happens in all cultural, ethnic and income groups. Abuse can be physical, emotional, verbal, sexual or through neglect. Child abuse may cause serious injury to the child and may even result in death.

Definition

Child abuse can be defined as 'a variety of abnormal, behaviors directed against children. It can take any forms.

Child abuse in general is a psychological problem or perversion of the abuser. The abuser is referred to as the perpetrator of abuse.

Child Abuse Includes the Following Conditions

- Child sexual abuse
- Pedophilia
- Physical abuse
- Child neglect
- Emotional neglect
- Failure to thrive (Munchausen's by Proxy Syndrome).

Predisposing Factors to Child Abuse

- *The Abused childhood:* Child abuse offenders were abused as children.
- *The abuser's substance abuse:* Atleast half of the child abuse case involves some degree of substance abuse alcohol, drug, etc. by the child's parent.
- *Family stress:* The disintegration of nuclear family and its inherent support system has been yield to be associated with child abuse.
- *Social forces:* Experts debate whether a postulated reduction (inherent supports system) in religious moral values coupled with

a increase in the depiction of violence by the entertainment and information media may increase child abuse.
- *The child:* The children at higher risk for child abuse include infants who are felt to be overly fussy, handicapped, children with chronic diseases.

Specific trigger events that occur just before many fetal prenatal hazards an infants and young children include an infants inconsolable crying, feeding difficulties, toddlers failed toilet training and exaggerated parental perceptions of acts of disobedience by the child.

Types of Child Abuse

Child Sexual Abuse

It includes any activity that uses a child to create sexual gratification.

Activities can include any conventional adult sexual activity with a child such as touching the child's genitals or fondling with intention of arousing sexual feelings.

Prolonged kissing, cuddling, French kissing, excessive touching and looking at children either without clothes with the intent to be sexually aroused can be also included.

Other forms of child sexual abuse include exposure of a child to erotic material in the form of live behavior, photographs, film or video.

The collection of any excessive number of photographs of naked children in any pose may draw the attention of law enforcement.

Sexual Abuse

The signs are:
- Child tells you he/she was sexually mistreated.
- Child has physical signs such as:
  - Difficulty in walking or sitting
  - Stains of blood in underwears or garments.
  - Genital or rectal pain, itching, swelling, redness or discharge
  - Bruises or other injuries in the genital or rectal area.
- Child has behavioral and emotional signs such as:
  - Difficulty in eating or sleeping.
  - Soiling or wetting pant or bed after being potty training.
  - Acting like a much younger child.
  - Excessive crying and sadness.
  - Withdrawing from activities and others.
  - Talking about or acting out sexual acts beyond normal sex play for age.

Pedophilia

It is a form of child sexually abuse, is an abnormal interest in children that is based on the intention by the perpetrator to be sexually aroused by children.

Someone with an erotic interest in children may collect material that show a child in sexual poses.

The person who seek interaction with children with the intention of satisfying an erotic or sexual desire or seek a sexual relationship with a child.

Adults who seek actual physical sexual relations with children are the most extreme and deviant of the pedophilia.

Using children to create erotic materials or for erotic acts with other adults is another form of child sexual abuse.

Pedophilia, if not resisted, repressed and treated will result in the most severe legal consequences.

It is imperative that any person who feels sexually attracted to children immediately seeks help from a qualified therapist.

People who use children to create sexual arousal for others are already involved in serious criminal activity.

Physical abuse:

- Physical abuse of children is defined as excessive intentional physical injury to a child or excessive corporal punishment of a child.
- Torture, beatings and assault of children are obvious forms of physical abuse.
- Punishments that leads to marks, that last for more than a few minutes can be interpreted as abuse. The use of any objects to strike a child like belts, peddles, sticks or any other objects (other than open hand) is wrong.
- Excessive physical, discipline is harmful and dangerous to children, young children can be killed by relatively minor acts of physical violence.
- Any severe beating with an object, forceful shaking, submersion in hot water, intentional burning and other forms of intentional infliction of pain are inappropriate and criminal behaviors.

Signs of Physical Child Abuse

- Unexplained or repeated injuries such as belts brusies or burns.
- Unreasonable explanation of the injury.
- Injuries that are in shape of an object like belt-buckle or electric cord.

- Injuries not likely to happen given the age or ability of the child, e.g. broken bones in child too young to walk or climb stairs.
- Disagreement between the child and parents explanation of the injury.
- Neglect of the child like dirty, under nourished in appropriate clothes for weather, lack of medical and dental care, etc.
- Fearful behavior.

Child Neglect

Child neglect in any form, when it concerns a child's welfare, is generally considered to be criminal behavior.

Child neglect is considered as possible diagnosis for children who are poorly cared for, not fed properly, improperly clothed, denied basic necessities, denied proper medical care, or treated with indifference to a degree that appears to cause damage or suffering.

Failure to continue, to get help for a child who is not doing well or who is improperly cared for may be interpreted as another form of neglect.

Emotional Neglect

- Emotional neglect is a condition in which children do not get adequate rebellious behaviors or become alienated from their parents.
- In more severe cases of emotional neglect, especially with babies or very young children, neglect can result in very abnormal behavior such as these:
  - Restlessness
  - Profound detachment from the parents
  - Poor bonding with other people
  - Aggressive or withdrawn behavior
  - Afraid to go home
  - Staying away from physical contact with parents or adults.

These abnormal behaviors in young children continue as they get older and can transform into other personality or mental disorder that can be difficult, if not impossible to treat.

Parents can avoid the consequence of emotional neglect through parental training courses reading and effort.

Failure to Thrive

- Failure to thrive is a condition in which children fail physically to develop together normal full genetic potential. It is caused most

commonly by medical conditions that can result in children not growing as expected.
- ❖ The diagnosis is made when a doctor compares the growth of a child on standard growth charts and looks of changes in the rate of growth of a child.
- ❖ Any decrease in the rate of growth of a child with respect to weight, height or head size will raise concern and force the doctor to consider the diagnosis of failure to thrive.
- ❖ Once failure to thrive is considered, parents must comply with their doctors recommendations regarding testing and any other investigation into child's failure to thrive.

Munchausen Syndrome by Proxy

Munchausen syndrome by proxy (MSBP): This is a serious psychiatric disorder of parents or guardians of children.

The parents or guardians referred to as the perpetrator, intentionally or unintentionally manufactures signs and symptoms of disease in the child they are caring for.

Other Forms/Types of Child Abuse

- ❖ Abandoned infants
- ❖ Non-accidental poisoning
- ❖ Substance abuse, etc.

Characteristics of Child Abuse in Family

- ❖ Abuse can happen in any family, regardless of any special characteristics. However in dealing with parents, be aware of characteristics of families in which abuse may be more likely.
- ❖ Families which are isolated and have no friends, relatives or any other support system like church, temple, mosque, etc.
- ❖ Parents who tell they were abused when they are as children.
- ❖ Parents of alcoholic addiction or drug addiction.
- ❖ Parents who are very critical of their children.
- ❖ Parents who are very rigid and discipline their children.
- ❖ Parents who show too much or too little concern.
- ❖ Who feel that they have a difficult child.
- ❖ Who are under a lot of stress, etc.

Diagnosis

- Through careful history and through examination of child
- Radiological investigations like X-ray, CT scan, ultrasonography, MRI, etc.

Management

- Treat physical injuries appropriately
- General education
- Social awareness
- Improvement of socioeconomic conditions
- Counseling and support of parents and other family members
- Take help from voluntary and social organizations like foster homes, placement in orphanages.
- Rehabilitation of the child in the same family is possible.

Preventing of Child Abuse

- Child abuse is prevented, first through awareness then by early detection and intervention.
- The education of children to recognize in appropriate behaviors and report possible abuse at its earliest behaviors and report possible abuse at its earliest stages to their parents or family will help children avoid being abused.
- Save families from dysfunctional interventions, identify real abusers and help in the identification of family members with abusive tendencies before a criminal act occurs.
- In an ideal world psychiatric help would be available to treat those who abuse children.
- To prevent abuse by changing the behavior of the abuser, tendencies to be abusive must be identified, before any actual takes place.
- Most child sexual abuse will ultimately be discovered and the perpetrator should be prosecute.
- Take care around children at all times to prevent activities that might be constructed as sexual abuse.
- To identify the physical signs of child sexual abuse take the child to the family doctor for examination.

- Children in day care, children cared by others or children who spend time alone with other people are at risk of sexual abuse.
- Change in behavior, including indiscipline problems, fecal soiling, bed wetting, insomnia, nightmares, depression, or other changes in the way a child acts can be sign of sexual abuse.
- Parents should discuss the possible reasons for such changes in behavior with professionals and explore the possibility of child sexual abuse.
- Any person who has been reared in an environment of violence may be more likely to inflict violence on others. Try to suppress their violent tendencies through conscious and diligent effort at all times.
- People who are physically violent generally demonstrate violence against at exalting levels, early interventions is the best strategy to avoid lifelong consequences.

CHILD LABOR

A child is a symbol of joy and his divine smile pleases everyone. Each and every child is an asset of the society and of the nations. Most of the under developed and developing countries are reporting the problems of child labor.

Definition

Any work done by the child in order to economically benefit their families or themselves directly at the cost of their physical, mental and social development.

The International Labor Organization (ILO) convention of 1973 set out a definition of unacceptable child labor which include:
- Dangerous work jeoparding the health safety and morals of children below 14 years of age.
- Normal work for children below 14 years of age.
- Even part time light work below the age of 12 years.

Different Forms of Child Labor

In rural areas the child laborers work in agriculture and cultivation. They will be engaged with non-domestic works.

In urban areas, the children work in market places, street corners as hawkers, shoe shine boys, waiters in restaurants, helpers in shops, carpet weavers, etc.

Factors Contributing to Child Labor

Family Factors

The main causes of child labor includes poverty, parental death, large family with more number of children and father's addiction and debt.

In these circumstances, the socioeconomic status of family will be very low and children will be compelled to go for occupation, in order to meet the basic needs of themselves and their family members. Thus it results in the formation, child laborers.

Child Factors

The factors are basically related to the child himself. They include the poor academic performance repeated failures in examinations, sense of economic independence and repeated birth of female child in the family.

Because of repeated failures and poor academic performance, sometimes children themselves stop their education and they go for employment in order to get the economic independence.

Social Factors

Social factors play another role in child labor.

Social factors include lack of access to schools, poverty, parental illiteracy, attitude of parents that skills more important than education, caste system, lack of child welfare scheme, economic advantage by cheap labor, migration of children from rural area to urban in search of livelihood, etc. may result in child labor.

Because of caste system, the scheduled caste children become laborers in their young age itself, the lower caste child are asked or forced to involve with certain working society members.

The lack of child welfare schemes is also result in child labor.

Hazards or Ill Effects of Child Labor

- ❖ Child labor has a vast number of ill effects on physical, social and psychological health of the victims. Most of the children go to work with inadequate food, clothing and shelter.
- ❖ Child laborers will develop wide range of diseases like diarrhea, viral and bacterial infections, general weakness, etc. Other than this they may prone to develop various occupational injuries also.
- ❖ Most of the children are working in their childhood and adolescent ages, this is the time, where maximum growth occurs, physiological changes takes place and their personality develops. During this time if they are not meeting the nutritional

needs and physiological work is more, they may be at risk of growth retardation, under nourishment, improper personality development.
- Child laborers who develop serious injuries will be treated poorly and it may result in various systemic disease, and permanent handicaps. It can alter their emotional status and they will be maladjusted to the society.
- The child laborers are lacking in their psychological requirements like love, securitry and emotional support from their parents, lack of independence and opportunity for personality development.
- Inadequate rest, sleep and emotional satisfaction may lead them to some of the antisocial activities like stealing, gambling, alcoholism, drug abuse, etc.
- Some of them become the child prostitutes, these children are at high risk to develop veneral diseases like HIV/AIDS.
- Because of their inadequate education, they will not get job opportunities in the future.

Prevention and Control of Child Labor

There are some specific measures given by the National Child Labour Project (NCLP) the main initiative of Government of India, for the prevention of child labor has been given below:
- The employers, who are engaging children for work should be motivated to have gentle and humor attitude towards children. They should provide minimum facilities, which are lacking in the working site.
- The environment and facilities in the work place should be improved.
- Separate area should be given for eating, proper drinking water facilities, toilet and washing area.
- Facilities for health check-up and treatment for medical problems like investigations and referral services should be provided.
- Recreational facilities and rest can be given by the provision of play grounds, recreation rooms with television and radio.
- Encouragement for formal or informal education during leisure time, street classes and night schools. Motivate them by giving incentives to those who perform well in the academic performance.
- Training children in banking, budgeting simple accounts and savings.
- Protect them from the alcoholism, smoking, substance abuse, sexual abuse and venereal disease. Providing sex education is also necessary.

- Teach morals and make them to lead a productive life with religious and social development implementations of these measures can be done in various child labor projects.

SUBSTANCE ABUSE

Substance abuse can be defined as using a drug in a way that is inconsistent with medical or social norms and despite negative consequences.

According to WHO

'Drug is defined as any substance that when taken into the living organism, may modify one or more of its functions.'

The problem related to the drug use are given below:

- *Legal:* The drug being taken is strictly prohibited by law and is accompanied by severe punishment for its use or possession.
- *Social:* The use of substance will produce disruptive or bizarre behavior that separates the use from the society. Thus it results in social problems.
- *Medical:* Continuous substance abuse may affect the physical and mental health of the users.
- *Individual:* Continuous drug uses diminishes that person's performance and greatly affects his productive life in the society.

Causes of Substance Abuse

The causes/factors can be divided into three. They are:

Biological Causes

- Family history of substance use disorder
- Personality disorders
- Co-morbid medical disorders
- Re-enforcing effects of drugs
- Withdrawal effects and craving
- Biochemical factors

Psychological Factors

- Curiosity
- Poor impulse control
- Low self-esteem
- Poor stress management skills
- Childhood trauma or loss

- To escape from the reality
- Psychological distress
- Usage as a relief from fatigue and boredom
- Social non-conformity
- Sensation seeking
- Reaction to neglect.

Social Factors

- Peer group pressure
- Modeling or limitation of behavior of important factors.
- Easy availability of alcohol and drugs
- Family conflicts
- Religious reasons
- Poor family support or social
- Unemployment
- Rapid urbanization
- Permissive social attitudes
- Strictness of drug law enforcement.

Commonly Used Substance

The commonly used substances which produce drug dependence are the following:

- Alcohol
- Opioids
- Cannabinoids, e.g. cannabis
- Cocaine
- Amphetamine and other sympathomimetics
- Hallucinogen, LSD, phencyclidine
- Sedatives and hypnotics, e.g. barbiturates
- Inhalants, e.g. volatile solvents
- Nicotine
- Other stimulants.

Alcohol Abuse

Alcohol dependence was known by the name alcoholism.

Alcohol becomes the drug of choice for adolescents, because of the peer group pressure, social acceptance and easy accessibility. Most of them take alcohol as a defense against depression, angry, fear and anxiety.

Harmful Effects of Alcohol

Physical and psychological effects:
- Cirrhosis of liver
- Gastritis
- Malabsorption syndrome
- Delirium tremors
- Suicide
- Head injury and fractures
- Alcoholic hypoglycemia and ketoacidosis.

Social effects of alcohol are the following:
- Accidents
- Divorce
- Marital problems
- Criminal behavior
- Financial problems
- Social disharmony.

Body Fluid Alcohol Levels and Effects

Blood and urinary alcohol concentration represents the behavioral changes and effects of alcohol.
- BAC 25–100 mg % : Excitement is present.
- BAC 80 mg % : The legal limit for driving especially in UK
- BAC 100–200 mg % : Presence of serious intoxicant, slurred speech, in coordination and nystagmus is seen.
- BAC 200–300 mg % : Very dangerous.
- BAC 300–350 mg % : Presence of hypothermia, cold sweats and dysarthria.
- BAC 350–400 mg % : May lead to occurrence of coma and respiratory depression.
- BAC > 400 mg % : Death can occur.

Opioids Use

Opioids are the substance that commonly produces dependence. The commonly used opioids are morphine, heroin, methadone, etc.

Chronic ill effect of opioids use include Parkinson, peripheral neuropathy, skin infections, AIDS, etc.

Cannabis Use

Cannabis is the substance which produce very mild physical dependence and mild withdrawal syndrome like fine tremors, irritability, restlessness, insomnia.

The active ingredient cannabis is marijuana. The ill effects of cannabis use include the psychiatric disorders like acute anxiety, paranoid psychosis, etc.

Cocaine Use

Cocaine is the other substance can be used orally, intranasally, by smoking or parentally.

The most common form available is cocaine HCl.

The ill effect of cocaine dependence are anxiety, impaired social and occupational functioning seizure.

Amphetamine Use

Amphetamine is one of the powerful Central Nervous System (CNS) stimulants and it has a peripheral sympathomimetics effect also.

It do not produce strong physical dependence and it can be withdrawn without much danger. Intoxication may produce tachycardia, hypertension, cardiac failure, seizures, etc. Chronic intoxication may lead to chronic compulsive craving for the drug.

LSD Use

Lysergic acid diethyl amide is a powerful hallucinogen.

Acute intoxication may produce depersonalization, illusion, halluncination and automatic hyperactivity like tachycardia, sweating, etc.

LSD use may produce psychiatric symptoms like anxiety, depression, and psychosis.

Barbiturate Use

Commonly the barbiturates have been used as sedative, hypnotics, tranquilizers, anesthetics and anticonvulsants.

Acute intoxication produces irritability, increased productivity of speech, slurring of speech, ataxia.

Benzodiazepines and other sedative hypnotic use:
- ❖ Benzodiazepines are the important drugs used in the treatment of insomnia and anxiety.

- Benzodiazepines produces physical and psychological dependence.
- Acute intoxication may resemble the alcoholic intoxication. Where chronic use may produce amnestic syndrome.

Inhalants/Volatile Solvents

The commonly used volatile solvent includes, petrol, varnish remover, glues, aerosols, etc. It is more common among the adolescents, inhalation may lead to euphoria, excitement, dizziness, slurring of speech. Death may be of respiratory depression, cardiac arrhythmias.

Phencyclidine Use

It is used by a number of people in the society. Intoxication may produce euphoria and dysphoria.

Other Substance Use

Other commonly used substances are caffeine and nicotine. These drugs may produce dependence, tolerance, intoxication, withdrawal symptoms.

Control and Eradication of Substance Abuse

Various methods can be used to control and eradicate the substance abuse.

Primary Prevention

- Provision of happy and healthy family life.
- Establishment of healthy parent-child relationship
- Provision of love and care to the children
- Have open discussion among parents and children
- Share the problem of child and teach him how to solve the problems
- Usage of peer pressure
- Avoid bad companionship to prevent bad habits
- Offer counseling to the teenagers.
- Reduce the availability of drugs.
- Legislation should be directed towards controlling the manufacture, distribution, prescription, price and time of sale and consumption of a substance.

- Physicians must be careful while prescribing the drugs of powerful action and if needed advise the clients to take drugs on prescription.
- Drug must be safeguarded to prevent the illicit use.
- Community approach by the provision of alternative activities to prevent drug abuse, e.g. teen centers.
- Provision of positive and negative reinforcement for the performance of the children.
- Women should actively participate in the movements which are working against the substance abuse because they are the real sufferers of the substance abuse of their male family members.

Secondary Prevention

- Closely monitor the changes in the behavior of an individual
- Early detection and treatment of addicts.
- Establishment of de-addiction centers, after care centers and day care centers which may assist the individual and family to overcome the problem of drug addiction.
- Proper treatment and specific therapies should be given to prevent complication of disease.

Tertiary Prevention

- Provision of treatment in the state of severe dependence.
- Provision of rehabilitation measures for the drug addicts.
- Involvement of family in the restorative and rehabilitation activities.
- Involvement of social agencies for the rehabilitation.

DRUG ADDICTION

Drug addiction and alcoholism are detrimental not only to the health and welfare of the individual, but to the family, community and society at large.

The word **drug** is defined as any substance that when taken by the living organism may modify one or more of its function.

When a drug can alter consciousness it is called 'psychoactive drug'. Drug may be divided into:

- *Stimulant:* These alter consciousness because, e.g. caffeine, nicotine, cocaine and amphetamines.
- *Depressants:* These are reverse to the stimulants. It alters the consciousness by depressing the central nervous system and make people more relaxed and less tense, e.g. alcohol, barbiturates, marijuana (pot or grass).

- *Hallucinogens:* Those are drugs which cause a person to have hallucinations or visions, e.g. LSD (lysergic acid diethylamide), hashish, ganja, bhang.

These psychoactive drugs act directly upon the brain. It can change our ability to focus attention, remember thing, use judgement, have sense of time, control our actions and emotions.

Definition

WHO defined drug addictions as 'A state of periodic or chronic intoxication detrimental to the individual and to society, produced by repeated consumption of a drug, either natural or synthetic.'

The characteristic of drug addiction are mainly:
- An overpowering or compulsive desire to continue the use of drugs.
- Adopting any method to procure it.
- The tendency to increase the dose.
- A psychic and often physical dependence on the drugs.

Do you know to call a person a drug addict, the following criteria must be satisfied:
- *Psychological dependence:* There is an overpowering desire (compulsion) to take the drug and obtain it by any means.
- *Physical dependence:* When drug is withdrawn, the patient shows withdrawal symptoms such as irrational and violent behaviors, nausea, diarrhea, watering from eyes and nose, etc.
- *Development of tolerance:* There is a tendency to increase the dose.

Causes of Drug Addiction

There are several causes for drug addiction. Some of which are the following:
- To get thrill and pleasure. To satisfy curiosity.
- To relieve tension and anxiety. To get rid of situations of problems.
- History of addiction is family, broken homes, family disorganization.
- Adolescence and youth are at higher risk of drug addiction.
- Strenuous work or studies affluent modes of life.
- Easy availability of drugs. To express independence or hostility.
- Force from peer group. Urban life with its anonymity.

Drug Addiction

It ruins one's life in several ways:
- Health
- Career
- Prestige and
- In fact total life
- Once the habit is established, it is very difficult to cure the problem and withdraw the habit.
- Hence, prevention is better than cure' is extremely important in respect of drug addiction.

Withdrawal Syndrome

If the drugs are stopped suddenly, patient suffer from severe physical and psychological problems like waning, sneezing, tremors, restlessness, sweating, anorexia, vomiting, diarrhea, fever, muscular pain, weakness, insomnia, headache, palpitation, delirium, manic symptoms and even collapse also occur when drug addict withdraw drug suddenly.

Preventive Measures

These can be explained under three headings.

Primary Prevention

Primary prevention is through two main methods.
- By limiting the availability of drugs.
- By educational measures.

In all countries, there is legislation to control the production, supply, sale, possession and export of drugs. These drugs should be guarded and controlled that no one can be diverted for illicit use.

The public especially youth should be warned of the danger of drug addiction and should be educated to use their time and energy in useful manners.

Secondary Prevention

- This is achieved through early identification of drug addicts, so that they can be treated promptly to prevent the development of complications.
- Remain of medicine, syrups, needles, pricks on the body, nervousness, restlessness and abnormal behavior of the young people should be watched closely.

Tertiary Prevention

- This is the treatment of the state of severe dependence.
- Many addictions centers, psychotherapies, social workers and social agencies are working to help the drug addicts.
- Help and support of family member is extremely important in overcoming the problem.
- Treatment of drug addicts is very important not only for themselves, but also for others.
- Nowadays there is additional danger of AIDS, because this can spread through contaminated syringes and needles.
- Simultaneously with medical treatment. Changes in environment (homes, school, college social circle) are important.
- Preventive measures include education of largest group and public through TV radio, leaflets and posters to create awareness of the problem. The government has promulgated an act called as 'Narcotic Drugs and Psychotropic Substances Act.' Which came into force in 1985 to combat this problem.

ALCOHOLISM

Alcohol like opium product is narcotic. But alcoholism constitutes a special problem.

In recent times alcoholic beverages are looked upon as a matter of course. They are regular part of a meal and an ever present means of stimulating social intercourse.

Meaning

Alcoholism means excessive consumption of alcohol and becoming addicted to it.

Effects of Alcohol

Alcohol if consumed in small quantities, does not cause problems. On the other hand a small amount of alcohol may be used as a tension releaser.

Alcohol relaxes the mind and sedates the brain especially to painful emotions and promotes a sense of pleasure and well-being.

But most people are not able to control the desire to drink. Once used to drinking, there is a tendency to fall into excessive consumption regularly.

Classification

Drinkers may be broadly classified into two groups:
- *Moderate drinkers:* Who consume alcohol moderately and their drinking habit does not cause much problem.
- *Problem drinkers:* Who consume alcohol in huge amounts which lead to addiction and causes physical, social and psychological problems.

What is Alcoholism?

Alcoholism is an insistent craving for alcohol and its effect. As that condition is characterized by relatively permanent, persistent desire for alcohol for the sake of its anticipated effects upon body and mind.

Causes

- *History drinking:* Alcohol serves as a temporary escape from situations and problems in life. Men start drinking in order to forget the miseries and problems of life.
- *Friendship:* Many drinkers are drawn into this habit by friends. People at first start drinking for company sake and slowly many of them addicted to it.
- *Fashion:* Drinking has become a fashion among many people and it is taken as a sign of modernity.
- *Weak personality:* Many weak minded people are not able to face the hard realities of life and they find an easy escape by drinking.
- *Sudden losses and frustrations:* Sudden loss of dear ones, ruin in life's ambition, frustration in love and fall in business all may lead people to drinking.
- *Ignorance:* Many of the hard physical laborers are under the impression that alcohol can give additional strength and vigor.
- *Unhealthy environment:* People living in slums or poor dilapidated conditions often find that they are surrounded by alcholics. Soon they also follow it.
- *Occupational factor:* Many men consume alcohol because of physical exhaustion.
- Alcohol gives a temporary boost in energy and this helps them to do hard physical labor without feeling of fatigue. Truck drivers, laborers and other manual workers indulge in drinking due to these reasons.

- *Business and profession:* In business and professions to increase their contacts, late night parties accompanied with alcohol have become a common feature.
- *New Elites:* Those people who become rich in short time have a tendency to take drinks. They think it as an additional means to improve their social status (symbol of status).
- *Urbanization:* Modern city life with its mechanized ways of life, high materialistic values and cut throat competition all create tensions, conflicts and alcohol is accepted as a natural ways of escape.
- *Sudden success in business:* Many cases of drinking arise after apparent success in business or professional life.
- *For companionship and fun:* Men drink for companionship for fun and for vitality.
- *Social inadequacy:* Crisis in life may create a feeling of inadequacy and inferiority complex in the individual. There is a feeling of incompleteness. These people start drinking to overcome their social inadequacy temporarily which later on takes on the form of habitual drinking.

Alcoholism is Characterized by Four Factors

1. Excessive intake of alcoholic beverages
2. Individual's increasing worry over his drinking
3. Loss of the drinker's control over his drinking habit
4. Disturbances in his social life.

Consequence of Alcohol Abuse

Excessive consumption of alcohol harm the human body in different ways.

By its action on the brain it blocks the functions like sensation, perception and reasoning by its action on the stomach, it causes gastritis, by its own action on the liver, it causes cirrhosis of liver and its action on the heart may produce hypertension and heart failure.

Consequences of alcohol abuse cause many social evils, such as crime, murder, prostitution, neglect of families, malnutrition disease, unemployment, indebtedness, child delinquency, road accidents, loss of friends and self-esteem.

Over the past fifty years, alcohol consumption has increased both in quantity and frequency. The age at which people start drinking has also declined. The population at greatest risk are those undergoing rapid socioeconomic and cultural changes. They view alcohol as a symbol of prestige and social status. Drinking by adults serve as a role model for the younger ones.

Stages of Alcohol

Elliot and Merrill have given five stages through which a person has to pass till he becomes a complete drunkard and his personality is completely disorganized. Those are:
- Morning drinking
- Escape drinking
- Increased consumption
- Drinking for social function
- Extreme behavior.

The first danger signal is when a person starts to drinking in the morning. He needs alcohol to push him through the day.

The second stage starts when a person feels he cannot face a difficult situation or escape from the difficulty with the help of alcohol.

The third stage starts when the amount of alcohol consumption increases in the course of every month or year. This is a serious sign of personal disorganization and the values of the person are changing.

The fourth stage may come when an alcoholic may feel that he has become so dependent upon alcohol and he cannot face an evening without it. Thus alcohol itself becomes much more significant than the company of human beings.

The fifth stage reaches where a person drinks excessively and behaves indiscriminately. It may be abusing, fighting, throwing away things, beating wife and children, playing absurd or even dangerous pranks and they can easily enter into pathological stage.

Dreadful Effects of Alcoholism

Drinking alcohol affects the health of the people adversely. With long use of alcohol it causes:
- Tremors
- Unsteady gait
- Lusterless eyes
- Haggard look
- Cirrhosis liver
- Crimes and lawlessness
- Taking bribe to purchase alcohol
- Loss of efficiency and self-control

- Loss of studies
- Unhappy families, problems and tension, finally family disorganization.
- Loss of money
- Poverty, misery, violent and abusive
- Alcoholics children become delinquent
- Beat up wives and children
- Commit crimes and anti-social acts
- Moral, ethical and spiritual value of society undermined which leads to social disorganization
- Gambling, prostitution and other vices.

Treatment

- Addiction cannot take place unless the individual willingly come forward and attend the de-addiction program.
- Unfortunately most alcoholics are not motivated to undergo treatment.
- Identification of risk factor is essential for prevention.
- Long term treatment is not only a medical problem and needs the cooperation of psychologists and social workers as well.
- There is also problems of high relapse rate with all treatment methods.

Suggestions

- As alcoholism is common in industrial workers and other laborers, the working conditions are to be improved, if the problem is to be eradicated.
- Mass education through various means of communication about evils of drinking.
- Recreational facilities should be provided.
- Brothels should be away from industrial worker's residence. It is said wine and women usually go together.
- Housing facilities should be provided for the workers either by management or government, high officials in administration should not indulge in drinking.
- The practice of serving drinks in parties should be banned.
- Women should undertake anti-drinking movement, because they are the worst sufferers if the menfolk drink and behave irresponsibly.
- Early detection and treatment of alcohol addicts. But without family support this cannot be achieved.

- ❖ The central, state government and as well as local self-government together with private agencies should see that complete prohibition is imposed by stopping the production sale and consumption of alcohol in any form.
- ❖ A prohibition enquiry committee was setup in 1954, in order to find out the effect of the previous efforts and also to suggest measures to make prohibition more effective.

JUVENILE DELIQUENCY

It is term which describes the breaking of law by youth. The age limit varies from country to country. The lower age limit is 7. It is believed that a child below 7 is incapable of committing crimes, because he/she cannot distinguish between right and wrong and he cannot realize the consequences of his action.

The upper age limit varies between 16 and 21.

Meaning

Juvenile delinquency is an anti-social behavior committed by young people. It is the most serious problem of modern industrial and urbanized society.

Definition

Delinquency is said to be a crime, when it is committed by adults. Therefore, juvenile delinquency can be called as a 'child crime.'

Juvenile delinquency is 'any act of a child which is against the norms and values of the society and which violates the law of the state.'

According to **Sethna**: Juvenile delinquency involves wrong-doing by a child or young person who is under an age specified by the law of the place concerned.

'Juvenile delinquency' includes peddling, begging, disorderly conduct, malicious mischief and ungovernable behavior.

According to **Newmeyer**: 'A delinquent person, underage, who is guilty of antisocial act and whose misconduct is an infarction of local.'

Causes

Poverty and child abuse, breakdown of joint family, breakdown of religious influences and moral values, illiteracy and lack of education, industrialization and urbanization, together with a large scale migration to cities. Absence of proper facilities for marriage and family counseling so as to have responsible and mature parenthood political problems and social changes.

Some of the causes that lead to juvenile delinquency are as follows:

Physical Causes

- **Hereditary:** If the father is a delinquent, this character may be transmitted to his offspring through hereditary. Thus, since his childhood he may have the tendency to be a delinquent and may express anti-social behaviors.
- **Physical disabilities:** Some societies do not accept the physically disable or handicapped children like blind and deaf children as they believe that they are good for nothing. Even some parents refuse to take care of these children. These problems can lead the child to become a juvenile delinquent,
- **Excessive physical strength:** The person who is physically strong may develop atheletic type of body built. There is significant relationship between athletic type of body built and anti-social personality. They may express impulsive behavior.
- **Other sexuality:** Due to sexual urge, develops in the very young age and they become sexually active. This may lead them to commit adultery in their early life.

Social Causes

- **Broken homes:** The children from broken homes, due to influence of their parents may be too disciplined or not all disciplined. These children do not get proper guidance from their family. This may mislead the children and can finally lead them to involve in some antisocial activities.
- **Parents attitude at home:** If the parents behavior at home is not good, the child also behaves in a socially unacceptable manner. This further lead him to be a juvenile delinquent.
- **Urbanization:** In modern families, the parents find less time to spend with their children. The parents go for their jobs at different times and they both do not find time to spend with their children. Due to lack of guidance, the child may lead an ideal life.
- **Criminal background of the family:** The children may get the criminal behavior if his or her siblings or close relatives are criminals.
- **Lack of proper education:** Improper education and lack of proper guidance during school days can increase the criminal activities.

- **Lack of religious and moral education:** Subjects like moral science and other religious education should be included in curriculum.
- From the childhood onwards the children should be told about many moral stories by their parents and teachers. It may increase the sense of moral values and prevent them from committing mistakes.

Economic Causes

- **Poverty:** Due to the poor economic status or due to the death of the bread winner of the family, the children are compelled to do some antisocial activities like theft for leading their life. When the parents are not able to meet the basic needs of the child he starts to involve in truancies.
- **Unemployment of parents:** The parents when they do not have any occupations or incapacitated to meet the needs of the child, this lack of fulfillment can lead the child to become a juvenile delinquent.
- **Child labor and child abuse:** Abusing and neglecting the children creates more number of juvenile delinquent.

Geographical Causes

- **Overcrowding and slum areas:** Children from slum area have more chance of developing criminal behaviors. These children at the age of learning good behaviors, learn how to steal and rob things.
- **Isolated areas:** people living in isolated areas do not have good socialization. The children of these areas may not able to interact with the society. Since there is no good socialization with the people, these children may develop antisocial attitudes.

Psychological Causes

Neglected children, children from broken homes and death of parents in the early childhood may lead the child to develop psychological defects. They may develop impulsive behavior. These situations make the child to develop physically and mentally aggressive and involve with antisocial activities.

Serious forms of juvenile delinquency in India
- Damaging and stealing property
- Murder, assault, suicide

- Sexual offences like rape and sodomy
- Escape from custody
- Ticketless travel in trains
- Gambling, etc.

Prevention and Control

The measures to be taken to control and prevent the juvenile delinquency are given below:

Probation

Probation office supervises and looks after the delinquents in order to establish a normal lifestyle. Through the advices and assistance of probation officer, juvenile delinquents are able to reform themselves. Thus, they will be able to lead a socially acceptable life after the probation.

Remedial Measures

- While treating a juvenile delinquent, the welfare of the child is given foremost importance.
- Since the juvenile delinquent is a minor, he cannot be held responsible for the offensive act he has committed.
- Our purpose is not to punish him, but also correct his criminal tendencies and make him useful citizen.
- The children act of 1960 passed by our parliament seeks to provide for the care, protection, maintenance, welfare training, trail and rehabilitation of delinquent and neglected children.
- The home is the natural environment for any child and all effort should be made to help him to continue in the same home as far as possible.
- Every attempt is made to correct his deviant behavior and also to equip him for a normal adult life.
- Proper assessment of the problem as per scientific principles of sociology.
- Improvement in economic conditions of the masses.
- Provision of better educational facilities.
- Training for parents in parental responsibility.
- Encouraging religion and morals.
- Facilities for proper treatment and reformation of juvenile delinquent with the provisions of juvenile courts, juvenile police and reformative centers.

Correctional Institutions for Juvenile Delinquents

Juvenile Courts

Juvenile courts for minor adults and young persons are to hear charges against children place them in the correctional institutions known as Borstals.

- The borstal schools act are in operation in Chennai, Kerala, Karnataka, Punjab, Uttar Pradesh, West Bengal and Madhya Pradesh.
- The reformatory school act of 1987 has been made applicable to all bigger states.
- At present there are 90 juvenile courts and child welfare board, 98 special school and 10 after care homes, 120 observations homes, offering institutional services to children.

Remand Homes

When a child is apprehended under the act, he is brought before magistrate within 24 hours, he is kept in the remand home until the final disposal of the case takes place.

Certified Schools

Certified schools are for the treatment of children with subnormal mental ability and they are sent for long-term treatment.

These are two types of school:
1. Junior schools: Under 12
2. Senior schools: Under 16

Auxiliary Homes

Delinquents are kept for some time and studied by a social worker and then sent to the certified schools.

Auxiliary homes are just like remedy homes, attached to certified schools for the reception of inmates of certified schools.

Foster Homes

These are for delinquent children under 10 years, who cannot be sent to approved or certified schools, unless the court is satisfied that they cannot be dealt with otherwise.

Fit Persons Institutions

These non-governmental institutions provide facilities for bringing up children in trusted to their care in conformity with their religious of birth.

These are specific institutions for specific type of children.

Uncared Children Institution

The children in the predelinquent or near delinquent stage, who are mostly found in a state of destitution or neglect are cared for in various orphanage and children's institution.

Reformatory School

These are meant for the education and vocational training of delinquent children with much regard to the type of crime committed.

The delinquent are removed from bad environment and places in the reformatory school for some time after which they can adopt some vocation learnt in the school.

Borstal Institutions

Social treatment is provided for adolescent offender between the age of 15 to 21 years (between 16 and 21 years of age where children act in force). There are two types of borstal institutions.

Close Institutions

- It is a converted prison building and security is provided when necessary.
- But the gates remain open and large part of the activities are carried outside the walls.

Open Institutions

- It is a camp or building in open country with no surround wall.
- The training is different for boys and girls such as mixed farming, building and engineering for the farmer and laundry, cooking and home use work for the latter.
- The term borstal is 2–3 years.
- The date of release is depend upon conduct and progress of delinquent and also decided by the borstal authorities like probation officer or borstal associate.

- Borstal schools are in Chennai, West Bengal, Mumbai, and Karnataka state at present.
- Juvenile jail is in Bellary for juvenile offenders under age of 21.

CRIME

Definition

Crime is an act forbidden by the law of the land and penalty is prescribed.

Factors Contributing to Crime

There are so many factors, which contribute to this major social problem. They can be classified as physical, social, economic, political, environmental, familial and psychological.

Physical Factors

Physical factors mainly the physical environment includes season, climate, population density, economy, culture and other ecological factors.

If he develops any physical defects in his life, he may turn into the criminal activities, e.g. a man living in a poor economic condition may commit some of the criminal activities like robbery, murder, etc.

Social Factors

- **Lack of social control:** Moral values are the indirect means of social control. It controls the human behavior and tendencies.
- **Advancements:** Availability of good transportation facilities help the criminals to escape after committing the crime. Remote control, e-mail, mobile facilities help the criminals for their criminal network.
- **Complexity and harassments:** If anybody wants to inform about the crime to the higher authority, they have to undergo the complexity and harassment given by police.
- **Political pressure:** Nowadays the punishment to the criminals became less or most of them escape with high political influence.
- **Education:** In olden days, the schools were considered as the temples of education because the olden education emphasize the moral values. But modern education just superficially emphasizes some of the formalities. The knowledge about science and technology can be utilized for constructive and destructive

purposes. The unemployment and under employment problems stimulate the youngsters to commit criminal activities.
- **Mass media:** Most of the cinema lights up the violence and all sorts of crimes in the society. Newspaper and TV also highlights the criminal activities in the society.
- **Religion:** Nowadays religion becomes the source of violence. The non-coordination and competitive nature of religious leaders leads to crime such as murder, burning, looting, etc.
- **Alcoholism and drug abuse:** Due to over usage of alcohol and drug the crime increases, individuals are losing their productivity and social respect.
- **Superstitious beliefs:** The people perform crime in the name of human sacrifice in order to please the god.
- Marriage and dowry system
- Misguiding of children by adults
- Disorganized community
- Bad friendship.

Economic Factors

- **Poverty:** History has the strong evidence, many socio-economically poor individuals, who become the member of terrorist group in the society.
- **Unemployment:** Unemployment becomes one of the major problem for criminal activity.
- **Industrialization:** Industrialization leads men in alcoholism and prostitution and finally they may perform crime like robbery, murder assaults.
- **Urbanization:** Urbanization is the result of industrialization. In cities, there is a lack of control over the individual so they may commit antisocial activities.
- **Political factors:** Constitution of India has given so many laws against crime. With the help of politics or political leaders, immorality and corruption of police departments false things can be proved as true and true things can be proved as false. Because of these causes crime became a great problem in the society.

Environmental Factors

More number of crimes are committed in hot tropical countries than the cold or sub-tropical countries. Seasonal climate has an effect on crime.

Familial Factors

- **Broken family:** Broken families include divorce, death of parents, or any one parents, absence of love and affection to children lead to crime.
- **Family size:** It is difficult for parents to control and supervise children in large families. This negligence leads to develop delinquent behavior.
- **Parent-child relationship:** Ineffective parent-child relationship may result in behavioral problems or crime.
- **Democratic home:** In this 21st century not only fathers but also the mothers becoming alcoholics. These demoralized conditions make the children to commit many form of crime.
- **Position of child in the family:** Surveys have been proved that the second child in the family will commit most severe crime.

Psychological Factors

Whenever the person's emotional or psychological need is not satisfied his behavior may change.

A person with mental disorders like neurosis, guilty feeling, conflicts, etc. may commit any form of crime.

Commonest form or Crimes

S. No.	Forms	S.No.	Forms
1.	Robbery	11.	Gambling
2.	Murder	12.	Pick-pocket
3.	Looting	13.	Stealing
4.	Communal riots	14.	Corruption
5.	Burning	15.	Black marketing
6.	Sex crimes/rapes	16.	Racketeering
7.	Adultery	17.	Smuggling
8.	Abortions	18.	Tax evasion
9.	Prostitution	19.	White collar crime
10.	Juvenile delinquency	20.	Terrorism

Prevention and Control Measures

Prevention of crime is mainly possible by two methods:

One aiming to reduce the number of crime and other is reformation Impairment is the common method using to prevent and control crime. Besides imprisonment some other punishment also helps to control crime.

Imprisonment

Prison is model setup where all opportunities have been given to develop their personality and make them useful citizen in the society.

In our India, some of the prisons have the facilities like reading room, canteen, hospital library, recreation room, etc. Welfare officers and teachers will educate the prisoners.

Probation

Some of the criminals are put down under supervision of probation officers, without sending them to prison. Mostly juvenile and minor offender's are put down under this probation.

Probation officers have some functions for treating these criminal's problems.

- To protect/keep the criminals under his personal care.
- To reform the criminals.
- To bring out life history of criminals and reduce their tendencies of crime thoughts.
- Help to find out solution for criminals problem.
- Provide relevant information to court regarding the criminals.
- To provide occupational assistance or rehabilitation to the criminals.
- Make the criminals as a good citizen in the society.

Parole

Parole is another form of reformation of criminals. Other than probation these will be a short period of imprisonment. During the parole, the criminals will be under the supervision of probation officer. This officer maintains contact with the criminal and tries to reform them.

Reformatory Home

Both juvenile and adult reformatory arrangement are available in the reformatory homes. The person who becomes criminal under the influence of circumstances will be kept in the reformatory homes.

Here the criminals will get the education in discipline, exercise, religion and principles of citizenship.

Borstal Schools

The criminals coming under the age group of 16–21 years kept in the borstal schools, where they are getting good education. The main aim of this school is to make the criminals as a good citizen in the society.

Nowadays the idea of crime and criminal has changed. The commitment of crime is becoming an illness of mind. By punishing the criminals, offensive behavior will not be controlled. But more than punishment the corrective actions will be required to change their criminal mentality.

Society has a great role in treating the criminals and making them as good citizens in our nation.

HIV/AIDS

AIDS means acquired immunodeficiency syndrome. A fatal disease caused by retrovirus known as human immune deficiency virus (HIV) which breakdown the body's immune system.

Causes

The AIDS is caused due to specific virus known as 'Human Immunodeficiency virus.'

Predisposing Factors

- Multiple sex partners
- Heterosexual/homosexual activities
- Unsafe sexual encounters
- Presence of sores in genital area/STDs
- Intravenous drug users
- Adult between age of 25–44 years are at high-risk.

Mode of transmission: HIV virus is transmitted by five major routes. They are:

Sexual Contact

The first and foremost transmission is through sex, vaginal or oral sex can spread AIDS. Risk will be affected by many factors like presence of STDs type of sexual act and stage of illness of the infected partner, women are more prone for HIV, because larger surface is exposed and semen contains high concentration of HIV than vaginal or cervical fluids.

Blood and Blood Products

AIDS is transmitted through the transmission of contaminated blood and blood products such as platelets, clotting factors, plasma, etc. The risk of HIV infection through transmission of one unit of blood is estimated at over 95%. In developed countries, the transmission of blood and blood products playing a minor role in the transmission of HIV.

Contaminated Needles

Transmission through the contaminated needles or syringes or any other skin piercing instruments are less compared to the sexual transmission and through blood transmission.

But in case of drug users who inject cocaine or heroin, chance of transmission is more because of frequent exposure, like several times in a day. This infects to the medical professionals because of their carelessness.

Transplacental and Perinatal Transmission

HIV can transmit from an infected mother to her fetus through placenta or the infant during delivery and by breastfeeding. The risk is highly in case of newly infected mother or those who already developed AIDS. About 1/3rd of children of HIV positive mothers get the infection through the above mentioned routes.

Organ Transplantation

It is one of the routes of transmission like blood and blood products. Carelessness of the medical professionals is the main cause for this mode of transmission.

Prevention and Control of HIV/AIDS

HIV/AIDS is not merely a medical problem to manner in which virus is impacting upon society reveals the intricate way in which social, economic, cultural, political and legal factors act together to make certain sections of society more vulnerable. The basic approaches for the prevention of HIV/AIDS include the following:

Education

Education can be given through mass media, propaganda or banner.

Educate public to avoid unsafe sex and avoid sharing razors and tooth brushes. Educate intravenous drug users, to avoid sharing needles and syringes to prevent the risk. Educate the HIV positive women to avoid pregnancy since the infection can be transmitted to the unborn or newborn.

Prevention of Blood Borne HIV Transmission

Blood donation can save the life of many people at the same time it can ruin their life. So the people those who are donating their blood should undergo test specifically for HIV/AIDS so that the blood born HIV transmission can be prevented.

Not only before the blood donation, donation of organs, sperm or any other tissue the donor should be screened for HIV separate syringes and needles should be used as far as possible.

Preventive Measures for Health Professionals

All staff of testing centers and hospitals, both in public and private sectors should be trained and sanitized to prevent the acquireness of HIV during test.

Before collecting the blood from the patients make sure that whether he/she is HIV positive or not.

All staff should follow the universal precautions while dealing with the patients.

Education of HIV Infected People

Education plays a vital role in the management of HIV/AIDS. The education of HIV infected people include the following.

Education about Mode of Transmission

Educate the client regarding various mode of transmission of HIV, like sexual contact, blood and blood products, sharing of needles, etc.

Ensure them to make sure that he/she is preventing the transmission of HIV/AIDS by safe sex with partners, avoidance of multiple sex partners.

Make them understand in detail about the prevention of these transmission sources.

Education about Family Planning Methods

Educate the partners regarding the family planning methods to prevent transmission through sex.

Educate them about use of condom during sexual intercourse.

If the partners are having one child or more, encourage them for permanent family planning method.

Emphasize HIV Positive Women to Test for HIV Infection for Her Children

There is a high possibility of transmitting HIV to infant from the mother during pregnancy. Therefore, encourage the mother to do the HIV test for her children.

If not positive, prevent transmission and if positive immediately get the medical consultation and go for antiretroviral therapy.

Educate or Refer the Patient to the Resources Like National AIDS Hotline and AIDS Action Council

Educate the patient regarding the national AIDS hotline or AIDS action council. Enumerate them they can get the help from the sources in order to understand more about HIV/AIDS, its transmission and prevention.

If they require counseling, they can get it from these resources.

Support System for AIDS Patients

Most of the AIDS patients are rejected by the family, neighbors, friends and colleagues due to fear. Here the family and community are playing a role in the form of support system.

Family Support

The family can help the patient in many ways:
- Helping them to reduce their fear by loving them or making them feel loved.
- Providing a suitable environment where the patient can talk and discuss freely.
- Supporting the client financially as much as possible
- Providing and helping them to have nutritious food.

Community Support

Friends, neighbors, voluntary organizations, colleagues, religious groups, youth groups, etc. are coming under the community. These organization are playing a vital role in the support/assistance as given below:
- **Spiritual support:** Many AIDS patient needs spiritual support for comfort and strength to cope up with feelings of guilt, fear and

emotional stress. The community can provide the support through common prayer, singing hyms and reading from scriptures or writing, etc. Spiritual care help the patient to face sickness and prepare for death.

- ❖ **Emotional support:** Feeling of rejection is the devastating experience for the person with AIDS. Here the community support can be given by explaining the patient or if the family members reject him.
- ❖ **Economic support:** Presence of chronic illness, loss of job and high expense treatment will lead to financial crises in the patient's family. Here the community can support the client effectively by providing financial assistance by giving job opportunity and by providing concession for treatment.

SOCIAL WELFARE PROGRAMS IN INDIA

Social welfare system is a set of initiatives created to help those individuals and families who are in need. The government's efforts enable this system to run. These social welfare programmes assist individuals and families by offering financial assistance and welfare services. The majority of social welfare programmes offer a set of prerequisites for people who wishes to receive financial aid. It is an ongoing process designed to address particular societal demands. These programmes typically offer support for housing, childcare, food, and medical expenses.

In order to raise Indian residents' living standards, the First Five Year Plan (1951-1956) acknowledged the significance of promoting social services. Accordingly, the Central Social Welfare Board was set up in 1955 with the objective of organizing welfare programs for women, children and disabled persons. Social welfare programs are designed for the weaker sections of the society so as to help them join the mainstream society. The two main characteristics of the social welfare programs according to Wayne Vasey, 1958 are:

- ❖ Meeting the basic needs of the family and strengthening family system through utilization of welfare services.
- ❖ Strengthen the individuals' capacity to cope with their life situations.

Social welfare includes services for women, children, youth, elderly, minorities, disabled, drug and alcohol addicts, economically under privileged such as destitute and unemployed, scheduled castes and tribes.

ROLE OF NURSE IN THE PREVENTION AND ERADICATION OF SOCIAL PROBLEMS

Nurses have important role to play in the field of social pathology. Since they are involving with public very closely, analyze the trends and problems of the public, they can suggest for solutions for these issues.

The difference of the nurses are listed below:

- Nurses should show interests to know the current social issues. They should not confine themselves only to the hospitals or their working areas.
- All nurses must get adequate opportunities to deal with public during their academic and occupational life.
- Nurses should apply the principle of sociology when they are dealing with the patients, public and co-workers.
- Nurses should prepare themselves to work in areas like industries, community and other areas apart from hospitals.
- Many nurses hesitate to study the subject sociology. Learning sociology is useful to deal with society effectively.
- Nurses who work in the community get the opportunity to undergo sociological issues.
- All nurses should be aware of the cultural patterns of patients, identify cultural factors associated with patient's sickness.
- Nurses should involve in political field, so that they can bring to the notice of government about the health practices and issues in the society.
- Nurses can work successfully in the rehabilitation of AIDS and substance abuse.
- Nurses should report to the government sector about the victims of social issues like child labor, child abuse, etc.
- Nurses should cooperate with voluntary associations to eradicate social issues like poverty, illiteracy and crime
- Nurses can offer counseling services for the victims of social evils.
- Nurses should take efforts to remove the superstitious beliefs and prejudices from the general public.
- Nurses should know about the basic rights of women, children, and the privileges of minority groups.
- Nursing students should get opportunities for more institutional visits to get exact picture of the society.
- Over all, all nurses should work to improve socioeconomic status of the society.

WOMEN WELFARE SERVICES IN INDIA

The department for women and child development (1985) was formed to implement policies and programs related to women and child welfare. These are the following are the various programs for women:

Social Legislations

- The new constitution of India accorded equality of rights to women with men.
- The acts related to women welfare are:
  - **The Hindu Marriage Act and Divorce Act 1955**: It legalized the marriage and divorce process
  - **Child Marriage Restraints Amendment Act, 1978**: It prohibited child marriage and raised the age of marriage for girls from 15 to 18 years and 18 to 21 years for boys.
  - **The Dowry Prohibition Act, 1961 and 1984**: This legislation imposes a penalty in case of exchange or demand for dowry.
  - **Protection of Women from Domestic Violence Act, 2005**: This law protects the women from all forms of abuse namely physical, emotional, sexual or verbal aggression.
  - **The Maternity Benefit Act, 1961**: Provides maternity benefits to women
  - **The Equal Remuneration Act, 1976**: It provides equal remuneration to men and women workers.
  - **Women Health Volunteers [Accredited Social Health Activist (ASHA)]:** Started during 2005-06 with an objective of providing health services in rural sector.
  - **Girl Child Protection Scheme (GCPS) 2005**: It provides welfare services to children and disabled.
  - The **Pre-natal Diagnostic Technique Regulation and Prevention of Misuse Act, 1994:** It regulates female child related abortions.

Employment Programs

- **Employment and Income Generation Production Program, 1982**: It was started to train women of weaker sections of the society and provide them employment on sustained basis.
- **Rehabilitation and Distress Scheme, 1977**: It was launched to rehabilitate women in distress and provide them vocational training cum employment.

- **Swarnajayanti Gram Swarojgar Yojana (SGSY)**: This scheme helps women to improve their professional skills and promote marketing.
- **Development of Women and Children in Rural Areas Scheme:** This scheme provides self-employment services.
- **Jawahar Rozgar Yojana Scheme**: It aimed to generate employment on productive works that are of substantial benefit to poor and contribute to the creation of rural infrastructure.

Other Programs

- **National Maternity Benefit Scheme:** It is aimed to assist expected mothers by providing them 500/- each for the first two live births.
- **Accelerated Rural Water Supply Programme**: Through this program women are trained so as to master enough skills in using and maintaining hand pump for the supply of drinking water.
- **Rashtriya Mahila Kosh Scheme:** It facilitates credit support in the form of microfinance to poor women for income generating activities.
- **Ujjawala Scheme**: Comprehensive scheme for prevention of illicit trafficking, rescue rehabilitation and reintegration of victims who were trafficked for commercial sexual exploitation.

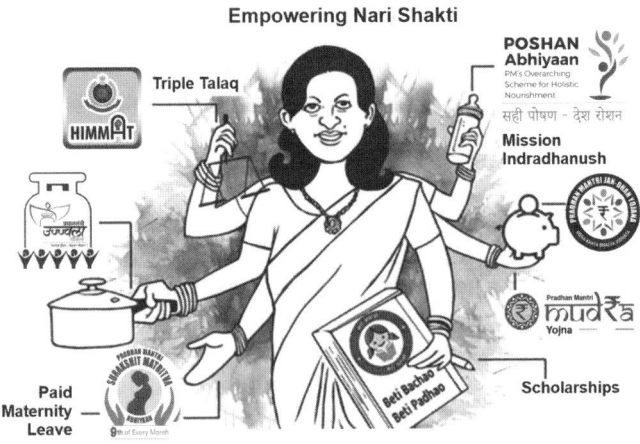

CHILD WELFARE PROGRAMS IN INDIA

Constitutional Safeguards for Indian Children

- Article 25 ensures that no child below the age of 14 years shall be employed to work in any factory or hazardous environment.
- Article 39 ensures that children are not forced by economic necessity to enter vocations unsuited to their age and strengths.
- Article 45 ensures free and compulsory education for all children up to the age of 14 years.

Welfare Programs Related to Children

- **Hindu Adoptions and Maintenance Act, 1956**: Laws related to adoption and maintenance of both boys and girls.
- **Pre-conception and Pre-Natal Diagnostic Technique Act, 1994**: Regulate the use of pre-natal sex determination techniques.
- **Child Labor Prohibition and Regulation Act, 1986**: Prohibits engagement of children in certain employment and regulates working conditions.
- **Juvenile Justice Act, 2002 and Amendment Act, 2006**: Laws relating to proper protection and care of juveniles in conflict with law.
- **Prohibition of Child Marriage Act, 2006**: Prohibits child marriages.
- **National Commission for Protection of Child Rights (NCPCR)**: It was set up in 2007 to protect, promote and defend child rights in the country.
- **National Institute of Public Cooperation and Child Development (NIPCCD)**: It focuses on maternal and child health, nutrition, positive mental health in children.
- **Integrated Child Development Services (ICDS), 1975:** This program is to improve nutrition and health status of children in the age group of 0-6 years. It provides supplementary nutrition, immunization, health check-ups, referral services, non-formal preschool education, health and nutrition education to all women.
- **National Health Policy for Children, 1974**: The provisions included in this policy are health, nutrition of children and mothers, education of mothers, free and compulsory education of children up to the 14 years, recreation, cultural and scientific activities.

- **National Institute of Co-operation and Child Development (NIPCCD), 1966:** The main functions are dissemination of information pertaining to women and child development and public co-operation through documentation and publications. Technical advice and consultancy to central and state governments in promotion and implementation of policies and programs for women and child development.
- **Mid-Day Meal Scheme:** Providing nutritional support to children in school.
- **Creche Scheme:** Overall development of children for working mothers.
- **Reproduction and child health programs:** To provide quality primary healthcare services to women in the reproductive age, family planning and immunization.
- **Immunization program:** Vaccinating all the children
- **Sarva Shiksha Abhiyan:** Focuses on compulsory education to all children
- **Integrated programs for street children:** Provision for shelter, nutrition, health care, sanitation, protection from abuse, education and recreational facilities for destitute and neglected children.
- **National Rural Health Mission:** Services are focused on women and child health, reduction in child and maternal mortality.

SOCIAL WELFARE PROGRAMS FOR OLD PEOPLE

- **Integrated Program for Senior Citizens:** Under this scheme, grant-in-aid are given for running and maintenance of senior citizen homes/old age homes, Mobile Medicare unit, etc.
- **Rashtriya Vayoshri Yojana (RVY):** This scheme provides physical aids, assisted living devices to senior citizens belonging to BPL category and suffering from age-related disabilities.
- **Senior Citizen Welfare Fund:** This welfare fund has been created to be utilized for such schemes, for promoting financial security of senior citizens, health care and nutrition of senior citizens, welfare of elderly widows, scheme related to old age homes and day care of senior citizens.
- **National Council of Senior Citizens (NCSrC):** It oversees the implementation of policy and programs for the aged.
- **Vayoshreshtha Samman:** This program recognizes the efforts made by eminent senior citizens and institutions involved

in rendering distinguished services for the cause of elderly persons.
- **National Social Assistance Program (NSAP):** Under this program old age pension is provided to old aged, widows, disabled persons and bereaved families on death of primary bread winner belonging to below poverty line household.
- **Annapurna Scheme**: Through this scheme senior citizens get food grains.
- **Antyodaya Anna Yojana (AAY):** Under this scheme rice and wheat is provided under subsidized cost to households headed by widows, terminally ill, disabled persons, senior citizens with no assured means of maintenance or societal support.
- **Pradhan Mantri Vaya Vandana Yojana (PMVVY):** Provides social security to elderly.
- **Income Tax Rebate:** Ministry of Finance provides income tax rebate to senior citizens.
- **Concession in fares and other amenities**: Indian railways have taken steps to provide concession in fares for senior citizens in addition to providing various welfare measures for the senior citizens.
- **National Program for Health Care of Elderly (NPHCE):** This provides dedicated healthcare services to the elderly people. This program is implemented through National Health Mission.

- Social organization is a state wherein various institutions in the society are functioning in accordance with their recognized or implied purposes.
- Social organization is a system by which the parts of society are related to each other and to the whole society in a meaningful way
- Goal, role, status, norms and mores and sanction are the elements of social organization.
- Voluntary organization is a group of persons organized on the basis of voluntary membership without state control for the furtherance of some common interests of its members. Indian Red Cross Society, Hind Kusht Nivaran Sangh, Indian Council for Child Welfare, Tuberculosis Association of India, Bharat Sevak Samaj etc are the examples of voluntary association.

Contd...

Contd...

> - Social role is a pattern of behavior expected of an individual in certain group or situation.
> - Social status is commonly thought of as the position which an individual has in the society.
> - Institutions are definite and sanctioned forms or modes of relationship between social beings in respect to one another or to soe external object.
> - Social control is an influence which is exercised by society for the promotion of welfare of group as a whole. It is considered important as it controls the member's behavior in society and is essential for maintaining continuity and uniformity in society.
> - Social control is a process by which, through the imposition of sanctions, deviant behavior is counteracted, and social stability maintained.
> - There are no of ways such as laws, customs, religion, folkways and mores.
> - Social disorganization occurs when various parts of society fail to adjust themselves to changing conditions.
> - Social problems are threat to society which need to be eliminated.
> - Nurse plays an important role in controlling social problems. She assesses the poverty level of people while doing home visits. She assesses overall social problems and do the activities to reduce health problems
> - Welfare activities for children, old people, disabled people, women and minority groups are carried out by government to improve the social life of people.

Review Questions

Short Answer Questions

1. Define social control.
2. What is social organization?
3. Write down the various characteristics of social organization.
4. Define voluntary associations.
5. What is social disorganization?
6. Write down the types of social disorganization.
7. Write down the fundamental rights of individual, women and children.

Long Answer Questions

1. Define social control. What are the means of social control?
2. Describe the various types of social control.
3. Write short notes on:
   a. Folkways
   b. Customs
   c. Mores
   d. Norms
   e. Laws
   f. Fashion
4. Define social system. Write down the characteristics of social system. Describe the elements of social system.
5. Define social problems. Write down the various social problems of India and its controlling measures.

7 UNIT

Clinical Sociology

 Chapter Outline

- Introduction to clinical sociology
- Use of clinical sociology in crisis intervention
- Sociological strategies for developing services for the abused

 Learning Objectives

After reading this chapter, students will be able to:
- Describe clinical sociology
- Explain the sociological strategies for developing services for the abused
- Understand the use of clinical sociology in crisis intervention

 Key Terms

- **Sociology:** Study of society
- **Clinical sociology is an applied practice that focuses on health intervention**
- **Crisis:** Condition of instability
- **Crisis intervention:** It is a technique that helps to understand and cope up with crisis.

CLINICAL SOCIOLOGY

Clinical sociology is the application of sociological theories, research/methods, and interventions to social issues and problems presented by clients. Thus, clinical sociology is the same as all sociology except that it adds intervention, prevention, and social amelioration components to its framework.

Meaning

"Clinical" means a problem-solving perspective. Clinical sociologists deal with what **Thomas Szasz** calls "problems in living" (Szasz 1970). Some sociologists prefer the term "sociological practice" or "applied sociology." Others refer to it as "doing sociology."

Definition

'Clinical sociology is the application of a variety of critically applied practices which attempt sociological diagnosis and treatment of groups and group members in the community.'
—**Glassner and Freedman (1979)**

'Clinical sociology is a kind of applied sociology or sociological practice which involves intimate, sharply realistic investigations linked with efforts to diagnose problems and suggest strategies for coping with these problems.'
—**Lee (1979)**

Nature of Clinical Sociology

Clinical sociology consists basically of the analysis of one human personality as a social unit with respect to the ingression into the psychic of various types of social experiences that emerge from the person's involvement with ecological structure, historical events, interpersonal relations, and cultural patterns. A social unit as used here, is always a personality which in its organization can be regarded as analogous to a miniscule social system.

The central concern, however, is always to obtain an explanation of the influence of these variables in accounting for the self-image, role style, behavior pattern and psychic orientation of a person who is part of a larger social system. In a most fundamental sense clinical sociology is a method for assessing the impact of the social process on human experience, and, in turn, of human experience upon the social process. In considering the nature of clinical sociology it would be a misconception to rely entirely on a medical analogy. In other words, because clinical medicine consists of the observation and examination of the person, it does not follow that clinical sociology studies an entire society. Nor does it follow that the employment of clinical sociology implies that society should be considered as "sick". Rather, clinical sociology consists of the observation, examination and analysis of an individual social unit, the personality.

Thus, the central objective is to arrive at a judgment, supported by evidence, concerning the nature and influence of the environmental factors —physical, social, and cultural —that contribute to an explanation of the organization and behavior of the personality under examination.

Functions of Clinical Sociology

- It interprets individual problems in a social context and helps the individual to change himself and the harmful aspects in the surrounding social environment.
- It applies sociological theories, research methods and interventions to social issues and problems.
- It focuses on health interventions by working with medical practitioners, community health services, social policy, and public health campaigns.
- It focuses on improving quality of people's lives.
- It is a practice-oriented specialty which works with individuals and groups, focuses on case studies and is change oriented. The aim is to bring a change in behavior and growth.

CLINICAL SOCIOLOGIST

'Clinical sociologists analyse social situations and reduce problems through interventions. Analysis includes critical assessment of beliefs, practices, and policies to improve the situation. Interventions include creation of new systems as well as change of existing systems based on continuing analysis.'

—**Fritz (2001)**

'Clinical sociologists may work as an individual, family or group counsellors, community organizers, consumer advocates, focus group facilitators, action researchers, administrators, or policy makers.'

Many clinical sociologists not only collaborate with medical practitioners, nurses, psychologists, psychiatrists, and nutritionists but also advocate and support health and mental health programs.

They also involve in counselling, interpersonal therapy, intervention programs with youth, substance abuse services and group grief counselling.

Clinical sociologists work in a variety of settings which include sociology and social work department of universities as a teacher or researcher, mental health care settings as a researcher or counsellor, community health centres, child guidance centres, juvenile institutions as a service provider

In all of these settings and roles, clinical sociologists have interpreted data obtained through various rese-arch techniques and approaches for the purpose of assisting their clients alleviate problems that inhibit growth and development, optimal activity and positive change.

Clinical Sociology in Crisis Intervention

Crisis

'Crisis is a state of disequilibrium resulting from the interaction of an event with the individual's or family's coping mechanisms which are inadequate to meet the demands of the situation, combined with the individual's or family's perception of the meaning of the event.'

—**Taylor**

Crisis intervention

Crisis intervention refers to the methods used to offer immediate, short-term help to individuals who experience an event that produces emotional, mental, physical, and behavioral distress or problems.

Crisis intervention is a short-term management technique designed to reduce potential permanent damage to an individual affected by a crisis.

Use of Clinical Sociology in Crisis Intervention

- Crisis intervention is a practice-oriented set of procedures designed to offer someone experiencing incapacitating stress emotional first aid.
- Concepts and ideas found in the sociological tradition are quite applicable to crisis intervention practice.
- What has been offered are alternatives to the traditional psychological and psychiatric positions.
- There are similar characteristics between crisis intervention and clinical sociology as change strategies and applicable at the individual level.

- ❖ Both interventions believe in the concept that individuals are social beings affected by social circumstances. Crisis is not experienced in a psychological vacuum. It is the social forces that are responsible for formation of crisis. Crisis event is a social act in that the individual experiencing the crisis is influenced through social circumstances.
- ❖ Crisis intervention and clinical sociology understand that social circumstances play a vital role in crisis development and crisis intervention.
- ❖ The ideas found under the sociological social psychology purview serve well when practicing crisis intervention.
- ❖ Crisis must be examined from a social perspective meaning the role of society and social forces which influence the individual must be recognized
- ❖ The interpretation of crisis events is a social act in that the individual experiencing the crisis is influenced through social circumstances.
- ❖ Social circumstances play a vital role in crisis formation and intervention. Intervention strategies are offered which integrate aspects of clinical sociology while using a case study for application.
- ❖ The crisis intervention steps include crisis assessment, information gathering, control, direction, progress assessment, and referral.

Through these procedures, the intervener may work with the client toward the goal of socioemotional stability.

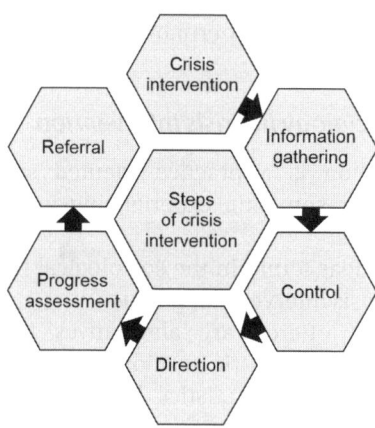

Crisis intervention steps

Use of clinical sociology in crisis intervention

SOCIOLOGICAL STRATEGY FOR DEVELOPING SERVICES FOR THE ABUSED

Abuse

Abuse is defined as any action that intentionally harms or injures another person. It is a form of behavior or an act that is intentional of imposing an authority over, intimidate, force, or hurt another person. It can be lack of proper activities or happening within any relationship where there is an anticipation of trust which causes harm or distress to a vulnerable person.

Clinical sociologists can do much to assure that the development of community resources and empirical research in this area precede hand in hand. The knowledge of sociological principles in the development of services for battered wives in a major metropolitan area. Major intervention strategies were employed in the committee setting provision of information about social structure and its consequences to enable members to develop more effective plans, use of sociological principles and data.

Types of Abuse

Abuse can be physical, psychological, sexual, financial, neglect, etc.
- **Physical abuse** may involve bodily injury. For example, slapping, pinching, kicking, choking, inappropriate use of physical restraints. The signs of physical abuse include bruises, lacerations, wounds, rope marks, fractures, etc.
- **Psychological abuse** refers to the deliberate causing of emotional pain. For example, bullying, threats of harm, abandonment, humiliation, blaming, harassment, isolating, use of silence, yelling, verbal abuse, etc. Signs of psychological abuse include being emotionally upset, agitated, extremely withdrawn, unusual behavior, nervousness, etc.
- **Sexual abuse** refers to unwanted sexual contact. For example, unwanted touching, rape, sexually explicit photographing. Signs

of sexual abuse include bruises around sexual organs, genital infections, vaginal or anal bleeding, torn, stained or bloody underclothes, etc.
- **Financial abuse** occurs when the resources or income of a vulnerable adult are illegally or improperly used by another person. For example, theft, fraud, exploitation, misuse of property, withdrawing money illegally, forging cheques, stealing valuables, etc.
- **Neglect** includes ignoring medical or physical care needs. It occurs when a person's action deprives a vulnerable adult of his basic needs. For example, not providing basic items such as food, water, clothing, safe living environment, medicines, or health care. The signs of neglect include dehydration, malnutrition, untreated bed sores, poor personal hygiene, unsafe living condition, etc.

Preventive Social Strategies of Abuse

The primary aim of safeguarding individuals from abuse is to keep in them in a safe and protected place and prevent further abuse. Some of the common strategies to prevent abuse are:
- Strengthening economic support to family
- Empowering the individual
- Informing about their rights
- Avoiding potential risk situations
- Awareness raising
- Providing information and advice Government programs to reduce abuse:
  - Beti Bachao Beti Padhao
  - Deendayal disabled rehabilitation scheme
  - Integrated Child Development Services
  - Integrated child protection schemes
  - Integrated Rastriya Madhyamik Shiksha Abhiyan
  - Janani Suraksha Yojana
  - Mahatma Gandhi National Rural Employment Guarantee Scheme
  - National Health Mission
  - National Mental Health Program
  - Scholarship Schemes
  - Pradhan Mantri Kaushal Vikas Yojana

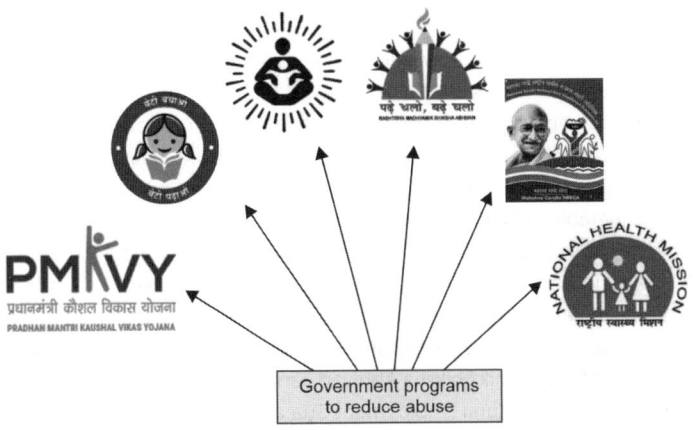

Government programs to reduce abuse

- Clinical sociology is the application of sociological theories, research/methods, and interventions to social issues and problems presented by clients.
- Clinical sociology is a kind of applied sociology or sociological practice which involves intimate, sharply realistic investigations linked with efforts to diagnose problems and suggest strategies for coping with these problems.
- Clinical sociologists analyse social situations and reduce problems through interventions. Analysis includes critical assessment of beliefs, practices, and policies to improve the situation. Interventions include creation of new systems as well as change of existing systems based on continuing analysis.
- Crisis intervention refers to the methods used to offer immediate, short-term help to individuals who experience an event that produces emotional, mental, physical, and behavioral distress or problems.
- Clinical sociologists can do much to assure that the development of community resources and empirical research in this area precede hand in hand.
- Major intervention strategies were employed in the committee setting provision of information about social structure and its consequences to enable members to develop more effective plans, use of sociological principles and data.

Contd...

Contd...

- Abuse is defined as any action that intentionally harms or injures another person. It is a form of behavior or an act that is intentional of imposing an authority over, intimidate, force, or hurt another person. It can be lack of proper activities or happening within any relationship where there is an anticipation of trust which causes harm or distress to a vulnerable person.
- Abuse can be physical, psychological, sexual, financial, neglect, etc.
- Government initiatives to reduce abuse-Beti Bachao Beti Padhao, Deendayal disabled rehabilitation scheme, Integrated Child Development Services, Integrated child protection schemes, Integrated Rastriya Madhyamik Shiksha Abhiyan, Janani Suraksha Yojana, Mahatma Gandhi National Rural Employment Guarantee Scheme, National Health Mission, National Mental Health Program etc.

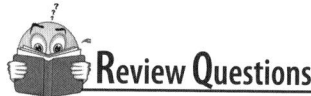

Review Questions

Short Answer Questions

1. Define clinical sociology.
2. What do you mean by crisis and crisis intervention?
3. Define abuse.
4. Briefly explain the types of abuse.

Long Answer Questions

1. Define clinical sociology. Describe the use of clinical sociology in crisis intervention.
2. Define abuse. What are its types? Elaborate the preventive social strategies for abuse.

Index

A

Abuse 343
    childhood 293
    preventive social strategies of 344
    types of 343
Abuser's substance abuse 293
Accessibility to community facilities 263
Accommodation 83, 86, 99
    and assimilation, difference between 86
    characteristics of 83
    different forms of 83
Accredited social health activist 331
Achieved status 219
    determinants of 220
Achievement role 218
Acquired immunodeficiency syndrome 325
    patients, support system for 328
    prevention and control of 326
Adaptation 99
Administration 211
Administrative region 123
Adverse climate and weather 259
Age minorities 290
Agrarian social system 216
Agrarian society 24
Agriculture 109, 110, 114, 259
    development of 252
    fields, improvement in 261
Alcohol 303, 307
    abuse 303
        consequence of 312
    effects of 310
    harmful effects of 304
    stages of 313

Alcoholism 310-312, 322
    dreadful effects of 313
Amphetamine 303, 307
    use 305
Anal stage 90
Anemia, prophylaxis against 277
Anganwadi workers 117
Anglo-Indians 292
Annapurna scheme 335
Antenatal nutrition 142
Anti-untouchability Act 235
Antyodaya Anna Yojana 335
Applied Nutrition Program 277
Arbitration 84
Architects 264
Art 233
    and literature 232
Ascribed status 219
Ashok Mehta committee 111
Assimilation 84, 86
    factors contributing to 85
Association 16, 18, 52, 85
Assumed status 219
Attitude 36, 101
Audience 73
Australoid 203
Authoritarian structure 156
Authority
    basis of 153
    role 218
Auxiliary homes 319
Awareness 35

B

Balwadi Nutritional Program 279
Banking 264

Barbarian social system 216
Barbiturate 303, 307
    use 305
Bathing 142
Bed sores, sign of untreated 344
Behavior, flexibility in 136
Behavioral stability 155
Belief 231
Beliefs regarding
    accepted behavior 231
    heaven and hell 231
    immortality and re-birth 231
    penances 231
Bernard classifies 230
Beti Bachao Beti Padhao 344
Bharat Sevak Samaj 214
Biological causes 257, 302
Biological factor 249
Biological inheritance 32
Bio-psychological causes 257
Birth 61
    not based on 56
    of child, customs related to 145
Blind Relief Society 215
Blindness 285
Blood
    and blood products 325
    no purity of 205
    relationship 157
Body fluid alcohol levels and effects 304
Bombay Devadasi Protection Act 273
Borstal institutions 320
Borstal schools 324
Breast feeding practices 142
Broken homes 316

C

Caffeine 307
Cannabinoids 303
Cannabis 303
    use 305
Capitalist 56
Caste 16, 59, 193, 220
    class and race on health and health
        practices, influence of 206
    endogamy 170
    meaning of 59, 188
    stratification 187
Caste system 109, 110, 115, 182, 188,
        191, 259
    changing trends in 63

during post independent period,
    changes in 65, 192
during pre-independent period,
    changes in 64
origin and development of 60, 190
special features of 61
Casteism 251
    and untouchability, elimination of
        252
Caucasoid 202
Central Social Welfare Board 214
Certified schools 319
Charles A Ellwood's classification 51
Child abuse 293, 317
    in family, characteristics of 297
    predisposing factors to 293
    preventing of 298
    types of 294, 297
Child factors 300
Child labor 299, 317
    different forms of 299
    factors contributing to 300
    ill effects of 300
    prevention and control of 301
    Prohibition and Regulation Act 333
Child Marriage
    Act, prohibition of 333
    opposition of 178
    Restraints Amendment Act 331
Child neglect 293, 296
Child sexual abuse 293, 294
Child Welfare Programs 333
Christians 291
Circumcision, customs related to 145
Civilization 138
Civilized social system 216
Class 53, 182, 193
    and caste 56
    difference between 193
    endogamy 170
    extremes 119
    stratification 188
    system 182
Clinical sociology 338-340
    crisis intervention 341
    functions of 340
    nature of 339
Clique 47
Club 47
Cocaine 303, 307
    use 305
Coercion 236

Collective functions 223
Common interest 39
Communication 43, 114
Community 16, 17, 26, 28, 29, 47, 51, 106
    and neighbourhood 28
    and society, difference between 29
    basic elements of 28
    characteristics of 106
    development
        important aspects of 114
        project and planning 114
    disorganization 251
    features of 27
    life
        benefits of 29
        participation of family in 263
    Nutrition Programs 278
    sentiment 27, 108
    size of 28
    support 328
    types of 107
Co-morbid medical disorders 302
Comparative sociology 10
Competition 76, 79
    advantages of 79
    and conflict, difference between 82
    areas of 78
    characteristics of 77
Compromise 84
Concept 31
Conciliation 84
Conflict 80
    advantages of 81
    characteristics of 81
    disadvantages of 81
    effects of 82
    groups 53
    important forms of 81
    theory 97
    types of 81
Congregate group 50
Conscious social control 229
Constancy of sex urge 168
Constitutional safeguards 333
Construction materials 264
Contaminated needles 326
Control social disorganization,
        measures to 251
Conversation 84
Cooley's classification 38
Cooperation 39, 74, 79, 89
    and competition, difference between
        79

    and social life 76
    classification of 74
    indirect 43, 75
    secondary 76
Coping ability 282
Cottage industries, establishment of 115
Council for Child Welfare 214, 279
Creche scheme 334
Credulity 71
Crime 32, 251, 321, 323
    factors contributing to 321
Criminals away from society 242
Crippled persons 287
Crisis 338, 341
    intervention 338, 341
        steps 342
        use of clinical sociology in 341,
            343
Crowd 50, 70
    acquisitive 73
    attack rage 72
    characteristics of 70
    classification of 72
    common interest 72
    escape 73
    expressive 73
    heterogenous 73
    homogenous 73
    panic 72, 73
    passive 72
    social aspects of 72
Cultural classes 55
Cultural competition 78
Cultural difference 170
Cultural diffusion 134
Cultural factors 102
Cultural invention 133
Cultural lag 103
Cultural problems 59
Cultural similarity 85
Cultural transmission 134
Cultural understanding and awareness
    145
Cultural uniformity 137
Culture 92, 110, 128, 130, 138
    and civilization, difference between
        137
    and health 141
    and social change, role of 102
    and socialization 138
    causes 257
    characteristics of 132
    diversity of 135

elements of 133
evolution of 133
homogeneity in 109
meaning of 129
nature of 131
on health and disease, impact of 142
uniformity of 135
Custom 232, 242
    and habit, difference between 245
    and laws, difference between 244
    characteristics of 242
    origin of 243
Cyclic poverty 257
Cyclical theory 97, 104

D

Danger of war, elimination of 252
Deafness 286
Death and grieving, fear of 283
Dedication Act, prevention of 273
Deendayal Disabled Rehabilitation Scheme 344
Dehydration, sign of neglect include 344
Delegate group 51
Democratic home 323
Dependency 28, 107
Dependent role 218
Depressants 307
Desert Development Programme 117
Devadasi system 273
Dharma, fulfilment of 174
Direct cooperation 75
Direct social control 228
Disabled minorities 290
Dispose property 253
Disruptive social change 250
Distributive role 218
District Primary Education Program 269
Diversity 128
Divisional endogamy 170
Divorce 250
    provision for 178
Dowry
    causes of 162
    Prohibition Act 162, 331
    system 161
Drink 32
Drinkers
    moderate 311
    problem 311
Drought Prone Areas Programme 117

Drug
    abuse 322
    addiction 307, 309
        causes of 308
    re-enforcing effects of 302
Durable relationship 39
Durkheim's classified 216
Dwight Sanderson's classification 50

E

Ecological factor 249
Economic 223
    causes 257, 317
    classes 55
    competition 78
    dependency 172, 281
    difference 54
    disparities, ending of 252
    factor 166
    independence 159
    institutions 26
    organization 212
    problems 281
    provision 150
    pull 121
    status, stability of 263
    structure 24
    support 329
Education 59, 115, 220, 223, 236, 321, 326
    about mode of transmission 327
    department of 270
    for children 118
    for diversity 141
    importance of 268
    lack of proper 316
Educational facilities 121, 261
Educational organization 212
Educational system, reforms of 252
Electoral law 255
Electrification 262
Emotional basis 152
Emotional neglect 293, 296
Emotional support 329
Employment and Income Generation Production Program 331
Employment programs 331
End social evils, collective efforts to 251
Endogamy 169
    causes of 170
    forms of 170
Endogenous forces 95

Index

Enforced celibacy 167
Engineers 264
Enriches human culture 11
Environment 92
Equal economical opportunity 85
Equal Remuneration Act 331
Equality before law 254
Equality of opportunity 254
Equilibrium 184
Escape drinking 313
Eternal relationships, concept of 172
Ethnic minorities 289
Ethnocentrism 49
Evolutionary theory 97
Exactivity 4
Excessive physical strength 316
Exogamy 170
    forms of 170
Exogenous forces 95
Experimentation 5
Exploitative and constructive methods 230
Expressive role 218
Extravagancy 259

F

Face care 143
Factors determining ascribed status 220
Failure to thrive 293, 296
Familial factors 323
Familial group 52
Familial system, changes in 115
Family 92, 118, 148, 149, 223, 234, 250
    and marriage 148
    on health, influence of 178
    broken 323
    changes in 162
    characteristics of 149
    conjugal 153
    consanguineous 153
    criminal background of 316
    disorganization 250
    distinctive features of 152
    endogamous 154
    exogamous 155
    extended 155, 157
    factors 300
    filo-centric 160
    functions of 151
    life 262
    matriarchal 154
    matrilineal 153
    monogamous 153
    organization 156
    patrilineal 153
    planning
        association 215
        methods, education about 327
    polyandrous 153
    polygamous 153
    position of child in 323
    reduced size of 163
    size 323
    smaller 159
    status of member of 156
    stress 293
    support 328
    types of 153, 259
    Welfare Programs 261
Fares and other amenities, concession in 335
Fashion 234, 243
    and custom, difference between 245
Female, earlier aging of 167
Feudal strike 81
FH Gidding's classification 50
Finance 264
Financial abuse 344
Financial organization 212
Financing, method of 213
Fit persons institutions 320
Fixing minimal wages 261
Folkways 231, 238, 239
    and mores, difference between 244
    arise spontaneously 239
    grow 232
    important feature of 239
Food
    customs related to 143
    supplies 276
Force 236
Ford foundation 215
Formal social control 120, 230
Formalistic school 1, 7
    criticism of 8
Formality 43
Formation, method of 213
Formative influence 152
Foster homes 319
Fractional strike 81
Franchise 47
Fraternal polyandry 166
Functional theory 97
Functionalist theory 105
Fundamental duty 254

Fundamental rights of
   children 255
   individual 253
      women, and children 253
   women 254

G

Gang 47
Gender and sexual minorities 290
General sociology 9
Genetic group 50
Geographic separation 170
Geographical causes 317
Geographical factors 249
Geographical location 136
Girl child
   no proper nutrition to 142
   protection scheme 331
Goals 34
   and means, conflict of 250
Gram panchayat 111, 112
Gram sabha 111, 112
Gross national product 260
Group 48-50
   accepted by 239
   classification of 36
   conflict 252
   control 35
   horizontal 50
   life-values of 227
   marginalized 289
   reference of 46
   secondary 41, 45
   structure 43
   types of 46
   vertical 50
   vulnerable 280
   welfare, concepts of 240
Growth 99
GVK Rao committee 111

H

Hair care 143
Hallucinogens 308
Handicapped 284
Handicaps, types of 285
Handwashing 142
Hazards 300
Health
   and disease 120
      influence of culture on 141
   and health practices 121
   and medical problems 282
   and nutrition 59
   and sanitation 115
   care delivery, improper 260
   education 261
   facilities, availability of 116
   individual 263
   problems
      and impact on 122
      region and 123
   professionals, preventive measures
      for 327
   services, equal distribution of 261
Heightened susceptibility 71
Hereditary 316
Hierarchical order 183
High and low, difference between 183
High emotionality 71
Hind Kusht Nivaran Sangh 214
Hindu Adoptions and Maintenance
   Act 333
Hindu Code Bill 223
Hindu Marriage 173
   Act 175, 235
      and Divorce Act 331
   aims of 174
   based on exogamy 176
   forms of 174
   modern changes in 177
Hindu Widow Remarriage Act 173
Historical sociology 10
History drinking 311
House for all project 265
Household 47
Housing 115, 262
   problem 264
   standards of 263
Human being, differences in 183
Human immunodeficiency virus 325
   infected people, education of 327
   infection, test for 328
   positive women, emphasize 328
   prevention and control of 326
   transmission, prevention of blood
      borne 327
Human praise 233
Human qualities 209
Human society 97
Human symbol method 229
Humane conditions at work 254
Humor and satire 233

Husband and wife, understanding between 168
Hypnotics 303

I

ICDS Program 280
Ideas, instability of 71
Ideology 231
Illiteracy 266
    and ignorance 259
    causes of 267
    effects of 268
Illness 142
Imitation 88, 91
Immoral Traffic in Women and Girls Act, suppression of 273
Immortality 71
Immunization Program 334
Impersonal competition 78
Impersonal ideals, conflicts of 81
Impersonality 43
Imprisonment 324
In group
    and out group, difference between 49
    characteristics of 48
Income tax rebate 335
Independence and self-esteem, maintenance of 282
Independent role 218
Indira Awas Yojana 265
Individual 18
    achievement of 220
        importance of 57
    and society 18
    group of 209
    heritage of 92
    number of 34
    regulate the behavior of 242
Industrial social system 216
Industrial society 25
    features of 25
Industrialization 322
    and commercialization 120
    regulated and planned 252
In-group and out-group affiliation, basis of 154
Inhalants solvent 306
Insanity 32
Institution 16, 17, 52, 222
    and association, difference between 52
    characteristics of 222

importance of 224
inter-relationship of 224
types of 223
Integrated Child Development Scheme 117
Integrated Child Development Services 333, 344
Integrated Child Protection Schemes 344
Integrated Program for Senior Citizens 334
Integrated Programs for Street Children 334
Integrated Rastriya Madhyamik Shiksha Abhiyan 344
Integrated Rural Development Programme 116, 117
Intelligence, lack of 71
Interaction
    and communication, system of 150
    system of 119
Inter-caste marriage 171
    permission of 178
Inter-generational social mobility 197
International Agencies Live Case 215
International disorganization 251
Intimacy 85
Intimate relation 108
Intoxicants, addiction to 250
Intra-generational mobility 198
Involuntary group 50, 51
Iodine deficiency disorders, control of 279
Isolation 86
    and contact 100
    and social life 87
    types of 86

J

Jajmani system 109, 110
Janani Suraksha Yojana 344
Jawahar Rozgar Yojana Scheme 332
Job opportunities 274
Joint family 155, 156, 167
    characteristics of 156
    demerits of 157
    merits of 157
    system 108, 110
Joint responsibility, ideal of 157
Juvenile courts 319
Juvenile delinquency 32, 315

correctional institutions for 319
serious forms of 317
Juvenile Justice Act 333

K

Kanyadan, ideas of 172
Kasturba Memorial Fund 215
Kitchen gardens 280

L

Labor, extreme divisions of 250
Land Acquisition and Development
    Schemes 266
Land alienation 59
Language 91
    group 53
Latency stage 90
Law 235, 241
    characteristic of 241
    prescribes uniform 235
Leader 235
    influence of 71
Leadership 235
    role 218
Learning
    disabilities 267
    simplifying process of 243
    skills 155
Legal status 107
Leopold's classification 50
Leprosy 288
Lifestyle 136
Linear theory 103
Linguistic conflict 252
Literacy within family, lack of 267
Literature 233
Litigation 81
Living
    common place for 150
    improving standard of 116
LM Singhvi committee 111
Local dais 117
Low income group housing scheme 265
Lysergic acid diethylamide use 305

M

Madras Devadasi Act 273
Mahatma Gandhi National Rural
    Employment Guarantee Scheme
    344

Malenesina 203
Malnutrition, sign of 344
Management 211
Manners and ceremonies 234
Manual labor 55
Marijuana 307
Marital and family problems 250
Marital system, flexibility in 116
Marketing facilities, improve 262
Marriage 118, 148, 164, 165, 177, 220
    aarsh 174
    anuloma 172
    asura 175
    basis of 153
    brahma 174
    characteristics of 165
    companionate 169
    contract, decreased control of 158,
        162
    customs related to 143
    daiva 175
    false hope of 272
    form of 150
    gandharva 175
    group 169
    legislations on 173
    outside
        gotra 170, 171
        pravara 171
        totem 171
    paisach 175
    prajapatya 174
    pratiloma 172
    rakshas 175
    restrictions on 63
    rites 176
    tribal 177
    types of 166
Marxian theory 104
Mass media 322
Materialism 119
Maternity benefit act 331
Mating relationship 149
Matrilocal residence, family of 153
Mechanical attitude 119
Mechanical social system 216
Medical measures 286
Medical practitioners 340
Members, responsibility of 153
Mental deficiency 32, 287
Mental disorders 287
Mental disorganizations 31
Mental Health Programs 340

Mental illness 271
Mental problems 287
Mentally handicapped 284, 287
Metropolitan region 123
Mid-day Meal Program 269, 277
Mid-day Meal Scheme 334
Middle class 56
Middle Income Group Housing Scheme 265
Miller's classification 50
Minority groups 289
    types of 289
Mob 47, 69
    characteristics of 69
Mobility 109, 119
Modern family 158
    emergence of 25
    feature of 158
    instability of 160
Mongoloid 202
Monogamy 168
    advantages of 168
Moral values 110
More 239
    characteristic of 240
    functions of 240
    important features of 240
    spontaneous social control 228
Morgan and other evolutionists 216
Morning drinking 313
Motivation 35
Motive 213
Multi-party system 67
Munchausen syndrome 297
Munchausen's by proxy syndrome 293
Muslim 290
    marriage 176
Muteness 286
Mutual behavior 89

N

Nail care 143
National AIDS Hotline and AIDS Action Council 328
National Child Labour Project 301
National Commission for Protection of Child Rights 333
National Council of Senior Citizens 334
National Goiter Control Program 277
National Health Mission 344
National Health Policy for Children 333
National Housing Policy 266
National Institute of Co-operation and Child Development 334
National Institute of Public Cooperation and Child Development 333
National Literacy Mission 270
National Maternity Benefit Scheme 332
National Mental Health Program 344
National Policy on Education 268
National Program for Health Care of Elderly 335
National Rural Employment Programmes 116
National Rural Health Mission 334
National Social Assistance Program 335
Natural calamities 258
Natural desire 233
Natural income 260
Natural resources
    destruction and lack of 259
    protection of 261
Neglect 344
Negroid 202
Neighbourhood, importance of 108
Net national product 260
Neutrality 27
New social values and attitudes, development of 251
Nicotine 303, 307
No physical proximity 43
Nonessential functions, separation of 159, 163
Non-fraternal polyandry 166
Nonpartisan 67
Non-sororal polygyny 167
Non-violence 234
Norms 34, 236
    importance of 237
    incorporate value judgment 237
    meaning of 236
Nuclear family 155
    characteristics of 155
Nurse 340
    role of 330
Nutrition programs 278
Nutritional anemia, prophylaxis against 278
Nutritionists 340

O

Occupation 54, 119, 220
    restrictions on choice of 63

Index

Occupational choice, no restriction on 115
Occupational role 218
Occupational subculture 26
Open class system 56
Open institutions 320
Opioids 303
    use 304
Oral hygiene, customs related to 144
Oral stage 90
Organ transplantation 326
Organic isolation 87
Organic social system 217
Organic theory, limitations of 22
Organization of government, improper 260
Organized social control 228
Our day-to-day behavior, determines modes of 240
Out group 48, 49
    characteristics of 49
Overcome housing problems, governmental approach to 265
Overcrowding and slum areas 317
Overpopulation 260

P

Panchayat 109
    powers and responsibilities of 112
Panchayat samiti 112
    block level 111
Panchayat system 110
    village level 111
Panchayat village level 111
Panchayati Raj, various committees on 111
Parent-child relationship 323
Parents
    attitude at home 316
    unemployment of 317
Parent-youth conflict 163
Park and Burger's classification 52
Parole 324
Parsis 292
    and jews 292
Participation classes 56
Patriarchal family 153
    causes of decay of 158
Patrilocal residence, family of 153
Pedophilia 293, 295
Peer group 46, 92

People, group of 27, 106, 108
Per capita income 260
Perinatal transmission 326
Permanent groups 51
Personal attainments 57
Personal competition 78
Personal disorganization 30, 250
    causes of 32
    classification of 31
    forms of 32
Personal resources, lack of 32
Personality disorders 302
Phencyclidine use 306
Physical abuse 293, 343
    signs of 343
Physical and emotional support 156
Physical causes 316
Physical child abuse, signs of 295
Physical deficiency 32
Physical dependence 308
Physical disabilities 250, 316
Physical disorganizations 31
Physical environment 100
Physical factors 249
Physical force method 229
Physical region 123
Physically handicapped 284
Political authority 220
Political classes 55
Political competition 79
Political corruption 251
Political factors 322
Political group 66
    important functions of 67
Political organization 212
Political part system, types of 67
Political pressure 321
Political subservience 249
Polyandry 166
    causes of 166
Polygamy 167
    causes of 167
    prohibition of 178
Poor housing, causes of 263
Poor personal hygiene, sign of 344
Population
    and house, proportion of 263
    changes 100
    check on 252
    density of 118
    explosion and industrialization 263
    factor 166
    type of 216

Positive social control 228
Posse 47
Poverty 251, 257, 267, 271, 317, 322
 absolute 257
 and indebtedness 59
 causes of 258
 elimination of 261
 measurement of 260
Pradhan Mantri Awas Yojana 266
Pradhan Mantri Kaushal Vikas Yojana 344
Pradhan Mantri Vaya Vandana Yojana 335
Praise 89
Pravaras 171
Pre-Conception and Pre-Natal Diagnostic Technique Act 333
Predictability 4, 5
Pre-Natal Diagnostic Technique Regulation and Prevention of Misuse Act 331
Prestigious life 271
Prevention and control measures 323
Preventive measures 286, 287
Primary and secondary group, difference between 45
Primary cooperation 75
Primary group 38, 45
 characteristics of 39
 functions of 41
 importance of 40
Primary inventions 134
Primary needs, fulfilment of 223
Primary social institutions 232
Probation 324
Procreation 174
Professional bodies 215
Progress 99
Prohibition Act 235
Proletariat 56
Proper guidance, lack of 260
Prostitution 270
 causes of 271
 classification of 273
 legal aspect of 273
 prevention and control of 274
 prohibitory measures for 275
 rehabilitation of 276
 types of 272
Prostitution Act 271
 preventing of 273
Protection 151, 262
Psychiatrists 340

Psychoactive drug 307
Psychological abuse 343
 signs of 343
Psychological causes 317
Psychological dependence 308
Psychological problem 282
Psychologically handicapped 284
Psychologists 340
Public opinion 233
 stronghold of 110
Punishment 89
Purdah system, customs related to 145

R

Race 199, 200, 203, 220
 characteristics of 200
 endogamy 170
 mixture of 205
 with culture and nationality, confusion of 205
Racial classification, classification of races-criteria of 202
Racial competition 78
Racial difference 170
Racial group 53
 traits for 201
Racial minorities 289
Racial purity, emphasis on 172
Racial stratification 188
Racial superiority, history believes theory of 205
Racism 204
 theory of 205
Rapid social and cultural change 119
Rashtriya Mahila Kosh Scheme 332
Rashtriya Vayoshri Yojana 334
Rationalization 84
Raw materials 264
Reciprocal relations 34
Recreation and play groups 234
Recreational facilities 121
Recruitment role 218
Red Cross Society 214
Reformation movements 173
Reformatory home 324
Reformatory school 320
Region, types of 123
Regional divisions 123
Rehabilitation 261
 and Distress Scheme 331
Rehabilitative measures 286
Relation 281

among family members, basis of nature of 153
regulation of 28
Relationship
cause and effect 5
of man and woman, changes in 158, 163
Relief fund in disasters, provision of 262
Religion 92, 223, 232, 322
customs, traditional mores, importance of 110
faith in 109
Religious
and moral education, lack of 317
belief 136
bigotry 251
competition 78
concepts 260
conflict 252
control, decline of 159, 163
differences 170
duties 174
factors 272
group 67
important functions of 68
minorities 290
organization 212
Remand homes 319
Rental housing scheme 266
Reproduction and Child Health Programs 334
Residence, basis of nature of 153
Responsibility in crowd, lack of 71
Retaining diversity 141
Retirement 281
Revolution 99
Reward and punishment 89
Right of property 253
Right to be protected 255
Right to constitutional remedies 253
Right to education 255
Right to equal opportunities 255
Right to free and compulsory elementary education 255
Right to freedom 253
Right to health 255
Right to identity 255
Right to leisure 253
Right to work 253
Right towards
culture and education 253
religion 253
Rights against exploitation 253

Rigid social customs, change of 274
Ritualized prostitution 273
Rockefeller foundation 215
Role 217
and status, comparison between 221
different types of 218
disintegration and confusion of 249
significance of 218
status and position 211
Rules and discipline 223
Rural and Employment Guarantee Program 116
Rural community 107, 116
Rural economy, changes in 116
Rural life, changes in 115
Rural Water Supply Programme 332
Rural youth for self-employment, training of 117

S

Sacredness, idea of 172
Sanction 212, 223
control by 229
Saptapadi 176
Sarva Shiksha Abhiyaan 270, 334
Satisfaction 36
Savagery social system 216
Schedule tribe 58
Scholarship schemes 344
School 92
School Mid-Day Meal Program 277
Scientific method 5
Scientific tests 205
Secondary group
characteristics of 42
importance of 44
Secondary invention 134
Sectional regions 123
Sedatives 303
Segmental roles 26
Self-identified classes 55
Senior Citizen Welfare Fund 334
Sensate 217
Sense of
consistency 155
inferiority 170
superiority 170
unity 108
Sentiment 107
Separation 250
policy of 170
Sex 32, 194

Index

differences coming under various legislation 273
   education 274
   relationships, laxity in 159
   tourism 272
Sexual abuse 294, 343
   signs of 343
Sexual contact 325
Sexual desires, over 272
Sexual need, satisfaction of 151
Sexual pleasure 174
Sexuality 316
   customs related to 144
Sharing responsibility 156
Shelter 262
Sikhs 291
Similar behaviors 35
Simple living 110
Single dominant party 67
Skilled labours 264
Sleeping habits, customs related to 145
Slum clearance scheme 265
Smoking, customs related to 145
Social adjustment
   easier 243
   helpful in 240
Social backwardness 267
Social base 242
Social behavior
   importance of 221
     law in 241
   influence of class on 56
Social causes 316
Social change 16, 93, 248
   community 94
   definite prediction of 94
   factor influencing 100
   forces of 95
   helpful in 240
   nature of 94
   process of 95
   role of nurse in 105
   speed of 94
   theories of 97, 103
   universal phenomenon 94
Social circumstances 342
Social class 53
   basis of 54
   system and status 192
   types of 55
Social competition 79
Social contract theory 20

Social control 223, 225-227
   aim of 226
   decline of 250
   formal means of 235
   importance of 226
   important agencies of 243
   indirect 228
   informal 109, 230
   lack of 321
   measures, role of nurse in 246
   nature and process of 226
   need for 226, 229
   purpose of 226
   types of 228
   unorganized 228
   ways of 230
Social disorganization 31, 208, 247-249, 252
   basis of 248
   characteristics of 248
   nature of 248
   types of 250
   unconscious 248
   unexpected 248
Social distance 119
Social dynamic 113
   deals 10
   meaning of 113
   society 113
Social education and propaganda 274
Social facilitation 71
Social factors 300
Social forces 293
Social group 16, 32, 33
   characteristics of 34
   importance of 35
Social heterogeneity 119
Social identity 36
Social institution 210
Social laws, lack of influence of 248
Social legislations 331
Social life 24
   and behavior, uniformity in 243
   homogeneity in 110
   importance of
     assimilation in 86
     house in 262
     role of community in 29
   uniform in 240
Social mobility 26, 196
   horizontal and vertical 196
   lack of 110
   meaning of 196
   types of 196

Index

Social morphology 9
Social norms 236
Social organization 16, 17, 208, 209
   basis of 108
   characteristics of 211
   elements of 211
   types of 212
Social physiology 9
Social problem 256, 282
   causes of 256
   classification of 257
   identify solutions of 11
   leading 249
   nature of 256
   prevention and eradication of 330
Social processes 73
Social reality 36
Social security schemes,
       implementation of 262
Social significance 221
Social status
   and roles 251
   characteristics of 219
   importance of 221
Social stratification 181-183, 185
   basis of 184
   biological basis of 184
   economic basis of 186
   factors of 183
   forms of 187
   political basis of 186
   religious basis of 186
   sociocultural basis of 185
   types of 182
Social structure 15-17, 101
Social suggestions 231
Social support 36
Social system 215
   horticulture and pastoral 216
   hunting and gathering 216
   types of 216
Social teaching 89
Social utility 243
Social welfare 115
   Programs 329, 334
Socialization 16, 87, 88, 139
   agencies of 91
   and education, control by 229
   elements of process of 92
   factors of process of 91
   process of 88
   stages of 90
Society 16, 18, 19, 29
   basic concept of 16
   collective aims of 210
   elements of 19
   hierarchical division of 62
   maintaining organization of 242
   nature of 20
   on basis of
      age, stratification of 185
      birth, stratification of 185
      sex, stratification of 185
   organic theory of 21
   planning of 11
   role and importance of custom in 243
   types of 22
Socioemotional stability, goal of 342
Sociological strategy 343
Sociology 1, 2, 4, 338
   importance of 10
   in nursing, importance and
      application of 11
   nature of 3
   scope of 6
Sorokin 217
Sororal polygyny 167
Special isolation 86
Special Livestock Production
      Programme 117
Special Nutrition Program 279
Specialistic school 7
Speech and expression, freedom of 253
Spiritual support 328
Spontaneous social control 228
Squad 48
Stability 39, 223
   and continuity 110
Stable environment 155
Stable family, contributes to 168
States region, group of 123
Status 16, 35, 194, 219
   achievement of 194
   system, social needs of 195
   types of 219
Street prostitutes 272
Structural mobility 198
Subcaste endogamy 170
Subsidized Industrial Housing Scheme 265
Substance
   commonly used 303
   use 306
Substance abuse 302
   causes of 302
   control and eradication of 306

Suicide 32, 250
Summer's classification 48
Superstitious beliefs 322
Supplementary Feeding Program 277
Surplus resources 120
Swarnajayanti Gram Swarozgar Yojana 332
Sympathy 88
Synthetic school 1, 8
Systematic and general sociology 10

T

Takhatmal Jain study group 111
Task motivation 36
Teaching 211
Team 48
Technological advancement 136
Technological factors 102
Temporary groups 51
Tension 250
Terminology 4
Territorial groups 53
Tertiary cooperation 76
Tolerance 85
    development of 308
Toleration 84
Tonnie's classification 51
Traditions and customs 259
Training 115
Transcultural society 140
Transition, time of 248
Transplacental transmission 326
Transport and communication, development of 120
Transportation 114
Tribal community, problems of 59
Tribal endogamy 170
Tribal society 22
    features of 58
    structure and features of 23
Tribe 57
    characteristics of 23
Tuberculosis association 214
Two-party system 67

U

Ujjawala scheme 332
Uncared children institution 320
Unconscious impulses, expression of 71
Unconscious social control 230
Unemployment 251, 322
    and poverty, end of 252
    and under development 259
Unequal distribution 259
Uniformity 128
Unity and solidarity 34
Universally practicable 168
Unsafe living condition, sign of 344
Urban community 118
    features of 118
Urban slums 122
Urbanization 121, 316, 322
Uttar Pradesh Naik Girls Protection Act 273

V

Validity 3
Values 101, 238, 249
Vayoshreshtha samman 334
Vertical social mobility, forms of 197
Village 24
    characteristics of 110
    community 107
        features of 108
    Health Guides Scheme 117
Vitamin A 278
    prophylaxis 277, 278
Volatile solvent 303, 306
Volition, lack of 71
Voluntary association 120, 212
    characteristics of 213
    functions of 213
Voluntary group 51
Voluntary health associations 214
Voluntary membership 43
Voluntary organization 213
Voting rights 255
Vulnerable groups, type of 280
Vulnerable person 343

W

War 81, 260
Wealth 220
Welfare programs 333
Wider ends 28, 107
Widow remarriage 172
    permission of 178
Withdrawal syndrome 309

Women and children in rural areas
    development of 117
    scheme, development of 332
Women conference 215
Women from Domestic Violence Act,
    protection of 331
Women health volunteers 331
Women in panchayats and
    municipalities, reservation of
    seats for 254
Women welfare services 331

Z

Zilla Parishad 111, 112